Salvador Cervantes Sala

Diseases of Senior Cats and Dogs

Diagnosis and Therapy

Second Edition

Forewords by

Albert Lloret

Andy Sparkes

edra
PUBLISHING

This book was originally published in Spanish under the title:
Manual clínico de geriatría canina y felina. Segunda edición

ISBN Spanish edition: 978-84-18706-35-6

Diseases of Senior Cats and Dogs. Second edition
Salvador Cervantes Sala

ISBN: 978-1-957260-10-5
eISBN: 978-1-957260-11-2

Book Publishing Manager: Costanza Smeraldi, Edra S.p.A.
Paper, Printing and Binding Manager: Paolo Ficicchia, Edra S.p.A.
Cover, Layout, Translation and Copyediting: Grupo Asís Biomedia S.L., Zaragoza, Spain
Project Manager: Jorge Viejo Adiego, Grupo Asís Biomedia S.L., Zaragoza, Spain
Scientific consultant: Enrico Febbo

Edra Publishing US LLC
3309 Northlake Boulevard, Suite 203
Palm Beach Gardens, FL, 33403
EIN: 844113980
info@edrapublishing.com
www.edrapublishing.com

edra
PUBLISHING

Printed by *"Rotomail Italia" S.p.A., Vignate (MI)*, Italy, April 2022

dedication

To my family: Anna, Salva, and Albert. Without you nothing would have made any sense. You are the cornerstone on which I have been able to build my life.

To my grandfather, Antoni Sala Casals, for teaching me that there is only one path, the correct path, and that effort is not an obstacle on this path that one must clear, but rather the salt that adds flavour to the journey.

To all my fellow veterinary surgeons who, after multiple editions and translations of the first edition, have provided me with their opinions, criticisms, and thanks. You make me a better veterinary surgeon.

acknowledgements

To Jorge Viejo and Tatiana Blasco, my colleagues from Servet–Edra who have guided me, provided suggestions, and corrected each page of this book. Without them, the quality of the final product would be markedly lower, and for this I extend my most sincere thanks.

To my colleagues and friends who have selflessly continued to collaborate by correcting my original versions, often in overly raw form: Antonio Peña, Cecilia Villaverde, Ana Prats, Elisa López, Isabel Gaona, Judith Herms, and Diego Esteban. Thank you all for your effort and patience and for continuing to put up with me after so many years together.

author

Salvador Cervantes Sala

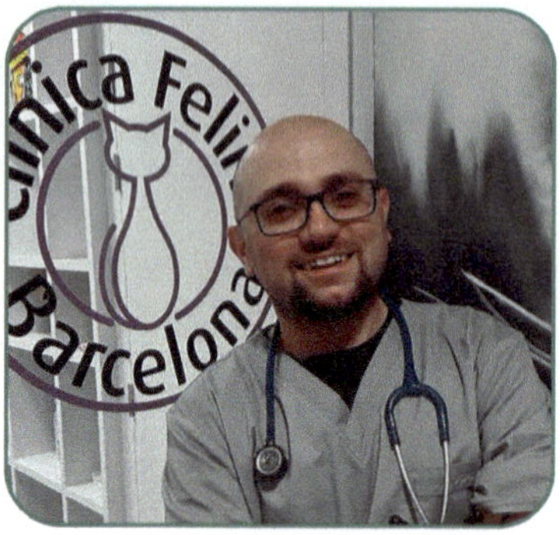

Salvador Cervantes Sala received his degree in veterinary medicine from the Autonomous University of Barcelona (UAB), Spain, in 1998. Between 2000 and 2002 he completed courses in feline medicine and surgery at the European School for Advanced Veterinary Studies (ESAVS) at the University of Zurich, Switzerland. In 2009, he completed the Feline Internal Medicine course taught by the Centre for Veterinary Education at the University of Sydney, Australia. In 2001, together with his wife, Anna Calvet, he founded S&A Veterinaris, a veterinary clinic in Barcelona. In 2016, he founded Clínica Felina Barcelona, a veterinary hospital specifically for cats, located in the same city.

Salvador is a member of the American Association of Feline Practitioners (AAFP), the International Society of Feline Medicine (ISFM), and the Feline Medicine Study Group of the Spanish Association of Small Animal Veterinary Specialists (GEMFE–AVEPA). He has participated in several congresses and is the author of multiple articles on feline medicine published in international journals, including an article on feline hypertension titled "ISFM consensus guidelines on the diagnosis and management of hypertension in cats", published in 2017 in the *Journal of Feline Medicine and Surgery*. In addition, he has co-authored the European edition of the GRAM (*Guidance for the Rational use of Antimicrobials*) guide, published by Ceva Santé Animale in 2016.

foreword

It gives me great pleasure to write the foreword to the second edition of this book on diseases of senior dogs and cats. Publishing a second edition implies that the first has been a success, and provides the opportunity to update concepts and contents in a discipline in which new studies continually provide further information. This edition includes new information on disease diagnosis and treatment that has come to light in recent years, as well as previously unpublished findings and an entire new chapter.

There are several important features of this book that I feel are worth highlighting. First, it is dedicated exclusively to diseases of senior dogs and cats. This approach is unusual in veterinary medicine, since most books focus on classic specialties or systems rather than a specific patient age range. Human medicine has distinct fields of paediatric and geriatric medicine. It is therefore of interest to use this same approach in veterinary medicine publications, especially in the field of geriatrics. The life expectancy of dogs and cats has increased considerably in recent years. This is thanks to advances in the diagnosis and treatment of many of the diseases that affect these animals. Moreover, owners are more willing not only to treat these diseases, but also to provide palliative and supportive care to improve their pet's quality of life. This was unthinkable a few decades ago.

Secondly, Salva combines his clinical experience and the top-quality care he extends to his patients and their owners with an unparalleled vocation for science and learning. This all-too rare combination makes for high level of clinical and scientific rigour: the information presented has been subjected to the strictest criteria for scientific evidence, while the information is presented in a practical, didactic, and direct writing style that the reader can easily understand. Numerous tables and figures serve as additional tools to help understand the concepts presented. Highlighting the clinical and educational vocation of the author, the book includes highly informative tables that summarise key points of interest to both veterinary practitioners and pet owners.

Lastly, I believe that this book is a truly vocational work. It has been created and written over countless hours with the sole objective of improving the clinical training of the author's veterinary colleagues. And this goal has been more than achieved. This book exudes scientific rigour and knowledge in a format, style, and presentation that is at once entertaining, practical, and easy to consult on the spot during a consultation.

Salva: congratulations on the second edition of this wonderful book. I will conclude this foreword by noting my admiration for your impressive capacity for work and your dedication to veterinary medicine and the training of your colleagues.

Albert Lloret
Ldo. Vet., MANZCVS (Feline Medicine), AVEPA-certified in feline medicine.
Internal Medicine Service, Clinical Veterinary Hospital,
Autonomous University of Barcelona, Spain

foreword

The saying goes "If you want something done, ask a busy person to do it!". Well that certainly applies to Dr Salva Cervantes Sala and what he has managed to achieve with this second edition of his book *Diseases of Senior Cats and Dogs*. This is a landmark edition, containing both new and updated information, and also being translated into new languages making this even more widely accessible.

This is a huge achievement – I have had the privilege of knowing Salva for many years and working alongside him on a number of projects. He has a passion for both high-quality veterinary medicine and for geriatric medicine, and that shines through in this book. He is an extremely busy clinician, but somehow has managed to find the time among all his activities to distil in this volume a highly informative and highly practical approach to geriatric medicine of the cat and dog. This, of course, is important both for the number of diseases that can affect older patients and also the high prevalence of comorbidities that we encounter among these patients.

Many veterinary books are destined to fill up space on a bookshelf, but rarely to be used – perhaps being too in-depth and complex for day-to-day reference, or too superficial in their approach to a subject. In this book, Salva has, I believe, struck an almost perfect balance – there is a wealth of helpful, practical information that is genuinely useful in the routine management of what are often complex problems in geriatric pets, but the information is presented in a highly accessible manner with practical tips, key points for owners and excellent use of illustrations, tables, and notes. The information is both current, and importantly concentrates on evidence-based case management.

I am deeply impressed with this book, and it deserves to be well read and highly used. I commend it to you without reservation and I have no doubt that it will be regularly used and referred to for the wealth of practitioner-orientated information it contains and the accessible way that information is presented. There is an ever-growing list of veterinary publications to choose from, and that is a good thing for all of us, but in terms of a book that will be of direct everyday benefit to clinical practice, there are few that could come with higher recommendation.

Andy Sparkes
BVetMed, PhD, DipECVIM-CA, MANZCVS, MRCVS
Editor, Journal of Feline Medicine and Surgery
Independent veterinary consultant
Former Veterinary Director, International Cat Care and International Society of Feline Medicine

preface

This book is a practical manual that comprehensively covers geriatric medicine of dogs and cats, and provides readers, whether veterinary surgeons working in routine clinical practice or students approaching the end of their veterinary medicine degree, with a different approach to clinically useful information on this topic. I did not discover any of the information presented in this book: my work is that of a clinician, not a researcher. However, I wish to emphasise that the task of updating the information in this book would be impossible without the work of veterinary researchers, who continually advance veterinary medicine and the veterinary profession.

It is thanks to the advances made in veterinary medicine in the last decade that we can present this new edition. All chapters have been rigorously reviewed and updated. New content has been added to the chapters from the first edition, and we have added an entire new chapter on endocrine problems in senior patients, a topic that was absent from the first edition.

Thanks to the effort of all those involved in this project, you have in your hands a reference manual for routine clinical practice that I hope will prove useful.

Salvador Cervantes Sala

table of contents

5 Environmental enrichment for cats and dogs 75

6 Chronic pain. Arthrosis 93

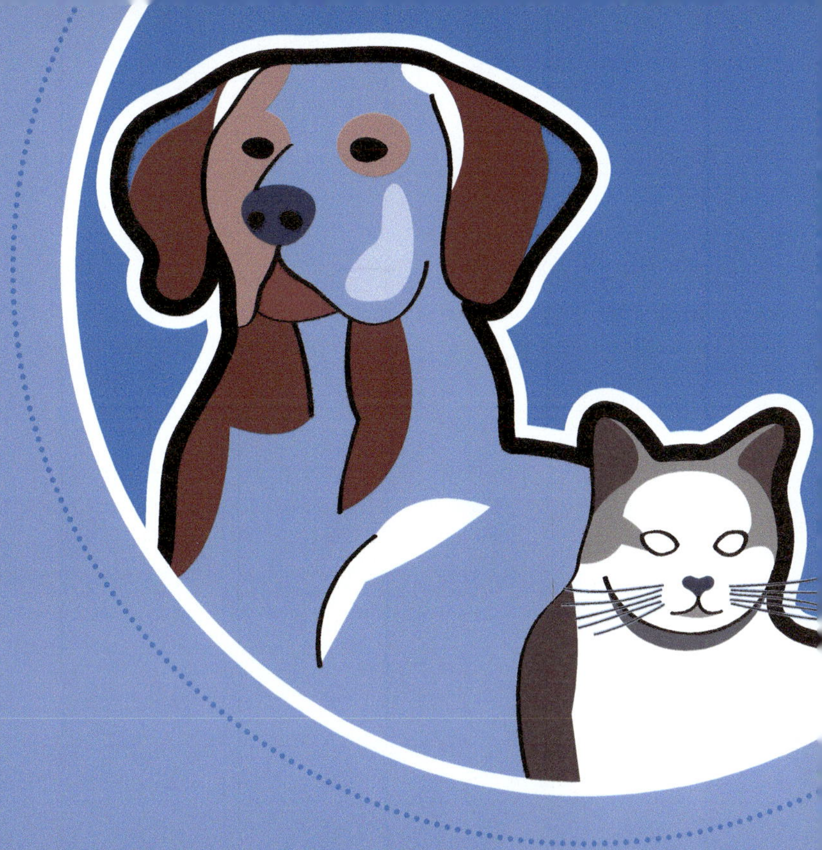

1 Ageing in small animals

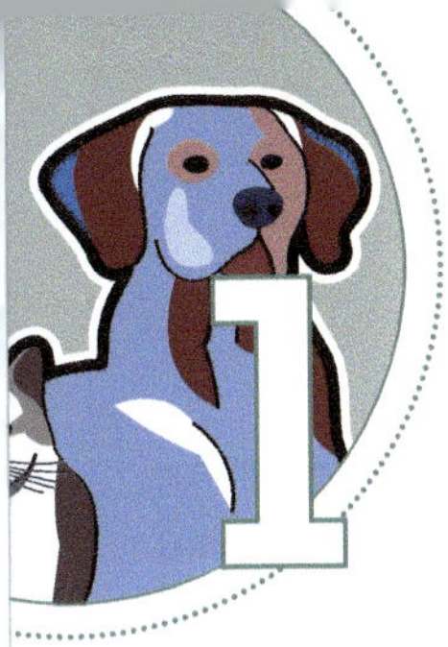

Ageing in small animals

The two most traditional small animal pets, cats and dogs, form an integral part of our homes, our families, and our society. The ever-increasing level of care and devotion shown by their owners is a reflection of this inclusion. A very important part of this care means owners must be willing to pay for professional veterinary attention.

For various reasons, both senior cat and dog populations are currently growing very dramatically; as is, therefore, the incidence of diseases associated with this age group. Some geriatric diseases are unique because they do not usually affect younger animals, but in others, it is simply a case of multiple interrelated and complex processes occurring in a single patient.

Ageing in numbers

One of the points that always comes up when talking about ageing is that it should not be considered an illness. All the experts highlight this fact at every opportunity. It is, however, a period or stage in life that transpires with a higher prevalence of diseases or pathological changes (Fig. 1). This means patients visit the veterinary clinic more often and need more complementary and diagnostic tests. Similarly, their pharmaceutical expenditure will increase, just as it does in human medicine. Figures 2 and 3 show how spending on medications and healthcare in Spain between 1998 and 2008 depended heavily on age group.[1]

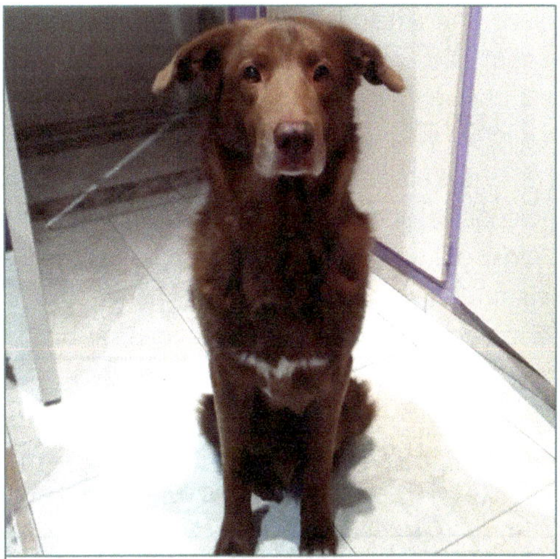

Figure 1. Twelve-year-old dog afflicted by pituitary hyperadrenocorticism and severe osteoarthritis.

- **Some specific cellular events:** one of the most notable discoveries was that as a cell divides and ages, the telomeres become shorter and shorter. Telomeres are protective structures that cap the ends of chromosomes in eukaryotic organisms. This represents a significant difference between prokaryotic and eukaryotic organisms, as it means bacteria can reproduce indefinitely. The main function of telomeres is to stop chromosomes from fusing together or undergoing abnormal recombination of their genetic material. As eukaryotic cells divide, the telomeres become progressively smaller until they practically disappear. This is precisely when cells enter into the stage of cellular senescence. When cells reach senescence, their ability to divide and perform other metabolic functions is decimated or even lost completely (Fig. 5).

  By contrast, the reverse transcriptase enzyme telomerase can catalyse the addition of segments of DNA to the telomeres, thus maintaining their length, which would translate into indefinite cell replication.
- **Mitochondrial mutations:** there is a third route that progressively diminishes cell integrity when mutations develop in the mitochondrial genome due to the continuous attack of free radicals generated during the univalent reduction of oxygen. The loss of regenerative capacity leads to a decrease in the number of mitochondria and a decline in ATP synthesis. This results in a loss of physiological function, which is the most apparent effect of ageing.[3]

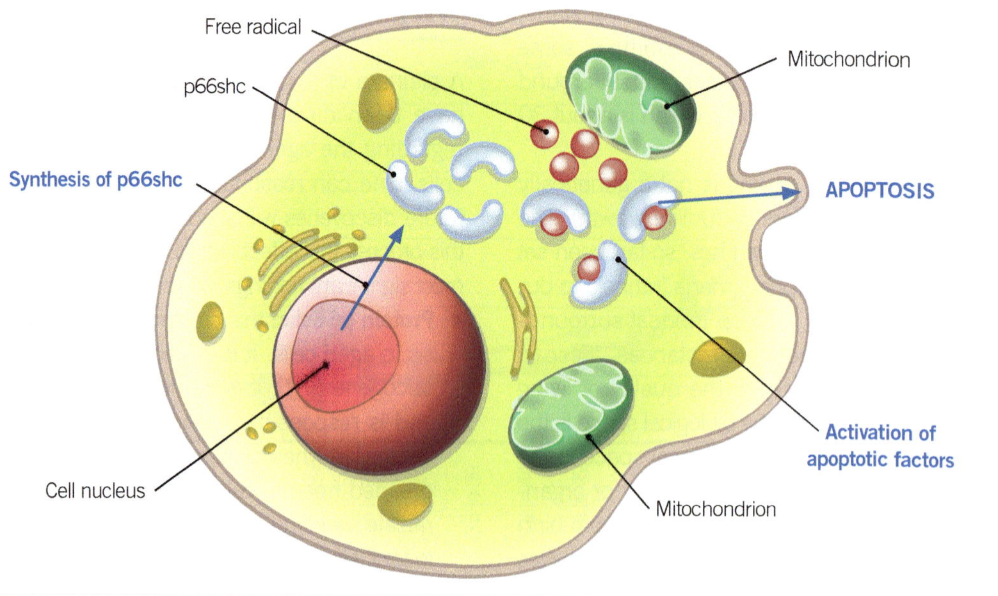

Figure 4. Synthesis and function of the protein p66shc inside cells.

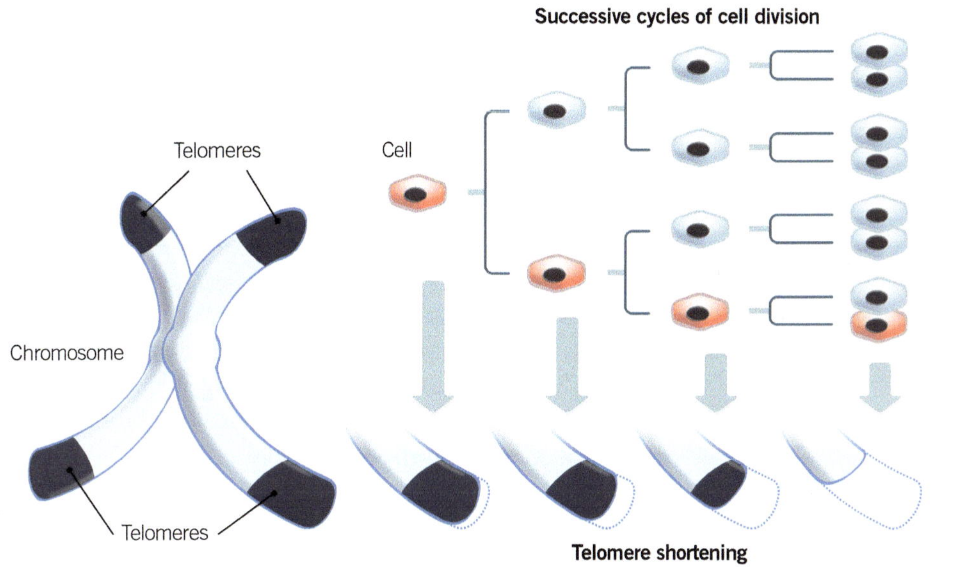

Figure 5. Shortening of telomeres following successive cycles of cell division.

THE DISCOVERY OF TELOMERES AND TELOMERASE

The Russian biologist Alexey Olovnikov first predicted the presence of a compensation mechanism in telomere shortening in 1973.[5] He also developed the hypothesis of cell ageing based on telomere shortening and suggested the relationship between telomeres and cancer. Telomerase was discovered in 1985 by Carol W. Greider and Elizabeth Blackburn in the ciliated protozoan *Tetrahymena*.[6] Along with Jack W. Szostak, Greider and Blackburn received the 2009 Nobel Prize in Physiology or Medicine for their discovery.

Consequences of ageing in cats and dogs

The repercussions of ageing in small animals are very similar to those observed in elderly humans. However, the prevalence of these consequences tends to differ between species, or at least this is what we believe. In fact, up until the mid-2010s, we still considered osteoarthritis an uncommon condition in senior cats.

Veterinary clinicians who are not involved in research may find it very hard to assess some of the effects of ageing. For instance, we all know that our pets lose their hearing as they get older, but how can we measure this decline? The list on the next page indicates some of the effects of ageing on our four-legged patients.

EFFECTS OF AGEING IN CATS AND DOGS

- Impaired hearing
- Changes in urination and hygiene habits
- Changes in dietary habits
- Respiratory problems
- Impaired vision
- Weight changes (either gain or loss)
- Changes in sleep–wake patterns
- Reduced capacity for exercise. Tiredness

Consequences for owners and veterinary surgeons

Consultations with senior patients should focus on preventive medicine to maintain their good health, prolong their lifetimes through the early diagnosis and preventive treatment of diseases, and improve their hygiene, environmental, and nutritional conditions.[7]

This may require a change of attitude, but owners are not always willing to make this change. Most owners now accept that their pet is prone to the effects of time, as we all are, and they recognise that the animal has some "special" requirements now it has aged. However, there are plenty of other owners who cannot or are unwilling to try and meet these needs. As vets and advocates of animal welfare, our work often entails having to persuade owners of elderly pets that anything which affects or will affect their furry friend can be resolved or treated palliatively in order to provide the best possible quality of life for the patient and an optimal pet–owner relationship. While this is not always easy, experience gained in our clinics has taught us that the best way of convincing owners is by implementing strict protocols during consultations or annual checkups throughout the patient's lifetime. So, if all the employees of a clinic always ask the same questions every time they examine a given patient, in addition to those necessary for the current diagnosis, then this will create habits that forewarn owners of the probable changes before they start to appear.

TIP

We need to get owners involved in observing age-related changes, as this will also increase their awareness of potential problems before they become chronic and untreatable.

In other words, if we present the owner of a 3-month-old kitten visiting the clinic for the first time with three different age-dependent health plans and we highlight the differences between plans for kittens, adults, and senior cats, when it comes to discussing the preventive medicine needs of their 10-year-old cat in the future, the owner will already be aware of the specific health plans for senior cats and that they are more expensive than plans for adult cats.

THE OWNER'S PERSPECTIVE

Owners of senior cats and dogs usually have a strong bond with their pet, they are concerned about its welfare and above all its quality of life. Vets should place an emphasis on explaining to owners that **preventive medicine** becomes **vitally important** in elderly pets so they are aware of what modern medicine can and cannot do.

It is often the owners who **ask for help** to treat their senior pets, and they may request a series of **services** which, for various reasons, are not available at the given clinic, such as geriatric checkups, reminders for six-monthly follow-ups, or monitoring of parameters. It is a good idea to **advertise the information** (according to each clinic's style) to ensure owners are **familiar with the services provided by the clinic**.

A lot of owners are **put off by the medication prescribed for their pets** after a geriatric checkup. Drug therapy is essential in many diseases; however, there is an increasing body of **scientific studies** which endorse the application of certain treatments but only at a specific moment. Medicating patients too soon tends to produce more problems than benefits. It is important owners understand that **their pet should only be treated at the right time**.

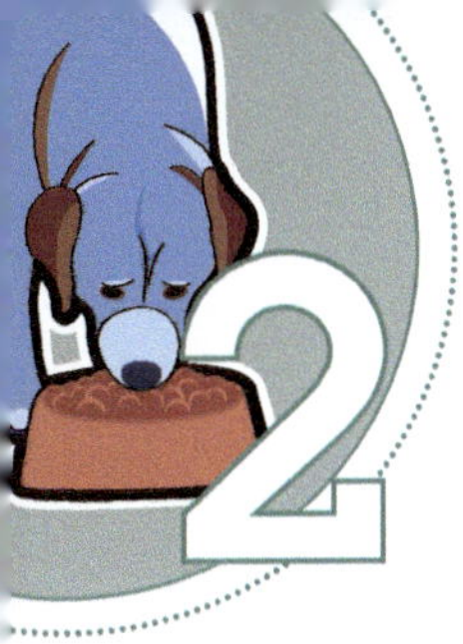

Nutrition in elderly patients

As veterinary practitioners, we often have to answer questions about pets' diets. For instance, "which is better, a dry or wet diet? Which is the best dry food on the market? When should I change my pet over to a senior diet?", and so on. These doubts can be answered easily enough when armed with the appropriate information; however, the problem is that most of us have only received relatively limited training or education on the matter. In recent years, we have accumulated a large amount of information on nutrition in cats and dogs. Some of it comes from commercial laboratories that develop high-quality pet foods, although we should not forget the wide array of scientific studies and sources containing more detailed information. You cannot rely merely on what is written on the product label, especially if you want to give the most professional answers possible to your client's queries.

Nowadays, we are all acutely aware of the importance of a healthy, complete, and balanced diet to maintain the body in optimal conditions, whether animal or human. It is said that Hippocrates (460–370 BC), who is widely considered the father of modern medicine, first underlined the relevance of good nutrition when he stated, "let food be thy medicine, and let medicine be thy food". The owner knows or perceives this, and they like watching their pet enjoy its food. Which is why we receive a constant barrage of questions about nutrition.

This chapter is organised into three main sections:

1. Assessing the patient's diet.
2. Nutritional imbalances in geriatric patients.
3. A brief review of conditions treated through nutrition (diabetes, obesity, and weight loss). (Note: you can find more nutritional information on some of the other diseases addressed in this book in the corresponding chapters).

Assessing the nutritional status of geriatric patients

This assessment is intended to detect food disorders and poor dietary habits as owners, for various reasons, might not report the full picture. At our clinic, we base the assessment of the patient's nutritional status on three key points: a dietary questionnaire (see page 29), a complete physical examination, and an assessment of the feeding regime.

Step 1: the questionnaire

We ask our clients to fill out the questionnaire in the reception area while they wait for their consultation with one of our vets. We hand it out whenever we notice a markedly overweight patient in the reception area, for consultations in which the diagnosed disease is highly sensitive to dietary treatment (chronic kidney disease, diabetes, hyperadrenocorticism, hypothyroidism, etc.), and every time an owner asks for information about changing their pet's diet. It ensures we have a systematically organised source of information, besides giving the visit a value-added touch of **professionalism**. Once the vet has all the information on the animal's diet, they should compare it to the patient's specific nutritional needs.

Step 2: the physical examination

Describing how to perform a complete, systematic physical exam falls outside the scope of this book. However, it is important to highlight some points that are very useful in these cases. The exam must, without fail, include weighing the patient (Fig. 1) and assessing their body condition (BC) score. Both increases and decreases in BC should be studied in detail and will probably require follow up with some more elaborate and complete complementary tests.

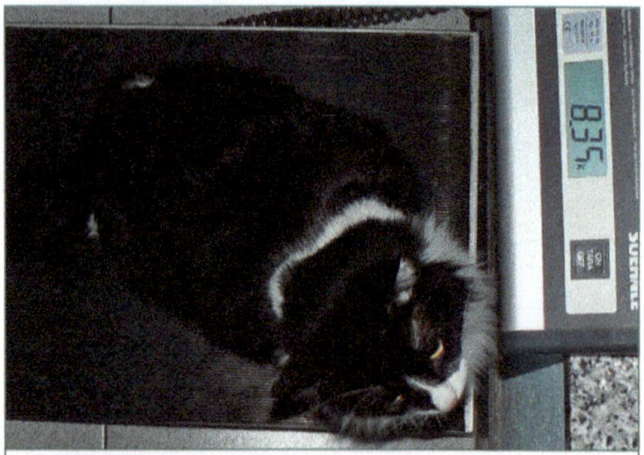

Figure 1. An obese cat on a balance in the consultation room.

Step 3: the dietary assessment

This involves assessing the patient's feeding regime. This point is important because knowledge of the patient's diet does not necessarily mean it is receiving the correct nutrition. The feeding regime is a basic factor and, in homes with more than one animal, each pet may eat more or less than it should because of its position in the social hierarchy. Such a piece of information is vitally important, not only when assessing the patient's current dietary situation, but also because it could influence future dietary recommendations when trying to achieve greater acceptance and stricter adherence from the owner (e.g. owners who fill their pet's bowl with dry food once a day may consider wet food three times a day to be an unnecessary inconvenience).

Effects of age on nutritional needs

Effects on energy requirements

I am sure we have all noticed that our canine patients tend to gain weight as they get older. Put rather crudely, it is because they eat too much.

This is because old age entails a reduction in their needs, so logically senior pets gain weight even though they eat the same amount. In more medical parlance, old age reduces a patient's **maintenance energy requirement** or **MER**. The MER is defined as the energy a normal animal requires to survive with a normal level of activity. Obviously, individual factors, such as genetic potential, overall health, and sterilisation status, can mean that the MER varies significantly between animals.

TAKE NOTE!

The MER must be calculated on an individual basis, as not all dogs gain weight with age. Some stay the same and others, however, lose weight.

Generally speaking, a dog's MER decreases as it grows older, just like it does in humans.[1] In one study that included English Setters, German Shepherds, and Miniature Schnauzers, the MER of 11-year-old dogs was approximately 25 % less than that of 3-year-olds of the same breed.[2]

TAKE NOTE!

Geriatric cats are remarkably different from dogs as their MER starts increasing again above the age of 13.

The MER calculation is based on the minimum energy expenditure of the organism's metabolically active cells. When considered as a whole, these cells are known as **lean body mass** or **LBM**. Lean body mass uses up 96 % of daily basal energy requirements.[3] The ageing body of both cats and dogs experiences a decline in LBM. And if this is coupled with less physical exercise in senior pets, then the reason for the decrease in the MER becomes much clearer.[4,5] By calculating these parameters we can appreciate why exercise that creates more muscle mass also increases the MER.

In cats, the MER also varies with age, but the pattern is slightly different. Studies conducted in cats aged 2 to 17 years demonstrated that the MER gradually fell at a rate of 3 % a year up to the age of 11.5 years. After this age it started to increase somewhat. This could be, at least partly, because a third of cats over 12 are less able to digest fat than they once were and 20 % of cats over 14 have a reduced ability to digest proteins (Fig. 2).[5]

This is why not all senior animals are overweight. In fact, proportionally there are more underweight dogs and particularly cats over 12 years old than in other age groups.[6] Which is why a full, patient-specific nutritional assessment is essential before making any changes to their diet.

Formulas for calculating MERs in cats and dogs (expressed in kcal):

$$MER_{dog} = 1.8 \times [70 \times (BW_{ideal})^{0.75}]$$

$$MER_{ster.\ dog} = 1.6 \times [70 \times (BW_{ideal})^{0.75}]$$

$$MER_{cat} = 1.4 \times [70 \times (BW_{ideal})^{0.75}]$$

$$MER_{ster.\ cat} = 1.2 \times [70 \times (BW_{ideal})^{0.75}]$$

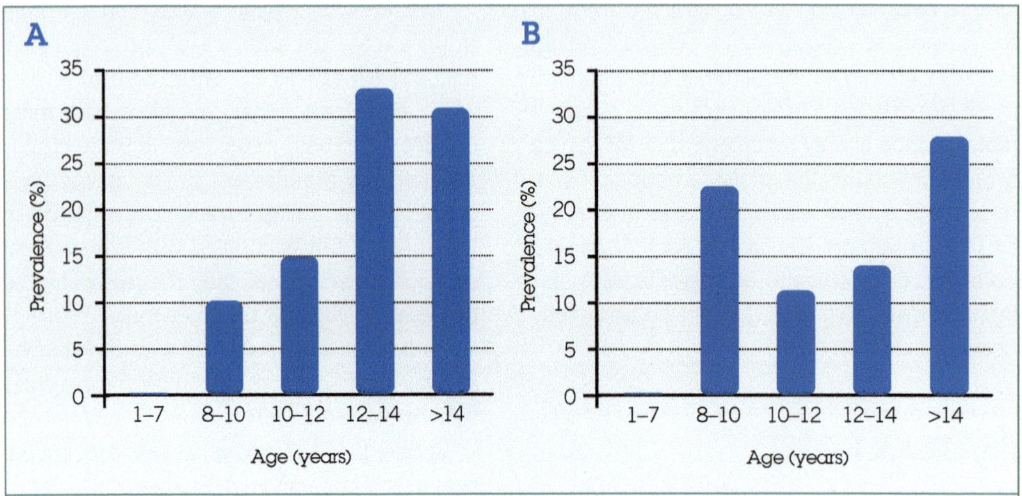

Figure 2. Graph A shows the number of cats with impaired fat absorption when its digestibility was reduced to less than 80 % (taking 90–95 % as a normal value). Graph B shows the percentage of cats with a protein digestion deficiency when its digestibility was reduced to 73 % or less (taking 85–90 % as a normal value).[5]

Effects on protein

Besides the number of calories or amount of energy we indicate for elderly patients, we must also worry about the correction provision of other nutrients. Of all the "major" nutrients, protein has easily received the most attention in articles and discussions. In the past, plenty of veterinary surgeons recommended a protein-restricted diet for geriatric patients with the intention of protecting kidney function. However, according to the data now at our disposal, there seems to be very little to gain by restricting protein intake in patients with good kidney function. Actually, as protein requirements typically increase at this age, senior dogs with normal kidney function should eat a diet with a higher protein content than adult dogs.[7–10] As long ago as 1966, Wannemacher and McCoy,[10] demonstrated that geriatric Beagles needed around 50 % more protein than young Beagles to maintain their body's nitrogen balance and optimise protein reserves.

While the nitrogen balance (the difference between nitrogen intake and its excretion) is still calculated today to help determine protein requirements, other methods, such as maintaining LBM or protein turnover measurements, are more accurate techniques.

TAKE NOTE!

Protein turnover involves the catabolism of endogenous proteins and the synthesis of new proteins required by the body at any given moment for use in enzymes, immunoglobulins, hormones, and so on.

WHAT HAPPENS IF A DOG RECEIVES LESS PROTEIN THAN IT NEEDS?

When dogs are fed a diet that does not provide enough protein, the body's initial reaction is to decrease the rate of catabolism and protein synthesis. The body also starts to mobilise protein from LBM so it can continue to synthesise essential proteins. At first, this situation does not pose any serious risk in a healthy animal, and it will adapt to the insufficient protein intake, thus maintaining the nitrogen balance. However, dogs that find themselves in such a metabolic state, even those which are outwardly healthy, have a reduced capacity to respond to threats, such as infections or intoxications.[10] The immune system seems to be weakened even in mild cases of protein deficiency.[11,12] If all of the above is coupled to the fact that senior patients will have a reduced LBM and slower protein turnover, then it is reasonable to expect that the side effects of a low-protein diet would only aggravate the consequences.

Over a decade ago, researchers at Auburn University (USA) found that dogs can maintain their nitrogen balance with just 16 % of their daily energy intake coming from protein. Yet the same study reported that the maximum protein turnover corresponded to a diet with 32 % of the energy intake from protein in both young and senior dogs.[11–13]

In summary:

- Daily protein requirements vary with age and, as explained earlier, they do not necessarily decrease.
- Individualised treatment is vitally important, as factors such as breed, lifestyle, health status, and, of course, each patient's metabolism can affect their requirements.
- Reducing the amount of daily protein in a healthy animal's diet does not offer any benefits and could even lead to potentially serious alterations.

TIP

Geriatric dogs should receive at least 25 % of their calorie intake from protein. In other words, a senior dog needs around 3.75 g of high biological value protein per kg of body weight per day.[10]

In the case of cats, as a strictly carnivorous species, not only are their daily protein requirements much higher than those of dogs, but they also need to consume protein of animal origin. Unfortunately, we are still waiting for studies that indicate the correct amount of protein for geriatric cats. But we do know that unless we increase the protein:calorie ratio, ageing cats are more likely to experience a loss of LBM or **geriatric sarcopenia**.

TIP

Adult cats should eat a daily diet containing 5 g of protein for each kg of body weight. That is, about 34 % of the calorie intake should come from protein.

Effects on other nutrients

We have already discussed MER and protein requirements. However, nutrition includes, as we all know, many more "other nutrients", with minerals and vitamins being the most notable. In contrast to their feline counterparts, there is scant evidence that a dog's daily requirements for these "other nutrients" vary substantially with age, especially in healthy animals. The age-dependent variation in cats is due to changes in protein and fat absorption. When a cat's ability to digest fat declines, it usually also suffers from malabsorption of B vitamins, vitamin E, potassium, and other minerals.[14]

Some of these "other nutrients" play a role in the fight against cell oxidation that occurs with ageing. Surely, all of us have heard that **oxidative damage** may be responsible for cell ageing and the development of certain age-related diseases, for example, osteoarthritis, cancer, and neurological and cardiovascular diseases.[15–21] It certainly seems to be the case, and deficiencies of nutrients with antioxidant activity, such as vitamin E,[22] can have negative effects on immune function and health markers.[15]

There are a myriad of reportedly antioxidant substances; notwithstanding, it should be noted that one of the most important ones in the body is **glutathione** (a small tripeptide protein formed by glutamic acid, cysteine, and glycine) and its synthesis in sufficient quantities requires an adequate daily intake of protein.[23]

The literature contains several studies that have assessed the reputed beneficial action of antioxidants in cats and dogs. Indeed, they seem to demonstrate a certain beneficial effect on oxidative markers in both species.[24–29]

Diets for nutrition-sensitive diseases

Many diseases are sensitive to changes in nutrition. However, do we know what a diet should contain in order to improve a patient's condition through their nutrition? There are plenty of commercial options, although the apparent tendency is to use these diets for organs rather than for diseases or in stages of illness where there is clear evidence they improve outcomes. For instance, we could prescribe a "renal" diet for a dog with early signs of kidney disease (IRIS stage 1 CKD) when there is no scientific evidence that a dietary change at this stage improves patient quality of life or survival.

The rest of this chapter describes some diseases that can be improved through diet.

Diseases that course with overweight or obesity

A lot of diseases either provoke or are due to overweight. Common examples are diabetes, hypothyroidism, and hyperadrenocorticism. Of course there is also primary obesity, in which case it is simply because the animal consumes more calories than it burns. Primary obesity includes cases related to the patient's age, overfeeding by the owner, castration, and so on, in the absence of any other reason for the tendency to accumulate fat (Fig. 3).

One study estimated that approximately 25 % of cats and dogs that visit a veterinary clinic in the United States are overweight or obese.[6] More recently, another study published in 2011 by the Association for Pet Obesity Prevention (APOP) concluded that 53 % of cats and 55 % of dogs in the US are overweight or obese.

At our clinic in the centre of Barcelona, although we observed slightly lower percentages, it is still a common problem in a lot of pets. Between September 2010 and August 2011, inclusive, 36 % of dogs and 40 % of the cats brought to our clinic were overweight or obese. In 2020, in the midst of the COVID-19 pandemic and with home confinement declared by the Spanish government, the prevalence of overweight and obesity in our patients was close to 50 % for cats and dogs alike. A lack of exercise and overfeeding where identified as the main causes of their excess weight.

TAKE NOTE!

Cats diagnosed with obesity can often suffer from stress or anxiety. These patients require comprehensive management in addition to dietary treatment to improve their body condition.[30]

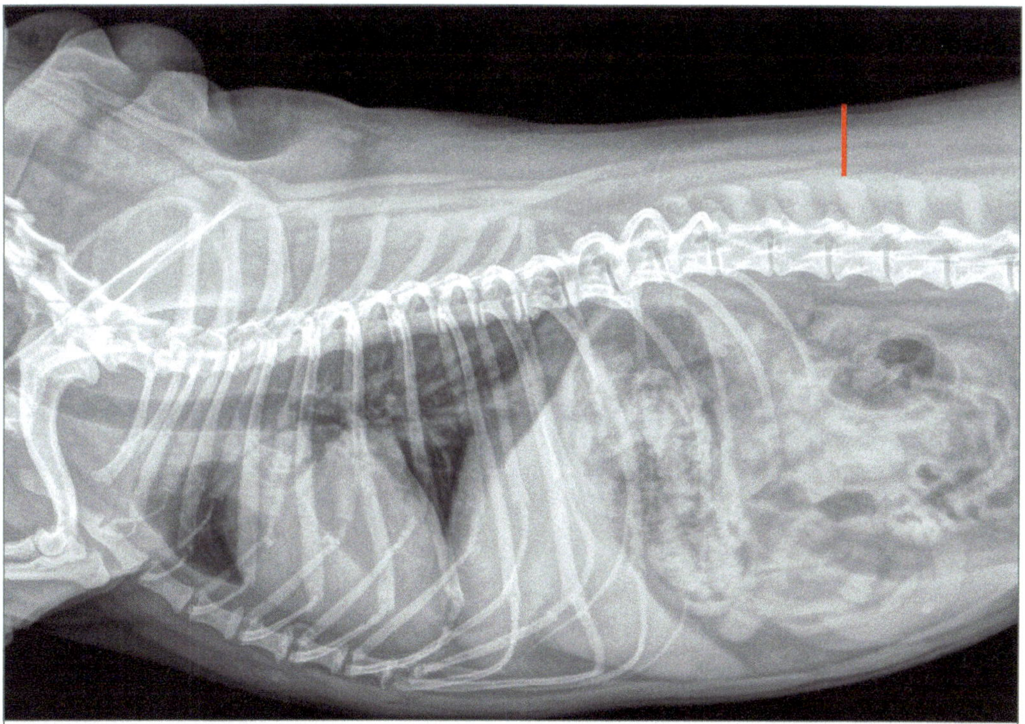

Figure 3. An 8-year-old female Dachshund with severe obesity (weight: 13 kg, ideal weight: <6 kg). Note the 3 cm thick layer of lumbar fat (red line).

As vets we can instinctively tell which patients are obese and which are slightly overweight. Nevertheless, we still need to calculate a patient's percentage over their ideal weight to decide if they are overweight, obese, or even pathologically or morbidly obese. This information is very clear in human medicine; physicians have tables and percentiles that readily illustrate our ideal weight based on a few parameters (age, height, sex, abdominal circumference, etc.). The line between overweight and obesity in humans is around 20–25 % over ideal weight. We can extrapolate this percentage to cats and dogs. It should be noted that the highest prevalence of obesity does not correspond to senior animals, but instead those aged 5 to 10 years.

TO COMMUNICATE WITH THE OWNER

One trick to help owners recognise their pet's degree of obesity is to calculate and then extrapolate it to a person with an ideal weight of 70 kg.

For example: a Yorkshire Terrier should have an ideal weight of 3 kg but actually weighs 4.5 kg. That equates to being 50 % overweight. The same level of obesity in someone with an ideal weight of 70 kg would correspond to an actual weight of 105 kg.

Why is achieving an ideal weight so important?

A lifelong study in Labrador Retrievers found that even slightly overweight subjects had a greater risk of morbidity and shorter life expectancy. In fact, dogs with an ideal weight lived 15 % longer than their overweight peers. The overweight dogs also spent longer periods of their lives taking long-term medications.[31]

The explanation for the poor health and shorter lifespans evidenced by this study may be due to the synthesis of different hormones in the adipose tissue, which was previously considered an inert tissue. These substances (tumour necrosis factor, C-reactive protein, and interleukins 1β and 6) have a proinflammatory nature[32–34] and are believed to be the cause of a persistent state of chronic inflammation secondary to obesity. This low-grade inflammatory state may be a predisposing factor for diseases such as osteoarthritis[35] and diabetes.[36] Furthermore, and linking with the end of the previous section, obesity has been associated with an increase in oxidative stress.[37] Researchers at Tufts University (USA) recently suggested that the shift in the oxidative balance may even play an important role in carcinogenesis (Fig. 4).[38]

Obese cats are also known to have an increased risk of suffering various diseases, including osteoarthritis, hepatic lipidosis, diabetes, and even premature death.[39]

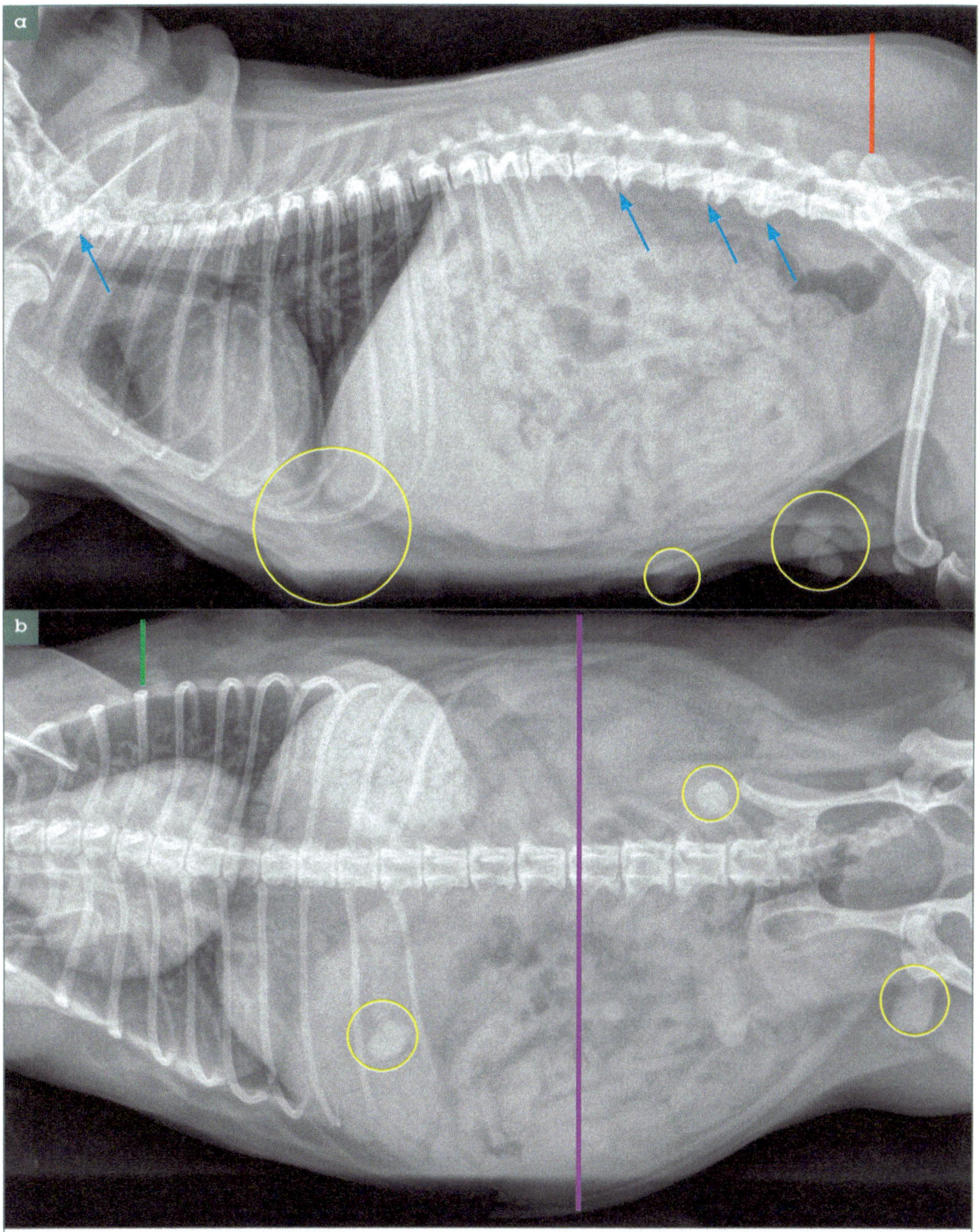

Figure 4. Lateral (a) and ventrodorsal (b) X-rays of a 16-year-old female dog with severe obesity. There is a 4 cm thick layer of fat in the lumbosacral region [red line in (a)], a large increase in the abdominal circumference [purple line in (b)], thicker layer of fat in the subaxillary costal region [green line in (b)], and, additionally, mammary tumours (yellow circles) and signs of chronic spinal instability (blue arrows).

Dietary treatment of obesity

The first step towards making owners of an obese animal aware of the need for their pet to lose weight is to show them that it is indeed obese (Fig. 5). Owners are often reluctant to recognise their animal is overweight, most likely because it implies that they either do not give their pet enough exercise or they overfeed it; either way, they feel responsible. So, you need to be tactful and avoid making them feel even more guilty than they probably already do.

A clear diagram of a 9-point body evaluation system can be a very useful tool when describing a pet's obesity.[40] Explain to the owner that each point on the body condition score (BCS) is equivalent to an increase of 10–15 % over their pet's ideal weight (BCS 4–5/9), and it helps to guide them through the reasons for their dog's BCS. For example, "can you see your dog's ribs easily near its armpits? Can you feel the spinous processes of your cat's lumbar vertebrae?", and so on. While illustrating their pet's excess weight problem, you can also explain the method, so the owner can repeat it at home in front of the rest of the family and throughout the treatment.

The next point to address is the patient's living environment and the owner's realistic means and capacities. It might be difficult for an 85-year-old client to take their dog out for runs, and it could prove impossible to control "extras" in a house full of children or other pets. The vet should be wary of being too ambitious. It is better to start gradually; ask the owner to be patient and trust in the weight loss plan that you are going to design, and which will require sacrifices from everyone involved. If we set and then fail to meet unrealistic goals, there is more chance of treatment dropout compared to when the first stages are simple and easily attainable.

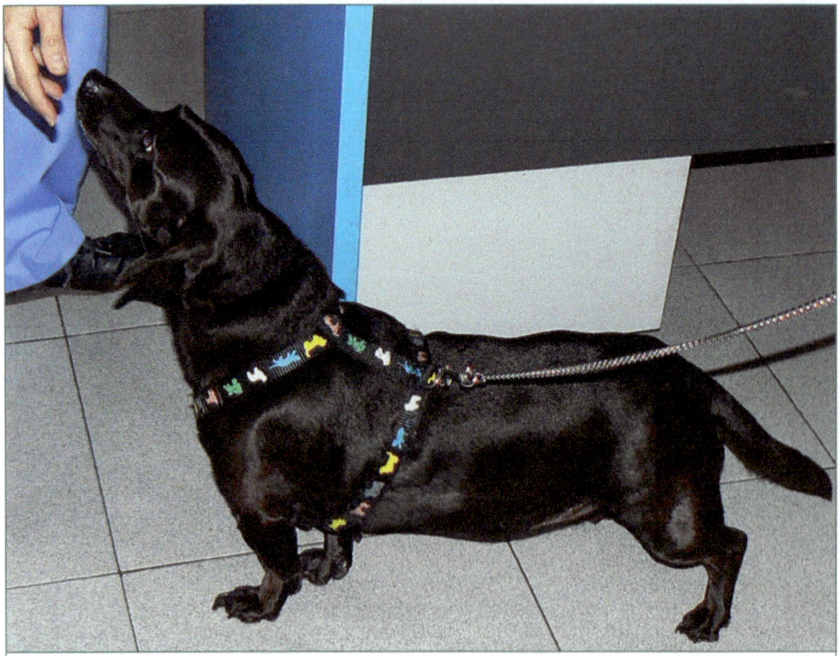

Figure 5. An obese mixed-breed female dog with hypotrichosis on the lateral aspect of the knee caused by rubbing against the floor.

Designing the plan is relatively straightforward. Basically, the patient's calorie intake must be less than its MER. However, there is a question commonly posed by owners or that we even ask ourselves, "which is better, giving the animal less of their usual food or changing to a low-calorie diet?" This time, while it may initially appear more complicated, the answer should be clear. The introduction of a hypocaloric diet with an increased **nutrient:calorie ratio** has an important advantage: it maximises the loss of adipose tissue, while also minimising the loss of LBM. This introduces the added complication of the patient having to accept a new diet, but you should explain that this means their pet will receive all the essential nutrients without developing any dreaded deficiencies. There is no need to rush the transition from the usual food to the hypocaloric diet.

TIP

Our closest ally in these cases should be flexibility. A serving size that helps one patient lose weight might not work for another one. One animal could get used to its hypocaloric diet in 2 days, another may need a month. Flexibility is especially important, and the main objective is the patient's health. It is never too late to achieve it.

The next step is to select a hypocaloric diet and, as always, the diet that works best is the one that is administered correctly. In general, low-calorie diets should be designed with a combination of one or more of the following characteristics:

- **Low fat:** reducing the diet's energy density. The food will have more volume and fewer calories.[41]
- **Relatively high fibre content:** this also increases the volume, which makes it more satiating, particularly for dogs. In addition, fibre prevents the rapid absorption of carbohydrates and fat, which helps maintain a more constant blood sugar level.
- **Slow digesting carbohydrates:** complex carbohydrates reduce spikes in blood glucose and help keep it at more stable levels.
- **Rich in high-quality protein:** the protein component is essential for the diet's palatability, to reduce the patient's BCS without losing LBM,[42,43] and it determines the price. Protein also has what is known as a thermic effect. This effect translates into an increased energy expenditure and a higher postprandial metabolic rate.[44] In other words, the body uses up more energy absorbing 1 gram of protein compared to 1 gram of fat or carbohydrates. This thermic effect is believed to make protein more satiating than other food components.[45,46]

Finally, owners need reminding that "extras" must also be considered a source of calories. If the owner cannot or does not want to eradicate the habit, then ideally, they should give their pet low-calorie treats and subtract the calories from its daily serving. Up to 5–10 % of the calories in the daily serving can normally be given as extras. Similarly, if we want the treatment to be a lasting success, it is important to stress that the patient must also get used to spending more energy through exercise. We need to be creative and flexible so that we may offer suitable options to all of our clients.

DOES L-CARNITINE HELP?

L-Carnitine is endogenously synthesised from lysine and methionine and is used in the β-oxidation of fatty acids. A study in dogs revealed that subjects given a diet supplemented with L-carnitine preserved their LBM better, but they also lost less weight than the control group fed on an unsupplemented diet.[47]

L-Carnitine supplementation appears to benefit humans and it may help prevent lipidosis and ketosis in cats.[48] It has been reported that obese cats given L-carnitine supplements loss weight more quickly than controls.[49]

TIP

Regular calls from the clinic's auxiliary staff to capture the clients' perceptions, to encourage them, and to clear up any doubts are key factors to the success of the weight loss plan.

General recommendations for weight loss are just 60 % of the daily calorie requirement in dogs, but the situation is not as clear for cats and their diet should start at 80 % of requirements or more. The aim is to achieve a weekly weight loss of 1–2 % for dogs and up to 1 % at most in cats. The patient's requirements can be calculated using the MER formulas explained at the beginning of this chapter. Bear in mind that the formulas correspond to the average requirements and each case must be monitored closely and the daily serving adjusted accordingly. The formulas, as it were, should only be used as a rough starting point, since the results can incorporate an error of up to 50 %.

Dietary treatment of diabetes

One in 400–500 dogs and 1 in 100–200 cats suffers from diabetes.[50,51] In contrast to cats, where most cases of glucose metabolism problems correspond to type 2 diabetes, dogs are more prone to develop type 1 diabetes due to an immune-mediated process. Consequently, the prototypical diabetic canine patient differs from a feline one. For example, diabetic cats are obese and over 8 years old. The classic model of a dog with diabetes is harder to define, but again patients tend to be over 8 years old, and it affects females more than males.

Cats aged between 7 and 10 years are eight times more likely to develop diabetes than younger cats. While cats over 14 have a 14 times greater risk of suffering from diabetes.[52] Similarly, an obese cat is four times more prone to manifest diabetes.[39]

Diabetes is generally a geriatric disease in both cats and dogs, although there is a rare form, juvenile-onset diabetes, which affects much younger dogs.

It would seem that obesity is not a predisposing factor for diabetes in dogs,[53,54] but this does not exempt diabetic dogs with overweight or obesity from losing weight to gain better control over their blood sugar levels.

The primary treatment goal in diabetes is to maintain blood sugar levels as close to the normal range as possible. Or at least low enough so the patient does not suffer any clinical signs of hyperglycaemia. This is achieved by administering **insulin**, **controlling concurrent diseases** (hyperadrenocorticism, hypothyroidism, hyperprogesteronism, acromegaly, and serious infections/inflammation, e.g. orodental problems), and through **diet**. Dietary control is crucial in all patients with diabetes[55] as it helps prevent spikes in glycaemic levels and reach an ideal BCS while preserving LBM, and it provides all the essential nutrients or can correct certain metabolic disorders secondary to the diabetes.

Even though type 1 diabetes is classed as being insulin-dependent, diet plays a key role in attempts to minimise both postprandial peaks in blood sugar and marked hypoglycaemia after receiving insulin. In type 2 diabetes, diet can reduce or even eliminate the need for exogenous insulin.[55]

SOLUBLE AND INSOLUBLE FIBRE

In very simple terms, we can say that soluble fibre is easily fermented, whereas insoluble fibre is fermented very slowly or not at all.

Fermentable fibre: pectins, gums, and mucilage, among others.

Nonfermentable fibre: cellulose and hemicellulose (although it is fermented to some degree in a dog's intestines).

Some of the most notable functions of dietary fibre are:

- It delays gastric emptying and alters bowel transit time, thereby decreasing and smoothing out any spikes in postprandial blood glucose levels.
- It determines faeces composition and volume.
- It promotes the growth of beneficial bacterial flora by lowering intraluminal pH.
- It helps control cholesterol levels by favouring the elimination of bile salts in the faeces.

What makes a good diet for diabetes?

- **Complex carbohydrates:** these are absorbed more slowly and steadily than simple carbohydrates, preventing peaks in blood glucose throughout the day. It has been shown that animals fed with simple carbohydrates that are absorbed rapidly need higher doses of insulin. Whole grains usually contain complex carbohydrates (e.g. whole wheat consists of bran and starch).
- **Fibre:** fibre can be found in whole grain cereals added to the patient's diet to prolong the absorption of sugars,[56–58] thereby smoothing postprandial peaks in blood sugar levels and in an attempt to improve our patient's blood lipid levels.[59] There are two types of fibre: **soluble** and **insoluble**. As mentioned, both types are known to help control blood glucose levels.[56,57,60] However, while it is clear that fibre is an excellent tool for controlling blood sugar levels in animals with diabetes, there is still some controversy about the correct amount and proportions of each type. In fact, a recent study reported that nonobese animals with well-controlled diabetes did not benefit from a high-fibre diet.[61] There are very few studies on the effects of dietary fibre on glycaemic levels in cats. Nevertheless, those which have been published appear to demonstrate that fibre in the diet improves blood glucose levels and reduces the amount of insulin required for cats with diabetes.[62,63] In any case, cats improve more with protein-rich diets low in carbohydrates and fibre than with high-fibre, moderate-carbohydrate diets.[64]
- **Protein:** protein is a good source of energy for animals with type 2 diabetes. In the case of type 2, a higher protein content has been shown to decrease insulin requirements and improve glycaemic control.[63,64] Unfortunately, and in light of the results from humans with type 1 diabetes, more protein might not be recommendable in animals with type 1 as it increases their exogenous insulin requirements.[65,66] In obese diabetic patients, however, a protein-rich diet helps maintain LBM while stabilising their weight and disease, as diabetes also results in increased protein catabolism.

DOES INSULIN FULFIL ANY OTHER FUNCTIONS BESIDES ALLOWING GLUCOSE TO ENTER CELLS?

Insulin performs several functions, and they are all related to energy metabolism. So, it would be a considerable oversimplification to say that insulin only helps glucose enter cells. Insulin also has an influence on fat and protein metabolism, because it inhibits protein catabolism and gluconeogenesis from amino acids, hence promoting amino acid uptake and protein synthesis. This is exactly the opposite of glucagon's effect on protein metabolism and gluconeogenesis. It is important to remember that the rate of protein catabolism is higher than usual, even in very well-controlled diabetic patients, so patients experience a net loss of protein.[67] Therefore, patients with diabetes must receive enough dietary protein to avoid catabolism and a loss of LBM.

- **Fats:** fat intake should be reduced in pets with diabetes and obesity, while stable, normal or underweight animals can consume regular or even high amounts, as long as there are no signs of pancreatitis. It should be noted that dietary fat plays a minor role in the onset and treatment of feline pancreatitis.

Dietary treatment of senior patients with weight loss

It is highly likely that a lot more owners worried about obese pets visit our clinics than those with underweight animals. Yet, there are more underweight animals in the senior age group than in any other, above all when considering cats and dogs over 12 years old.[6] When treating such a patient, the first step is to find out if they are eating more, less, or the same as usual. You can often come across elderly patients that have changed to a senior diet and eat more than before. This is due, in the absence of another diagnosis that explains the weight loss, to the reduced protein content and caloric density that is so typical of commercial senior diets.

The malabsorption of nutrients is not very common in dogs, but in cats, by contrast, 1 in 3 suffer fat malabsorption and 1 in 5 have protein malabsorption.[5]

Weight loss can be down to a wide range of chronic systemic, hepatic, renal, gastrointestinal, endocrine, or neurological diseases, among others, that generally affect appetite (Fig. 6). It is essential to diagnose and treat the underlying cause in order to correct the energy imbalance (each chapter on these diseases includes specific information on their dietary treatment).

TAKE NOTE!

Weight loss in cats appears to be a good indicator of chronic disease.

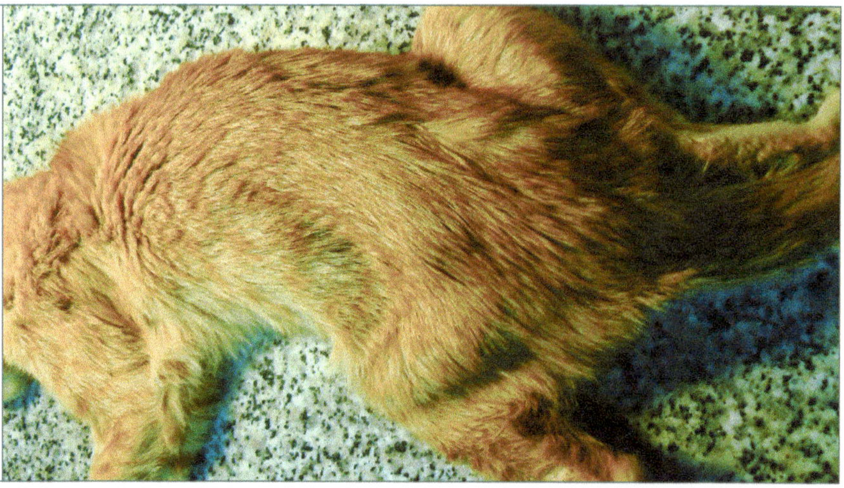

Figure 6. Emaciated cat due to a tumour. A lack of musculature in the femoral region and protruding ribs are clearly visible.

In a retrospective study of 258 cats, weight loss preceded death for various reasons. Cats with kidney disease, hyperthyroidism, or cancer started to lose weight 2.5 years before their death. In the first year they lost around 6 % of their weight and in the second year, before death, they had lost over 10 %.[5]

Notable gastrointestinal alterations related to weight loss include dental health problems (see Chapter 7) and malabsorption.

Dietary management of malabsorption

The closing section of this chapter discusses the dietary management of malabsorption due to **exocrine pancreatic insufficiency (EPI)**, **lymphangiectasia**, and **liver disease**. All of these processes course with weight loss as they result in the malabsorption of fat from the patient's diet. The digestion of fats, principally **long-chain triglycerides** (LCTs), requires the presence of hepatic bile acids and pancreatic lipase. Without them, the absorption of LCTs falls by up to 50–70 % if there is a lack of bile acids and it is practically nonexistent in the case of pancreatic lipase. Even if the owner does not describe their pet's faeces as being steatorrhoeal, the animal may still be digesting less fat due to malabsorption.

TAKE NOTE!

Undigested fat in the colon causes watery diarrhoea. This is due to the hydroxylation of fat by the colonic microflora.

Dogs with malabsorption should eat a low-fat diet, but it should not be zero fat. As such, LCTs can contribute up to 5–10 % of the total dry weight. **Medium-chain triglycerides** (MCTs) hold an advantage over LCTs because they can be absorbed without the need for pancreatic lipase or bile acids. They enter directly into the portal circulation, rather than the lymphatic vessels, at least in theory; hence they are particularly useful in the treatment of lymphangiectasia. Unfortunately, MCTs do not contain any essential fatty acids and therefore they should not represent more than 50 % of the fat consumed in the patient's diet.

Cats with pronounced malabsorption should be fed a diet with a moderate fat restriction to prevent the clinical signs from recurring. Such diets must also provide a normal or limited amount of fibre, as a high fibre intake has been shown to reduce enzymatic activity in the pancreas.

TIP

Appetite is rarely a primary problem in dogs. However, dogs with reduced appetite can be stimulated to eat more by adding warm water to the food, changing it frequently, and instructing the owner to encourage their pet while eating.

Lastly, in cases of weight loss for which all other causes have been ruled out, the first treatment option should be a calorie-dense, nutrient-rich diet.

DIET DATA SHEET

Owner's information:

Name and surname(s): ______________

____

Tel.: ______________

Email: ______________

Pet's information:

Name: ______________

Species: ________ **Sex:** M ☐ F ☐ CM ☐ SF ☐

Age and weight: _____ years and _____ kg

Body condition score: _____/9 (to be completed by the vet)

Level of activity: High ☐ Moderate ☐ Low ☐

Patient's dietary history:

Type of food: Dry diet ☐ Wet diet/cans ☐ Homemade food ☐

Amount and frequency of each type of food:

	Never	A small amount	Half	Mostly	Only this one	Approx. daily amounts	Brand (if applicable)
Dry diet							
Wet/cans							
Homemade food							

If you use a homemade diet, please list its main components:

Types of rewards or treats:

	Yes	No	Daily amount	Brand or composition
Commercial treats				
Human food/leftovers				
Dietary supplements				

Have you changed your pet's diet recently? No ☐ Yes ☐ Previous brand:

When did you change the diet? And why?

How would you describe your pet's appetite? Good ☐ Fussy ☐ Poor ☐

When does your pet eat? Morning ☐ Midday ☐ Evening ☐

For how long is food available to your pet? ___ minutes ___ hours He/She always has food ☐

How many times a day does your pet defaecate? 0–1 ☐ 2–3 ☐ 4 or more ☐ Not sure ☐

How would you describe the stools? Consistent ☐ Formed but not solid ☐ Soft, loose ☐

What about your pet's lifestyle? Does not leave the house ☐ Always outside ☐ Half and half ☐

How much exercise does he/she get each day? <30 minutes ☐ 30–60 minutes ☐ 1–3 hours ☐ >3 hours ☐

Does your pet live with any other animals? Yes ☐ No ☐

Please use this space to ask us any questions or add any relevant comments about your pet's diet:

Author's note: summarised example of a diet data sheet.

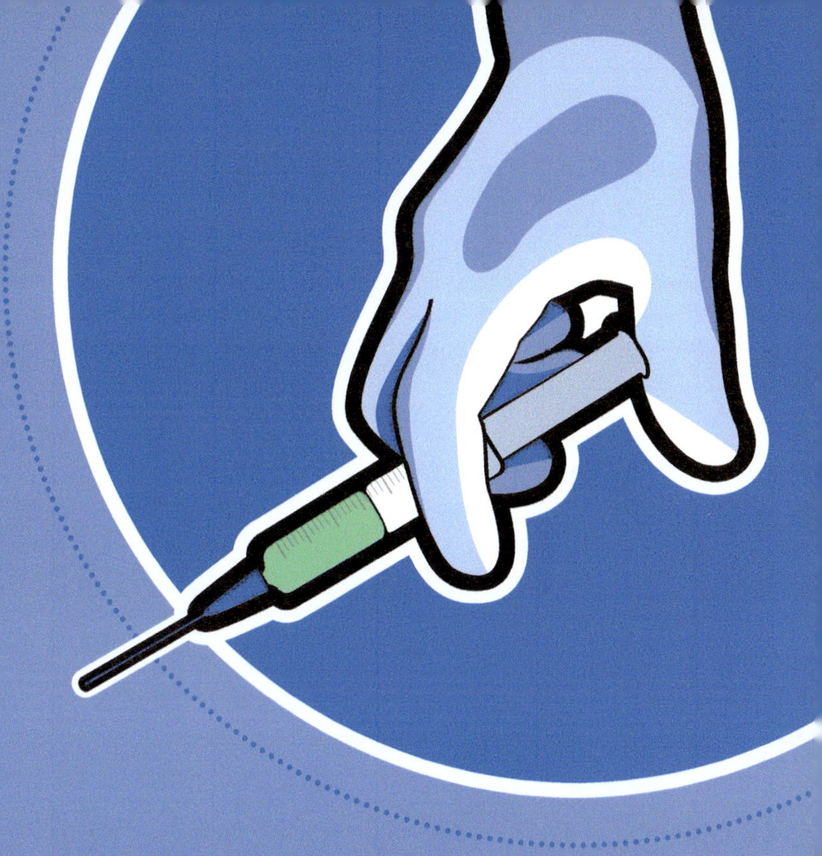

3 Pharmacological treatment of geriatric patients

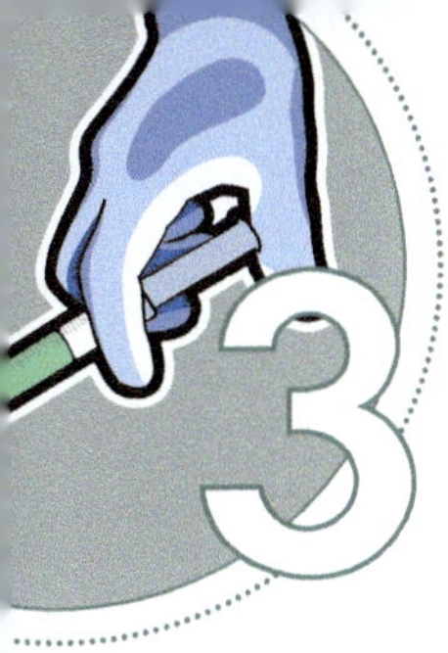

Pharmacological treatment of geriatric patients

As we mentioned earlier and will continue to discuss throughout this book, animals that have already enjoyed 85 % of their life span are more prone to diseases. Accordingly, owners often visit their veterinary clinic for diagnostic services, the results of which may indicate that we need to start treating the patient.

As we shall see in subsequent chapters, many of the conditions affecting this age group are chronic diseases that also require chronic treatment. A good veterinary clinician should be very familiar with the patient and the drugs they will prescribe. Besides explaining the patient's expected improvement to the owner, they should also describe the signs that owners should be aware of in case the medication causes any side effects.

We cannot go into all the drugs available, but we can set out some general guidelines to improve our confidence when prescribing drugs to elderly patients and when modifying the dosage regimen.

Basic concepts in pharmacology

Before delving into the details, let us clarify a few basic notions so we can advance with a solid understanding. We have all heard of these concepts, yet their infrequent application during regular veterinary activities means they are easily forgotten and seen as somewhat ineffective or distant.

The first principle is that of **pharmacodynamics**, which is the study of the biochemical and physiological effects of drugs, as well as their mechanism of action and the relationship between a drug's concentration and its effect on the body. In other words, pharmacodynamics is the study of the drug's action on the body.

On the other hand there is **pharmacokinetics**, which is the study of what the body does to the drug. Pharmacokinetics includes different stages from the drug's initial absorption, followed by its distribution and metabolism, and up to the elimination of the medication and/or its metabolites. Although when explained like this they may seem to be separate concepts, actually they are closely related (e.g. the effects of a drug, i.e.

its pharmacodynamics, depend on its concentration when it reaches the target organ or system and this concentration depends on the rate of absorption, metabolic capacity, etc., i.e. its pharmacokinetics).

We are also interested in the **volume of distribution (V_d)**, which is the volume of body fluid in which the drug is actually dissolved. However, the parameter "real V_d" is very hard to measure so we use the "apparent V_d", which is given by the equation:

$$V_d = dose/C_{plasma}$$

The apparent V_d is of limited value; above all, it indicates whether the drug tends to accumulate in blood plasma or elsewhere and therefore whether its concentration is high enough when it reaches the target organ.

Figure 1 shows how drug pharmacokinetics and pharmacodynamics change in elderly animals.

The methods described below can be used to adjust a drug's dose or dosing interval appropriately for geriatric patients.

Dose adjustments for geriatric patients

The aim of this section, and one of the key points in this chapter, is to explain how to individualise each patient's drug therapy in order to minimise the occurrence of adverse reactions, side effects, and, as much as possible, any drug–drug interactions. A drug's dose and dosing schedule can and should be modified so that it can be administered with the least possible risk for the patient. The best means of adjusting a drug's dosage is by measuring its blood concentration, as we regularly do with phenobarbital, potassium bromide, cyclosporine, and aminoglycosides. However, sometimes this is unfeasible because of the cost or a lack of laboratories that analyse other drugs. Accordingly, we need a method with a more affordable benefit–cost ratio and which is valid for most drugs. One such option is to make dose adjustments based on **creatinine clearance**. This technique relies on the fact that the elimination of creatinine and many other drugs via tubular secretion occurs in parallel to each other.[1]

Nevertheless, creatinine clearance testing is not used very often in veterinary medicine, primarily because it is hard to collect 24-hour urine samples. So in daily practice, therefore, we tend to measure the blood creatinine level and replace the creatinine clearance with this value in the formulas. The linear correlation between blood creatinine and creatinine clearance no longer applies for creatinine concentrations over 4 mg/dl.[2]

TAKE NOTE!

This dosage adjustment method does not consider V_d, the degree of protein binding, and other nonrenal routes of drug excretion.

Consequently, the dosage should be adjusted using the serum creatinine concentration as a guide, which in turn should be monitored to assess the effectiveness and for any signs of toxicity or side effects.

By adjusting the dosage according to the blood creatinine level, the vet can either reduce the amount of drug administered or increase the dosing frequency. The aforementioned formulas are:[2]

$$Dose_{corrected} = Dose_{normal} \times \left(\frac{Crea_{normal}}{Crea_{patient}}\right)$$

$$Interval_{corrected} = Interval_{normal} \times \left[1/\left(\frac{Crea_{normal}}{Crea_{patient}}\right)\right]$$

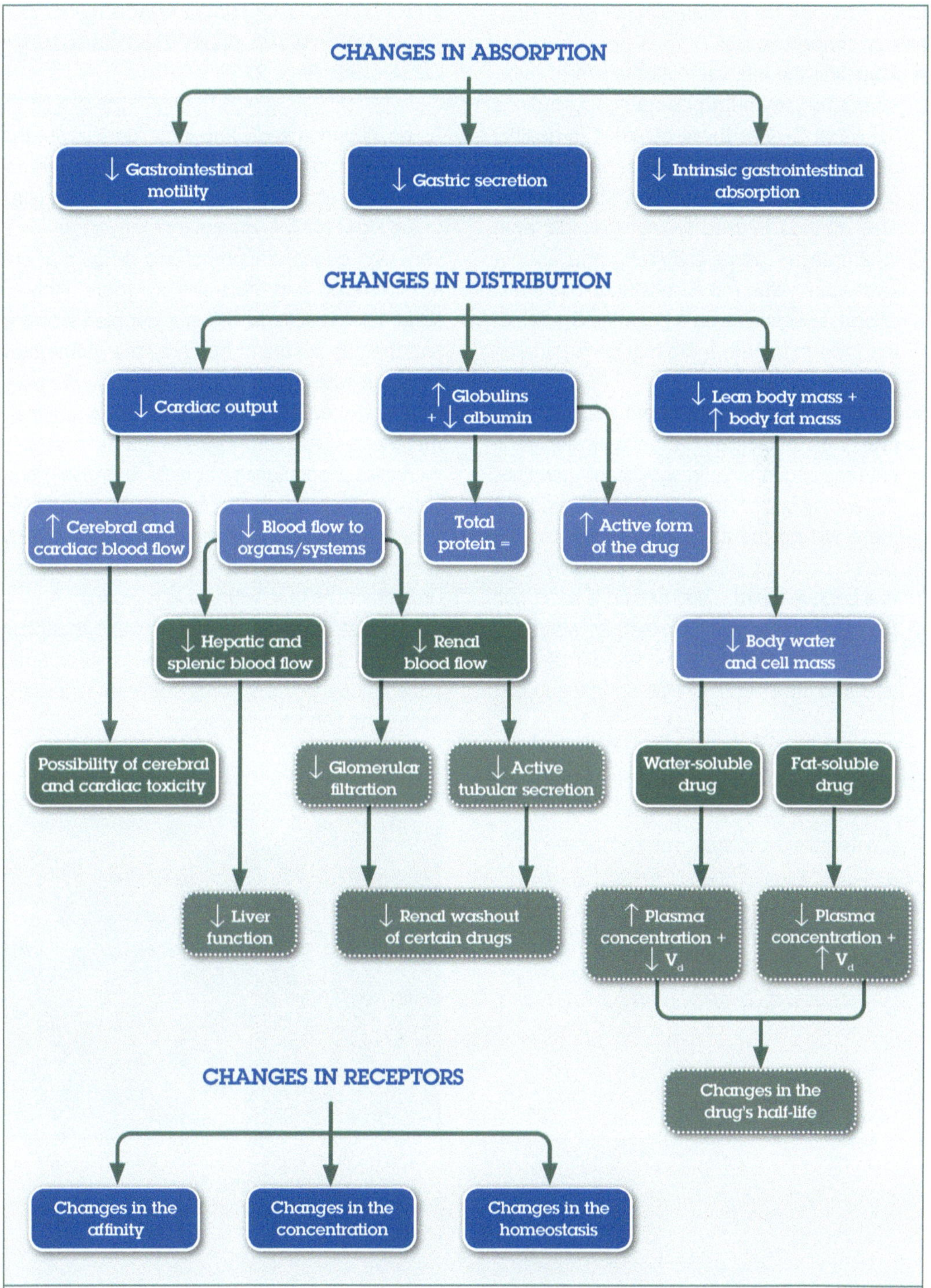

Figure 1. Pharmacokinetic and pharmacodynamic changes due to age.

Both methods try to maintain constant drug plasma concentrations:

- **Adjusting the interval** results in similar maximum and minimum plasma concentrations (C_{max} and C_{min}) as those obtained in healthy patients. However, the concentrations are occasionally subtherapeutic for short periods. This method is used for nonsteroidal anti-inflammatory drugs (NSAIDs) and aminoglycosides,[7] where their postantibiotic effect extends over time even though the C_{min} is less than the minimum inhibitory concentration (MIC) for the pathogen.
- If we use the **dose adjustment** method, however, then the active pharmaceutical ingredient may accumulate in significant quantities depending on the drug, but unlike previously, there will not be any periods at subtherapeutic concentrations once a steady state has been reached. This method is used with β-lactam antibiotics, for example, when C_{min} needs to be kept above the MIC for the bacteria and the drugs are relatively innocuous.[3]

TAKE NOTE!

The veterinary clinician must choose one of the two methods depending on what is more important for the drug – C_{max}, C_{min}, or the mean dose – and what is best for the patient.

Pharmacological changes in patients with chronic kidney disease (Fig. 2)

As we all undoubtedly know, the kidneys are the body's main organs of excretion. Under normal conditions, around 25 % of cardiac output goes to the kidneys. This means that they experience very high concentrations of any drugs that are administered and are therefore more likely to suffer toxic reactions. If this is coupled with the fact that, as occurs in humans, the **glomerular filtration rate** (GFR) in pets probably declines with age, then the tendency for drugs (or their metabolites) to accumulate in the kidneys also increases proportionally, at least for those medications which use this route of elimination.[4] This is believed to be one of the reasons why elderly humans experience 3 to 10 times more adverse drug reactions than younger age groups.[4–7]

It is also important to bear in mind that drug toxicity is greater than expected in azotaemic patients due to the synergy between azotaemic toxins and certain medications.

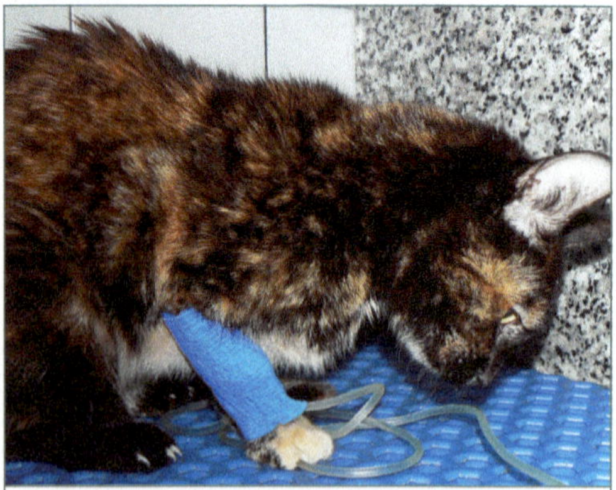

Figure 2. Nineteen-year-old female cat with severe hypokalaemia during the course of diabetic ketoacidosis. The patient also suffers from IRIS stage 2 kidney disease.

TAKE NOTE!

Besides the age-related decline in GFR, it is important to note that the rate of chronic kidney disease can exceed 15 % in geriatric dogs; this figure can increase up to 30 % in elderly cats.[8]

As explained earlier, the GFR and **renal clearance (CL_R)** of certain substances decrease in parallel to each other. The term CL_R is always for a given substance and is defined as the volume of plasma (in ml) that is cleared of the substance in unit time (in minutes) due to the effect of renal function. From this moment on, the cleared substance becomes part of the urine.[9]

Renal clearance can be calculated from the formula:

$$CL_R = CL_{GF} + CL_{TS} - FR$$

Where CL_{GF} is the clearance due to glomerular filtration, CL_{TS} is the clearance attributable to tubular secretion (mainly by the proximal tubules) and FR is the fraction of reabsorption from the tubules back into the systemic circulation (mainly occurs in the distal tubules). Tubular reabsorption is a passive process for many drugs but, by contrast, an active one (requires energy) for electrolytes, vitamins, and glucose.

Thanks to this formula, we know that if $CL_R > CL_{GF}$, for example, then the drug undergoes tubular secretion (CL_{TS}). If, by contrast, $CL_R < CL_{GF}$, in this case there is a significant fraction of reabsorption (FR).

Alterations in drug bioavailability and absorption

Azotaemic patients often develop vomiting and diarrhoea, and, logically, this alters the absorption of oral medicines. However, it is not the only factor that alters drug absorption rates; gastric emptying is slower[3] and the small intestine has a lower intrinsic absorptive capacity in patients with azotaemia.[1,10] The bioavailability of any pH-dependent drugs changes whenever they are coadministered, for instance, with antacids, which are often given to animals with a tendency for uraemic gastritis.[11,12]

Alterations in drug distribution

The V_d for a lot of drugs is altered in dogs with chronic kidney disease (CKD). Patients with CKD often suffer fluid retention which increases the V_d for any drugs that are principally distributed in extracellular fluid. There is also a reduction in the amount of albumin-bound drug; this is believed to be because albumin molecules alter their conformation in the presence of uraemic toxins.[13] Furthermore, studies have shown that there is a shift in the site where acidic drugs bind with albumin, whereas there is no change in how basic drugs bind with this protein.[13,14]

Alterations in hepatic metabolism

Some hepatic metabolic pathways function more slowly in patients with azotaemia, namely, acetylation, hydrolysis, and conjugation; on the other hand, methylation, sulphoconjugation, and glucuronic acid synthesis are unchanged.[15] This means a lot of drugs which would be eliminated, instead accumulate in the blood due to the reduced rate of their metabolic pathways. Contrastingly, sometimes there is a change in which organ eliminates the drug, so what was previously filtered by the kidneys starts to be excreted by the liver. One such example is the metabolism of tolfenamic acid. In this case, a reduction in plasma half-life, rather than an increase, has been reported in dogs with experimentally induced CKD. This seems to be because of an apparent increase in hepatic metabolism and excretion.[16]

HOW SHOULD WE DEAL WITH A SUSPECTED ADVERSE REACTION OR TOXICITY TO AN ACTIVE PHARMACEUTICAL INGREDIENT?

1 Replace it with another, equivalent drug that uses a different main metabolic pathway (e.g. enalapril and ramipril, which are primarily eliminated via the kidneys and liver respectively).

2 If it cannot be replaced:

- Reduce the dose or change the schedule without losing efficacy. The pharmacokinetic data help in this respect (e.g. gentamicin is better administered once a day SC rather than three times a day IV).
- Help reduce the workload on the excretory organ (e.g. by administering acetylcysteine or S-adenosylmethionine for the liver or fluid therapy for the kidneys).

3 Withdraw any medications with no clear benefit and stimulate the patient's appetite. It has been shown that patients who do not eat properly tend to endure more pharmacologically toxic events.[4,18]

Table 1. Drugs of interest for geriatric patients.

Drug	Reason for adjustment	Adjustment method	Monitor levels?	Notes
Aminoglycosides	Nephrotoxicity	EI	Yes	-
Penicillins	Can accumulate in patients with CKD	DR	No	Monitor Na and K if using IV administration Broad therapeutic window
Sulphamides	• Nephrotoxicity • Bone marrow depression • The concentration of protein-bound drug decreases in patients with azotaemia	DR	No	-

Table 1. Drugs of interest for geriatric patients (continued).				
Drug	**Reason for adjustment**	**Adjustment method**	**Monitor levels?**	**Notes**
Tetracyclines	• Nephrotoxicity, can accumulate in patients with CKD • Exacerbate azotaemia	DR, EI	No	Better to use doxycycline as it is less toxic
Fluoroquinolones	• Can accumulate in patients with CKD • Macrolides, lincosamides, and metronidazole do not need adjusting	EI	No	Broad therapeutic window
Carprofen	• Hepatic metabolism with metabolites in faeces and urine • Idiosyncratic hepatotoxicity	EI, DR	No	-
Meloxicam	• Its half-life gets longer with chronic use • All NSAIDs can produce hepato-/nephrotoxicity • Almost all undergo hepatic metabolism • The amount of protein-bound NSAID decreases in patients with azotaemia	EI, DR	No	-
Corticosteroids	• Increase the number and sensitivity of α-adrenergic receptors • Hepatic metabolism decelerates in CKD, exacerbating azotaemia • Can worsen hypertension	Avoid adjustments if possible	No	-
Furosemide	• The effect and absorption decrease over time, while the half-life increases • Azotaemia reduces protein binding	Individualise according to the effect	No	-

Table 1. Drugs of interest for geriatric patients (continued).

Drug	Reason for adjustment	Adjustment method	Monitor levels?	Notes
Pimobendan	Hepatic metabolism, eliminated in the faeces	Monitor effects and total bilirubin in hepatic patients	No	-
ACEI	• The hepatic metabolism of its active metabolite may decline • Increased hypotensive effect • Reduced renal clearance in CKD	Monitor effects and blood creatinine	No	-
α-Adrenergic blockers	• Increased bioavailability and half-life in elderly patients • Decreased hepatic metabolism	EI, DR	No	-
Digoxin	• Accumulates in patients with CKD • Decreased V_d due to a loss of muscle mass • Exercise precaution when coadministering with furosemide as it increases the toxicity	EI, DR	Yes	-
Phenobarbital	• Azotaemia reduces protein binding • Decreased hepatic metabolism and it may be hepatotoxic	Avoid its use in patients with liver disease	Yes	-
Potassium bromide	Renal metabolism, start with half the recommended dosage in cases of CKD	DR	Yes	-

EI: extend the dosing interval; DR: dose reduction.

THE OWNER'S PERSPECTIVE

Adherence to therapeutic dosing regimens is generally **low** and as more medications are added and the schedule becomes more complicated, it **declines even further**.

It is advisable to **select the medications** that are most likely to **make a difference** and giving the client a detailed **explanation** of **your actions** so they can **understand** the importance of these drugs.

You should also **describe any side effects** and **what to do in case they develop**. If the owner notices and considers a given drug is counterproductive, it can easily be discontinued. The vet must explain what to do under such circumstances.

Chronically ill geriatric patients often **require more medications** which implies more cost, sometimes significantly more. **Expressing the price** as the **cost per month** rather than per container of tablets often makes the **treatment seem more affordable**.

Daily/weekly pill boxes may be a big help for clients who do not have the best memory or find it hard to administer the prescribed fractions of tablets. Pill boxes are divided into seven smaller sections for each day of the week, and in some boxes, these are also divided in two for morning and evening medications. Auxiliary staff can fill the client's pill box each week and split any tablets correctly, if necessary. **Clients really appreciate this added-value service** and it ensures there is **very close contact and monitoring of the case**.

We are often keen to learn but fail to find enough time to learn. As veterinary practitioners, we regularly complete Herculean working days, so upon getting home it can be very hard to read a book or article on anaesthesia which assumes we can remember everything there is to know about pharmacology and animal physiology.

Lastly, please bear in mind that this chapter is written from a purely practical clinical perspective. It attempts to explain the basic and more advanced concepts of anaesthesia in a straightforward, comprehensible, and above all pragmatic manner.

How to design a personalised protocol for each case

Besides a good knowledge of anaesthesia and veterinary medicine, vets must also be able to interpret the clinical signs and any changes in laboratory values, as well as being aware of their own capacities.

Familiarity with the patient

Obviously, the patient will be either an elderly cat or dog. As we all know, geriatric animals tend to have more underlying diseases, or their systems and organs have lost some of their "reserves". The increased incidence of diseases and/or organ dysfunction is, to a certain degree, to be expected. However, the debilitation of elderly organs is not as obvious and is almost automatically embedded within the term **geriatric** or **"normal ageing"**. The deficit in reserves may or may not be apparent until the patient undergoes anaesthesia, surgery, or a period of hospitalisation.[1]

Systems most affected by ageing

The organs or systems that debilitate the most with age, and with most relevance for anaesthesia, are:

1. **Cardiovascular system:** geriatric patients have a reduced cardiac capacity. This limits their ability to compensate for the cardiovascular changes that will occur during anaesthesia. Senior pets suffer from a decline in baroreceptor function, blood volume, cardiac output, and blood pressure, whereas vagal tone increases.[2] In humans, the cardiac conduction system is also known to change as we age, which predisposes elderly patients to cardiac arrhythmias provoked by the anaesthesia.[3] The risk of progressive degeneration of the myocardium increases with age in both cats and dogs, and it is often associated with heart valve disease in the case of dogs. The myocardium has to work harder in the presence of these diseases and therefore consumes more oxygen, which may ultimately mean it is particularly sensitive to hypoxia. It should be noted, as occurs in elderly humans, that the walls of the great vessels develop thicker elastic fibres and accumulate collagen fibres and calcium. These changes translate into an increase in the peripheral resistance, thus reducing the capacity to adapt to hypotension.[4]
2. **Respiratory system:** as our patients grow older, the functional reserve of their respiratory function also wanes. This is because the respiratory muscles lose strength, the rib cage loses some capacity for distension, and the lungs lose elastic recoil.[5] One study conducted in Beagles concluded that ageing was accompanied by a reduction in lung elasticity, respiratory rate, tidal volume (amount of air moved within a normal respiratory cycle), minute volume, oxygen consumption, and carbon dioxide production. The authors also found a diminished presence of the airway protective reflexes.[6] Poorer reflexes means that our elderly patients may be more susceptible to aspiration pneumonia in the immediate postoperative period.[7]

3. **Liver:** as the years go by, the hepatic microsomal enzyme system experiences a decline in its functional capacity. This reduction in capacity is present even though the hepatic biochemical parameters are within normal values.[8] Furthermore, it is important to remember that elderly animals often receive less blood flow to the liver because their level of cardiac work has fallen. So it follows that the half-life will increase in any drugs that depend on hepatic metabolism, conjugation, or excretion. Reduced liver function can also result in a tendency for hyperproteinaemia, reduced activity of blood coagulation factors, and an increased susceptibility to hypoglycaemia.[1]
4. **Kidneys:** as occurs with the liver, an aged pair of kidneys receives less blood, again partly due to the reduction in cardiac work. Additionally, the number of functional glomeruli is known to dwindle with age. The renal tubules also go through changes (atrophy, hypertrophy, or a reduction in diameter, among others). Glomerular filtration can diminish by as much as 50 %. The inability to concentrate urine and excrete hydrogen ions (H^+) is due to alterations in the distal tubules. Consequently, the concentration of antidiuretic hormone (ADH) increases,[2] and so senior pets are more prone to acidosis. This results in patients who are more sensitive to dehydration and any fluids administered in excess. These changes mean that some of the drugs excreted by the kidneys have a longer half-life.

TAKE NOTE!

Anaesthesia can reduce renal blood flow and glomerular filtration by up to 40 %, which is why elderly patients are more susceptible to kidney failure after undergoing an anaesthetic procedure.

After developing a sound understanding of the characteristics of geriatric patients in general, the next step is to study each patient in a little more individual detail. This involves a series of preoperative phases, each more important than the previous.

The preoperative visit and tests

Senior cats and dogs frequently suffer from a range of diseases or lesions. These problems must be detected before surgery and none of them should be underestimated; the true value in such cases is to know they exist, then assess whether they entail any risk and how to minimise it accordingly. So, for instance, depending on the position we place a given patient during surgery, their hip osteoarthritis could cause more pain than the area operated on.

A comprehensive preoperative examination is essential and should include a special focus on the patient's cardiovascular system (thoracic auscultation, blood pressure, capillary refill time [CRT], femoral pulse measurement, presence of jugular pulse, etc.), hydration status, body condition, and an estimation of their ideal weight. If there are any clinical signs of systemic diseases, they must be studied further before subjecting the patient to anaesthesia or surgery.

TIP

One of the things owners value the most before an anaesthetic procedure is when the vet reexamines the patient. It is advisable to record all the information from this examination and hand a copy to the owner, together with the intraoperative monitoring data, after the operation.

CLASSIFICATION OF PATIENTS ACCORDING TO THEIR ANAESTHETIC RISK

(FROM THE AMERICAN SOCIETY OF ANESTHESIOLOGISTS, ASA)

Category 1 (ASA 1): healthy patient with no detectable diseases.

Category 2 (ASA 2): patient with mild systemic disease.

Category 3 (ASA 3): patient with severe systemic disease that limits their activity but does not incapacitate them.

Category 4 (ASA 4): patient with incapacitating systemic disease that is a constant threat to their life.

Category 5 (ASA 5): moribund patient who could die within 24 hours with or without the operation.

With regard to blood tests, it is quite hard to decide which tests to request and which to omit. There is no magic potion; the more parameters assessed, the easier it is to identify any alterations, if they exist. It is worth designing a series of test panels or packages, including a list of the tests each one contains and its price. Of course it is the owner who will assume the cost, but we should make sure they have all the information required to make the appropriate choice. Table 1 shows the preoperative panels we recommend at our clinics.

Table 1. Preoperative test panels recommended at the S.A. Veterinaris and Clínica Felina Barcelona veterinary clinics.

Type of panel	Tests included
Basic preoperative	Blood count + ALT + ALP + TP + Glu + Crea + Urea
Advanced preoperative	Blood count + ALT + ALP + TP + Glu + Crea + Urea + Alb + Na + K + Cl
Comprehensive preoperative	Blood count + ALT + ALP + TP + Glu + Crea + Urea + Alb + Na + K + Cl + Chest X-ray
Cardiac preoperative	Blood count + ALT + ALP + TP + Glu + Crea + Urea + Alb + Na + K + Cl + GGT + P + Ca + NT-proBNP* + Chest X-ray + ECG

* NT-proBNP is the amino-terminal fraction of brain natriuretic peptide.
Note: T_4 should always be determined in all geriatric cats and a fructosamine test is highly recommendable.[4]

REASONS FOR RECOMMENDING PREOPERATIVE TESTS

Advantages for patients, since the results can be used to:

- Personalise the anaesthesia.
- Predict possible peri- and postoperative complications.
- Collect some baseline values for the patient which are particularly helpful if complications arise and for future comparisons.

Advantages for owners:

- Many clinics offer discounts on preoperative tests. This could be the ideal moment for the owner to check on points that have never been analysed before.
- They minimise the risks associated with anaesthesia. Nevertheless, it is important to emphasise the tests only reduce the risks – they do not eliminate them completely.

Advantages for vets (besides the above, from which we also benefit):

- Increase in direct income. Evidently, more tests equals more income.
- Increase in indirect income. The detection of alterations or even the diagnosis of "silent" diseases will probably entail more tests and checkups that are far from insignificant.
- They help pay for the extremely expensive equipment required of a modern clinic.
- It reinforces our image as promoters of our patients' health and demonstrates we run a modern, up-to-date clinic.

TAKE NOTE!

No preoperative test or panel can replace a thorough preoperative exam.

Recognising our options and materials

We just wish to add a small point of reflection. Elderly patients have less capacity to adapt to the changes they will endure while under anaesthesia, or in other words, geriatric patients should be anaesthetised with a more guarded approach than that of a healthy 1-year-old whose organs and systems are all fully functioning. For example, no one would consider performing a thoracotomy without an automatic ventilator or at least an assistant working a manual ventilation mask, well nor should we anaesthetise the patient if we do not know how to calculate the tidal volume correctly or whether the ventilator is a pressure- or volume-cycled model. Put another way, your clinic could possess the best equipment available, but if no one knows how to interpret or, worse still, operate it correctly, it is going to serve very little purpose.

TIP

Spending some time familiarising yourself with the anaesthetic materials will allow you to get the most out of them and improve your anaesthetic procedures at no extra cost.

Just as we mentioned that it is difficult to decide which parameters should be analysed in the preoperative examination, it is also hard to affirm which of the monitoring parameters are most important. Therefore, the more parameters we monitor, the more information we shall have about the anaesthetised patient.

If we had to choose just one monitor, we find **waveform capnography** to be one of the safest and most reliable devices. Furthermore, **capnography** becomes almost indispensable when considering many of the complications that occur during anaesthesia are due to insufficient gas exchange. Unfortunately, it is still more expensive than **pulse oximetry** or **apnoea monitors**, but the investment is worth it.

Anyone interested in learning more about the subject can find an informative review article on capnography in dogs in reference 9.

TAKE NOTE!

No monitor or digital parameter should replace an intraoperative examination: check cardiac auscultation, mucous membrane colour, CRT, temperature, and blood pressure (invasive or noninvasive) every few minutes.

PARAMETERS THAT SHOULD BE MONITORED

Plane or depth of anaesthesia (ocular position and reflexes, pedal or anal reflexes).

Cardiocirculatory function (normal or oesophageal auscultation, femoral pulse assessment, mucous membrane colour, CRT, urine production, blood pressure, and ECG).

Respiratory function (pulse oximetry, capnography, and blood gas analysis).

Temperature (oesophageal is better than rectal).

Familiarity with the drugs used

Modern anaesthesia is founded on two concepts that have been incorporated in recent years. These approaches are **balanced multimodal anaesthesia** and **preventive analgesia**. Balanced multimodal anaesthesia works on the notion that a little bit of many is better than a lot of just a few, while the second concept involves treating pain before it arises.

BY DEFINITION ANAESTHESIA INCLUDES:

- Loss of consciousness
- Muscle relaxation
- Analgesia
- Amnesia

An example of unbalanced anaesthesia for a dog is something like:

- Induction with propofol: 7 mg/kg IV.
- Maintenance with isoflurane: 2–2.5 %.

An example of balance anaesthesia in the same patient is:

- Sedation with medetomidine: 2 μg/kg IV.
- Analgesia with methadone: 0.5 mg/kg IM or SC.
- Induction with propofol: 1–3 mg/kg.
- Maintenance with isoflurane: 0.5–1 %.

Below we present a brief summary of each group or specific drug normally used in veterinary anaesthesia.

TIP

It is important to remember the dose–effect relationship. We recommend preparing the full dose, injecting it slowly in subdoses of around 25 % of the total, and pausing when the correct effect has been achieved.

Sedatives

Phenothiazines

This group basically consists of **acepromazine** and **chlorpromazine**. They are potent drugs with an antihistaminic, antiemetic, and anxiolytic action. Their sedative action is due to depression of the reticular activating system and the anti-dopaminergic effect on the CNS. Suppression of the sympathetic nervous system reduces catecholamine secretion. They are strong hypotensive agents through vasodilation and should only be used in normovolaemic patients. This is because phenothiazines have an antagonist effect on α_1-adrenergic receptors. It has been suggested that this antagonism at a cardiac level reduces the risk of arrhythmias.[10] Lastly, it has always been believed that phenothiazines lower the seizure threshold in animals with epilepsy but in fact this relationship remains to be proven.[11,12] They undergo hepatic metabolism, so their use should be avoided or normal doses reduced in very elderly patients or those with liver disease.

Benzodiazepines

Benzodiazepines increase the activity of inhibitory neurotransmitters in the CNS (γ-aminobutyric acid and glycine). The three most commonly used benzodiazepines are **diazepam**, **midazolam**, and **alprazolam**. The first two are available in an injectable format, but alprazolam is not. They are good anxiolytics, sedatives, and muscle relaxants.[13] They produce a mild and sometimes unreliable sedative effect and can even cause paradoxical excitation in healthy animals if they have not been administered any other type of sedative (e.g. opiates). They have an excellent cardiorespiratory profile,[14] as they hardly depress either myocardial contractility or respiratory rate. Diazepam must be administered intravenously and slowly because of its diluent (propylene glycol). Its effect appears to last longer than that of midazolam at equipotent doses. As midazolam is water soluble, it can be mixed with other aqueous drugs and administered intravenously, intramuscularly, or subcutaneously. Alprazolam can be given orally as preventive treatment at home to calm anxious animals before the anaesthetic procedure. Its main effect is as an anxiolytic and it is believed to induce a certain degree of amnesia, although the amnesiac effect may apply to all three benzodiazepines described here.[15] Diazepam and midazolam also have anticonvulsant properties. Although rarely needed, their effects can be reversed using **flumazenil**.

α_2-Agonists

This a very large group of drugs. From the first to be marketed for veterinary use in Germany

Table 2. Sedatives for cats and dogs.

Drug	Dose	Route	Peak action time	Duration of action	Reduction of the anaesthetic	Analgesic	Muscle relaxant
Acepromazine	0.01–0.05 mg/kg	IM, SC, IV	IM: 35–40 min IV: 15–20 min	6 h	25–40 %	No	Yes
Diazepam	0.2–0.4 mg/kg	IV	5 min	2 h	10 %	No	Yes
Midazolam	0.1–0.4 mg/kg	IM, SC, IV	IM: 10–15 min IV: 5 min	1–1.5 h	10 %	No	Yes
Medetomidine	2–10 µg/kg*	IM, IV	IM: 15–20 min IV: 2–3 min	Sedation: 2–3 h Analgesia: 1 h	40–70 %	Yes	Yes
Dexmedetomidine	1–5 µg/kg*	IM, IV	IM: 15–20 min IV: 2–3 min	Sedation: 2–3 h Analgesia: 1 h	40–70 %	Yes	Yes

* Low doses for IV administration and higher doses for IM. Note the units of µg/kg.

used for induction in single doses.[1] The dose of thiopental should be down-titrated, and boluses should not be repeated.

Propofol

Propofol, which is a phenol derivative first synthesised in the early 1970s, has become a typical component of our anaesthetic protocols. Some well-defined pharmacokinetic and pharmacodynamic properties, together with a fall in its price and the need for lower doses when coadministered with opiates and/or α_2-agonists, have made propofol more affordable, and it has now displaced barbiturates as the most popular inducer. We shall not examine the effects of this drug in too much detail, just highlight the points of interest for geriatric animals. The main advantage of propofol is its rapid metabolism and the absence of any clinically significant accumulation following total intravenous anaesthesia (TIVA).

One study in elderly dogs showed that the induction dose (5 mg/kg) should be lower than the dose normally used in younger patients (7 mg/kg). The study also suggested an increase in the propofol clearance time.[18] However, used as an anaesthetic inducer (single dose), it does not hold a clear advantage over thiopental. In fact, in a comparative study, propofol seemed to provoke more hypotension and without sufficient compensatory reflex tachycardia,[19] as well as a greater reduction in cardiac output than thiopental.

Alfaxalone

The hypnotic effects of steroid products related to progesterone were first investigated in 1941. The early studies found that, besides their hypnotic action, these progesterone derivatives also cause muscle relaxation and a certain degree of analgesia.[20] Alfaxalone was originally marketed as a mixture with alfadolone and diluted in castor oil. This strange mixture was created because of the need to dilute alfaxalone in water. However, the excipient has a strong allergenic action,[21] so the mixture is now practically obsolete. Nowadays, alfaxalone is available in a crystalline aqueous solution thanks to the use of cyclodextrins. Cyclodextrins are carbohydrates with a conical structure produced when starch is broken down by bacteria. The outside of the cone is hydrophilic and the inside hydrophobic. The addition of cyclodextrins makes alfaxalone 375 times more soluble in water[22] and there are infinitely fewer anaphylactic reactions. Alfaxalone is a good hypnotic agent with rapid anaesthetic induction. The maintenance and recovery periods are characterised by excellent muscle relaxation. Cardiorespiratory system depression increases proportionally to the dose administered, although the change is insignificant at the recommended dose (<6 mg/kg IV). Respiratory depression and apnoea are the most common side effects. However, their risk can be minimised by injecting alfaxalone slowly and administering the dose based on the effect.

TAKE NOTE!

In anaesthesia, a slow injection is over the course of at least 2 minutes. Very small volumes should be diluted.

Alfaxalone is a viable alternative to the injectable anaesthetics available for veterinary medicine when administered for short surgical procedures.[23] It can be given intravenously, intramuscularly, or subcutaneously, but the low concentration of the commercially marketed solution means a large volume has to be administered, which complicates its subcutaneous use in medium to giant dogs. In cats, alfaxalone is a significant competitor for ketamine when given in intramuscular or subcutaneous anaesthetic mixtures.

Etomidate

Etomidate is a carboxylated imidazole derivative with no relation to barbiturates.[24] It is supplied as a transparent, water-soluble solution for use as an intravenous anaesthetic. There are two formulations: the first etomidate product marketed contains 35 % propylene glycol, which makes it an extremely hyperosmolar solution,[25] and the second is etomidate emulsion prepared with a creamy solution similar to the one used for propofol. It mainly has a hypnotic effect, as it suppresses the neocortex. Etomidate's function is mediated by suppression of the GABAergic system.[26] As mentioned earlier, γ-aminobutyric acid (GABA) is the main inhibitory neurotransmitter in mammals.[27] Etomidate does not act as an analgesic.[28]

Etomidate has some interesting actions and properties:

- The cerebral perfusion pressure remains more stable with etomidate than with thiopental or propofol because it hardly affects systemic blood pressure.[29]
- Etomidate is the anaesthetic that causes the fewest cardiac alterations with the initial doses. One study found there was no change

in heart rate, systemic blood pressure, left ventricular pressure (end-diastolic and peak pressure), left ventricular contractility, and myocardial oxygen consumption after administering etomidate.[30]

- In the respiratory system, anaesthetic doses of etomidate increase respiratory rate and reduce tidal volume, which translates into the same minute volume as before administration. From the information available, its respiratory depression effect is dose dependent. As occurs with other inducers, slow injection followed by constant rate infusion (CRI) reduces or avoids this slight depression.[30]
- As for its effects on the endocrine system, etomidate stops adrenal hormone synthesis by inhibiting 11α- and 11β-hydroxylase metabolism, as well as that of the cholesterol side chain reductase enzyme.[29] This suppression affects cortisol, aldosterone, and corticosterone production. It is known to occur in both dogs[31] and cats.[32] The inhibition has very little clinical significance, as it has not been linked to an increase in perioperative mortality. In the aforementioned studies, the adrenal suppression did not exceed more than 6 hours. In critically ill human patients sedated with etomidate via CRI over several hours there was an increase in mortality due to addisonian crises.[33]

Etomidate has emerged as the safest anaesthesia inducer available compared to barbiturates, propofol, or alfaxalone. It is the first choice in patients with liver problems or cardiac contractility and heart rhythm disturbances.[29,34] The induction and arousal stages, however, are not ideal with etomidate, and to avoid tremors and myoclonus, the patient should be well sedated (e.g. midazolam or midazolam–fentanyl).

Table 3 shows the induction dose of the five intravenous anaesthetics discussed here and Table 4 compares their properties and effects.

Agents used for maintenance

Historically, maintenance anaesthesia has predominantly been performed with halogenated gases (halothane, isoflurane, etc.), but these days, total intravenous anaesthesia, or TIVA, is also becoming very accepted. This chapter does not deal with the latter method, since it is easily applied and based on knowledge of the drugs described here and their dose for CRI.

Isoflurane and sevoflurane are the only two inhaled anaesthetic products currently approved for use in small animals in Spain. However, there is a wealth of references and literature that discuss them or compare them with their predecessor halothane. Before briefly describing these three products, we should quickly review some relevant concepts in the physics of anaesthesia.

Physics of anaesthesia

Solubility and partition coefficients

The solubility of an anaesthetic gas is defined as its capacity to dissolve in a liquid or solid. However, solubility is normally expressed as partition coefficients. These coefficients describe the ratio of concentrations of an anaesthetic gas in two inhaled solvents. The most relevant coefficients in anaesthesia are (Table 5):

- **Blood:gas partition coefficient.** Anaesthetics with a high coefficient are readily soluble in

Table 3. Induction dose of intravenous anaesthetics used in geriatric cats and dogs.

Anaesthetic	Induction dose
Thiopental	2–6 mg/kg
Propofol	2–6 mg/kg
Alfaxalone	0.5–2 mg/kg
Etomidate	0.5–1.5 mg/kg
Ketamine	3–5 mg/kg

Table 4. Comparison of the effects of some of the main injectable inducers (1 is the best effect, 4 the worst).

	Characteristics of induction	Characteristics of recovery	CNS effects	Therapeutic window	Cardiovascular effect	Respiratory effect
Thiopental	1	2	1	3	3	3
Etomidate	4	2	3	1	1	1
Propofol	1	1	2	3	4	4
Ketamine	2	3	4	2	2	2
Alfaxalone	1	1	2	2	2	3

Based on Ilkiw J. Injectable anesthesia in dogs - Part 1: Solutions, doses and administration. In: Gleed RD, Ludders JW, eds. *Recent Advances in Veterinary Anesthesia and Analgesia: Companion Animals.* Ithaca, International Veterinary Information Service (www.ivis.org), 2002.
Author's note: the evaluation of the effects of alfaxalone were not taken from the same source, but rather based on the literature and author's experience.

blood, while those with a low coefficient are poorly soluble and therefore act more rapidly. As such, the blood:gas partition coefficient can be considered a measure of the rate of induction, change of plane, and anaesthetic recovery.

- **Oil:gas partition coefficient.** This coefficient correlates with an anaesthetic gas' potency. In this case, agents with a high coefficient are more oil soluble (most of the brain consists of lipids).

Minimum alveolar concentration (MAC)

The MAC of an anaesthetic gas is the minimum concentration that prevents purposeful movement in response to a standard painful stimulus in 50 % of anaesthetised patients (Table 6). The standard stimulus is pinching the interdigital webbing or tail. A higher MAC equals a more potent anaesthetic. If gases are used without any other drugs for anaesthesia during surgery (which is not recommended), the concentration should be 1.2 to 1.4 times the MAC. On

Table 5. Blood:gas and oil:gas partition coefficients of some inhaled anaesthetics.

	Halothane	Isoflurane	Sevoflurane	Desflurane	N_2O
Blood:gas	2.36	1.41	0.69	0.42	0.49
Oil:gas	224	91	47	19	1.4

Table 6. Minimum alveolar concentration of inhaled anaesthetics in cats and dogs.

MAC	Halothane	Isoflurane	Sevoflurane	Desflurane	N_2O
Dogs	0.87	1.28	2.34	7.20	188–297
Cats	1.19	1.63	2.58	9.79	255

the other hand, when using a good combination of sedatives and/or analgesics, the amount of anaesthetic gas dissolved in oxygen can be reduced to 0.5 times the MAC. The MAC is influenced by various factors including hypothermia, hypotension, hypoxaemia (PaO_2 <40 mmHg), hypercapnia ($PaCO_2$ >95 mmHg), pregnancy, and age (as in the present case).

TAKE NOTE!

A drop in body temperature is a common side effect of anaesthesia and often causes the most complications.

How do you determine the ideal concentration of anaesthetic gas for each patient?

Unfortunately, it cannot be calculated with a formula. To find the ideal minimum concentration for each patient, after inducing anaesthesia with one or more injected agents, start with a concentration of at least 2 % isoflurane for small animals. After allowing the phases to equilibrate (usually a few minutes, less than five), start diluting the gas by reducing the amount in steps of 0.1 or 0.2 %, while remaining alert for signs of a superficial plane of anaesthesia (tachycardia, recovery of ocular reflexes, etc.). Upon observing signs of the superficial plane, immediately return to the previous concentration of anaesthetic gas. This routine must be applied for each patient, as it ensures a state of anaesthesia with the least possible depression of the cardiovascular system. The side effects of inhaled agents should not be underestimated, above all because they are all strong hypotensive agents.

Inhaled gases

- **Isoflurane:** a highly stable isomer of enflurane. It is not as potent as its predecessor halothane, but the induction and recovery are quicker. Unlike halothane, isoflurane is not arrhythmogenic and provides more cardiovascular stability. It is eliminated via pulmonary clearance (99.8 %).
- **Sevoflurane:** thanks to its low blood:gas partition coefficient, it produces even quicker induction and recovery, which improves control over the anaesthetic plane. However, it has a higher MAC. It can react with soda lime to produce **compound A**, which can cause nephrotoxicity. Isoflurane is preferred over sevoflurane for inhaled induction because its odour is less unpleasant.

Analgesics for acute or postoperative pain

Pain management should be a leading priority from the outset of any intervention on an elderly animal. Uncontrolled pain stimulates acute catecholamine secretion or chronic cortisol secretion and can lead to surgical/anaesthetic failure or even death of the patient. Therefore, it is important to apply a preventive, multimodal approach to pain management that covers both intra- and postoperative pain.

Nowadays, it is inconceivable to design an anaesthetic plan without a good analgesic. Five different types of drug, described below, can be combined to obtain the most effective multimodal analgesia possible.

Nonsteroidal anti-inflammatory drugs (NSAIDs)

NSAIDs inhibit cyclooxygenases, which are enzymes responsible for producing prostaglandins from arachidonic acid, although they are believed to act in other locations as well. There is a lot of information in the literature discussing their use, classes, and COX-1/COX-2 selectivity, yet there are no studies that indicate which is the best or safest NSAID.

TAKE NOTE!

NSAIDs can be considered the cornerstone of veterinary postoperative pain management.

Tables 7 and 8 (for dogs and cats respectively) show the recommended doses for each of the NSAID active pharmaceutical ingredients marketed in Spain. Note the following four points when using NSAIDs to avoid their associated problems:

- Never administer to dehydrated animals or those with kidney disease or electrolyte disturbances.
- Monitor intra- and postoperative blood pressure.
- Advise the owner of the animal given an NSAID that if the patient does not eat or drink properly after surgery, they should inform you as soon as possible.
- To avoid NSAID-induced gastric problems, the preventive agent of choice has traditionally been misoprostol (a semisynthetic prostaglandin E_1 analogue), although proton pump inhibitors, such as omeprazole, have proven to be as or more useful than misoprostol.

Opiates

The use of opium derivatives in veterinary operating rooms has gained supporters over the last 20 years. This is because of the need to counteract the harmful effects of pain in patients undergoing surgery and because opiates allow for the use of lower doses of anaesthetics. Opiates can be classified according to the receptor upon which they act, their relative potency, or their half-life, among others. However, to simplify matters, as a general rule we should use a **pure agonist (μ/OP_3)** (morphine, pethidine, methadone, fentanyl, etc.) to ensure a strong level of analgesia. **Partial agonists** (buprenorphine) can be administered for moderate pain. Butorphanol (an **opioid agonist-antagonist**) should be used as a sedative and mild analgesic. It has a short duration of analgesic action but works well for visceral pain (Table 9).

α_2-Agonists

The analgesic effect of this group of drugs is well known, but until recently it was not used in the immediate postoperative period. This is because it was hard to guarantee they were used safely. With the appearance of dexmedetomidine, which is much more reliable and has a more reproducible effect, their use has increased considerably thanks to constant rate infusions.

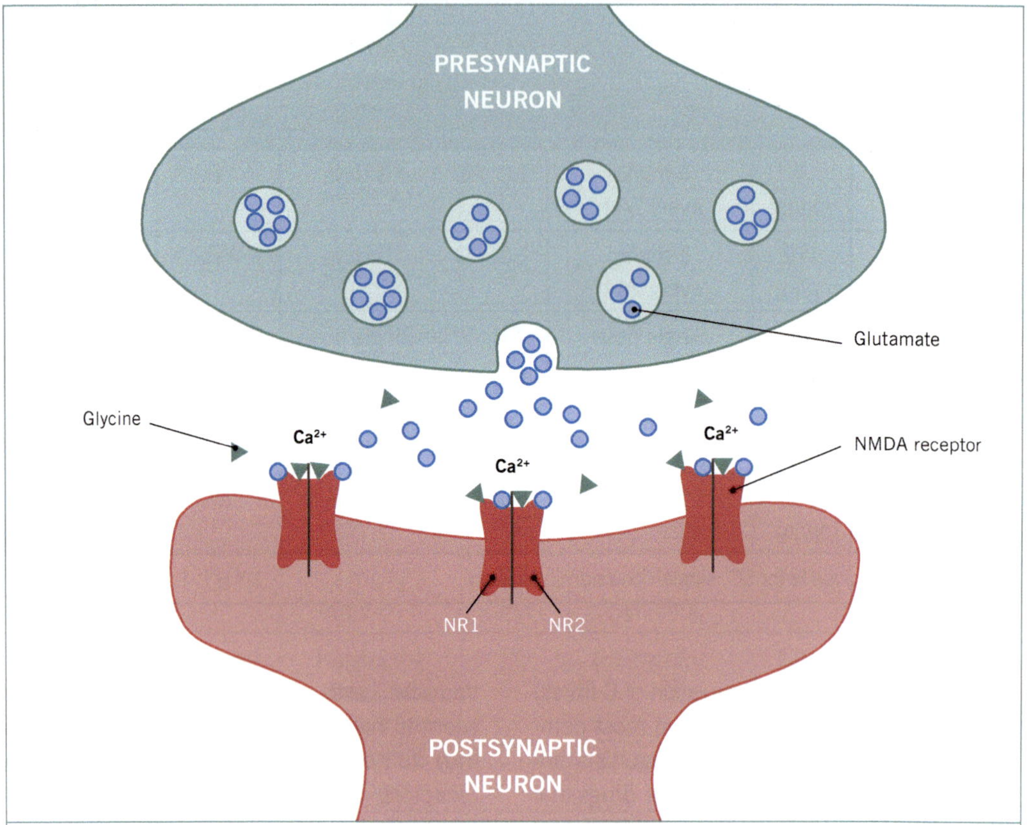

Figure 1. The NMDA receptor.

Local analgesics

Besides local anaesthetics, we can use opiates and α_2-agonists for a localised action, although generally only for epidural use. Similarly, there are also reports on the epidural use of ketamine and NSAIDs, but such use is still very restricted.

Local anaesthetics

Local anaesthetics are considered as the only true analgesics. They do not compete for receptors or block the release of neurotransmitters, rather they directly cut off the painful nervous stimulus and prevent the signal from reaching structures in the upper central nervous system. Various techniques can be applied when administering local anaesthetics and they require some practice. Nevertheless, they should not be undervalued given they are very effective and can be exploited to perform even the most painful operations without having to reach anaesthetic planes so deep that they endanger the patient's life. This section explains some locoregional, continuous/intermittent catheterisation[37] (see pages 68 and 69), and epidural anaesthesia techniques (Tables 10 and 11).

Some of the most used local anaesthetics belong to the amino amide family (lidocaine, bupivacaine, etc.).[38] They are safer and less allergenic than products from the amino ester family (benzocaine, tetracaine, etc.).

Table 10. Analgesics administered epidurally to cats and dogs.			
Drug	Dose	Onset of action	Duration of effect
Lidocaine (2 %)	• 3–5 mg/kg • 1 ml/7.5 kg for analgesia of the rear third • 1 ml/6 kg for abdominal analgesia	10–15 min	1–2 h
Lidocaine (2 %) + adrenaline (5 mg/ml)	As above	As above	2–4 h
Mepivacaine (3 %)	• 3–4.5 mg/kg • 1 ml/7.5 kg for analgesia of the rear third • 1 ml/6 kg for abdominal analgesia	10–15 min	1.5–2 h
Bupivacaine (0.5 %)	• 1–2.5 mg/kg • 1 ml/7.5 kg for analgesia of the rear third • 1 ml/6 kg for abdominal analgesia	20–30 min	4–6 h
Morphine	0.05–0.15 mg/kg	30–60 min	12–24 h
Meperidine	0.5–1.5 mg/kg	5–10 min	1–4 h
Fentanyl	0.001–0.01 mg/kg	5–20 min	2–4 h
Buprenorphine	0.005–0.015 mg/kg	60 min	16–24 h
Morphine + bupivacaine (0.5 %)	0.1 mg/kg of morphine + 1 ml/7.5 kg of bupivacaine for the rear third, or 1 ml/6 kg of bupivacaine for the abdomen	Same onset of action as for each drug separately	Same duration of effect as for each drug separately

Note: the volume should never exceed 8 ml. It is good practice to reduce the dose of the drugs by 25 % in geriatric, juvenile, or pregnant patients.

Table 11. Local anaesthetics for nonepidural use.					
	Commercial strength	Maximum dose in dogs (mg/kg)	Maximum dose in cats (mg/kg)	Duration of analgesia (min)	Onset of action (min)
Lidocaine	0.5–2 %	8	6	60–120	10–15
Mepivacaine	1–2 %	5	4	90–180	5–10
Bupivacaine	0.5–0.25 %	2	2	150–360	20–30
Etidocaine	0.5–0.75 %	3	2	120–360	5–10
Ropivacaine	0.50 %	3	2	150–360	5–15

PLACEMENT OF AN INTERMITTENT INFUSION CATHETER FOR LOCAL ANAESTHETICS

These catheters can be purchased or easily custom made with a little practice. Figure 2 shows which materials are required: some orange rubber tubing, mosquito forceps, scissors, stopper with injection port, and a lighter.

First measure a suitable length of rubber tubing and then cut off the excess (Fig. 3). Bear in mind the full path the tubing most follow, from the deepest point of the wound to its most superficial layer.

After cutting, clamp the end with some mosquito forceps (Fig. 4).

Heat over the flame (from a lighter or Bunsen burner) (Fig. 5).

The rubber will melt and seal the tube at one end (sometimes this step has to be repeated a few times) (Fig. 6).

Next, use a small-calibre needle (25 gauge) to puncture small holes every 5 mm that are evenly spaced along the full length and all the way around the tube that will be buried in the wound (Figs. 7 and 8).

Attach a stopper with a rubber injection port (Fig. 9).

Inject saline or air to check the stopper is watertight (Fig. 10).

If it works correctly, small drops of local anaesthetic should emerge from the holes punctured in the tube (Fig. 11).

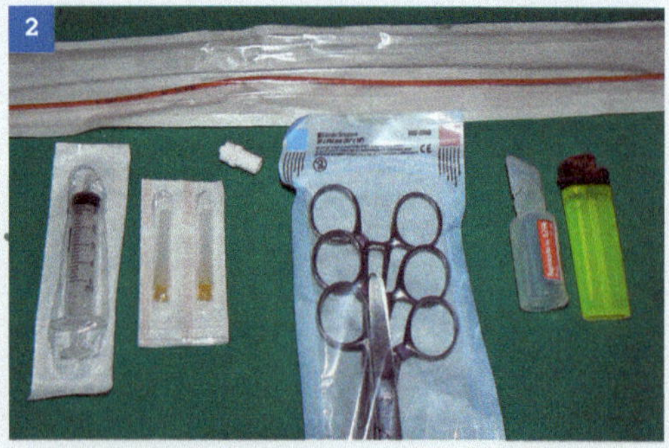
2

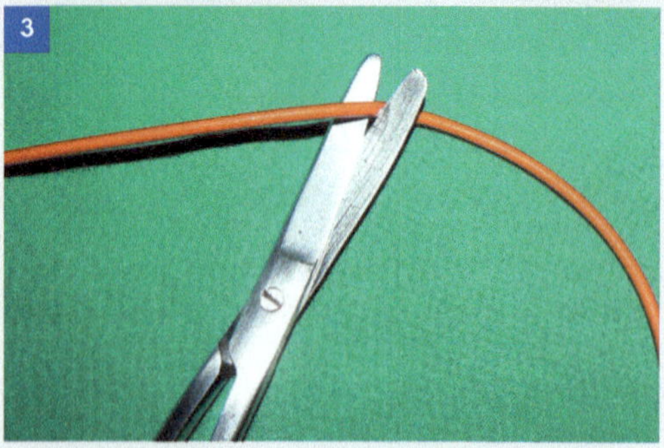
3

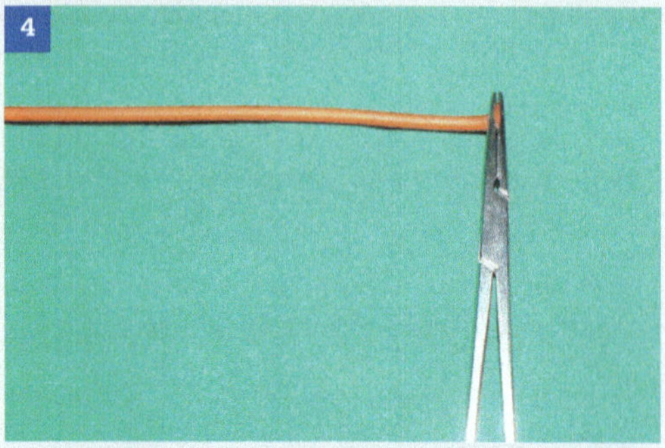
4

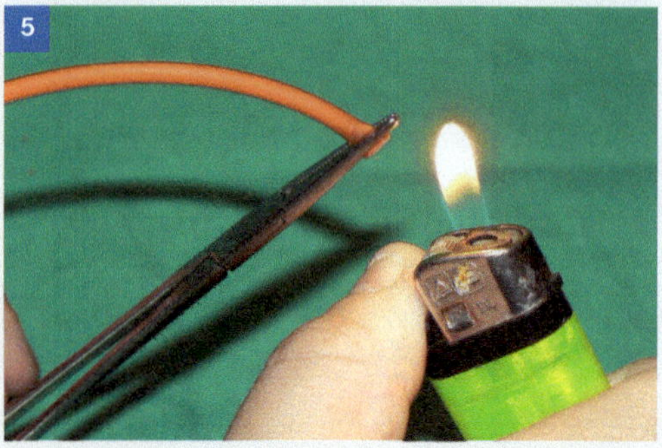
5

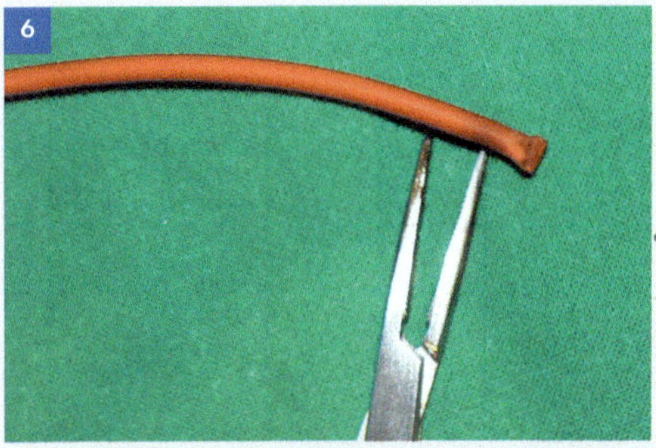

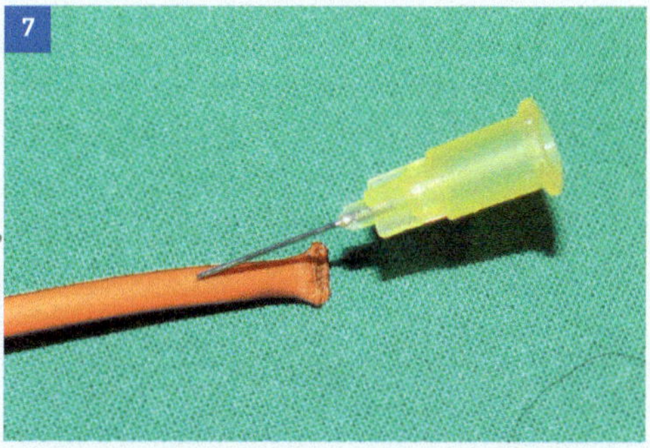

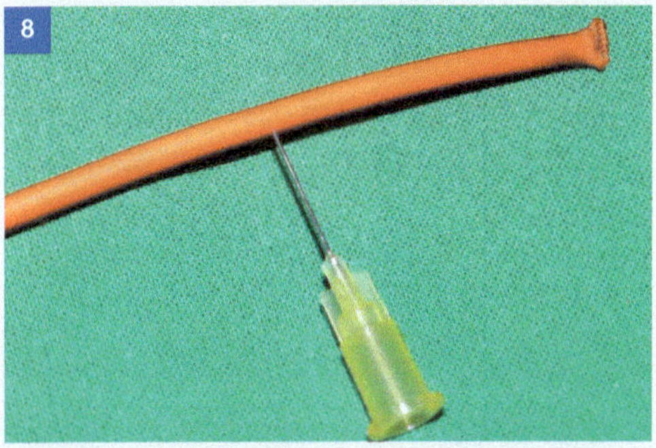

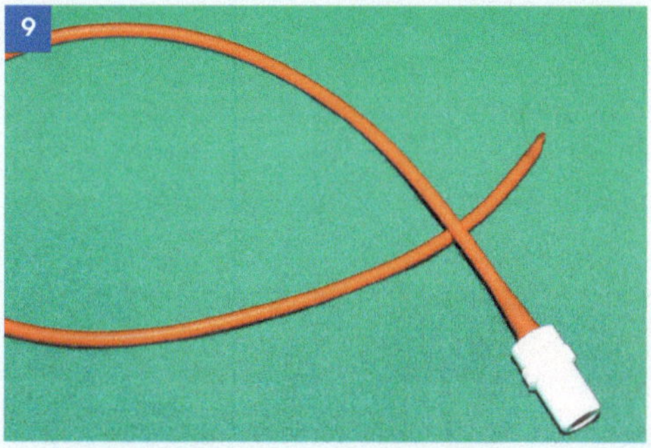

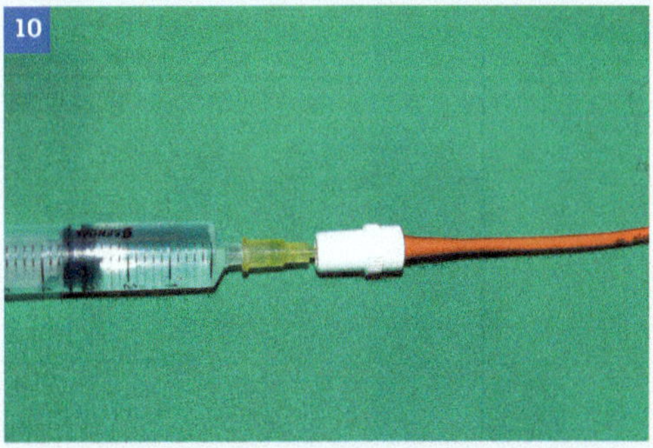

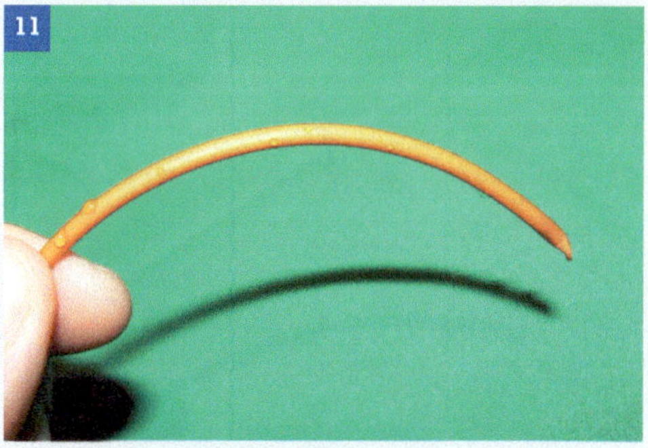

NOTE

It is important to remember that this tube should not be attached or pierced with any stitches so that it can be withdrawn at any time. It can be prepared prior to surgery and sterilised later, or the whole process can be done under aseptic conditions. The first dose of local anaesthetic can be given before the animal awakens after surgery; by doing so, it eliminates the initial burning sensation.

There is a delay between their administration and the onset of action. This time varies according to the active substance, and it must be respected before starting the intervention to ensure the patient does not feel any pain. The box on the right contains some practical advice on the use of local anaesthetics.

Opiates in epidural anaesthesia

When injecting into the epidural space, patients will not feel any pain, but they maintain motor function in the rear third. The most popular opiate in Spain to achieve this effect is preservative-free morphine. The onset of action is 1 hour after injection, but it may last for up to 24 hours following its administration. Another opiate commonly used in dogs is buprenorphine and it is just as effective as morphine, yet the duration of epidural buprenorphine in cats is much shorter.[39,40]

TIP

You can avoid waiting an hour before performing surgery by using an epidural combination of lidocaine and morphine since the lidocaine is effective within 5–10 minutes and when it wears off the morphine will have started acting.

Besides its effects on pain, a combination of morphine and bupivacaine is also known to reduce the neuroendocrine response to post-operative stress.[41]

PRACTICAL ADVICE FOR THE CORRECT USE OF LOCAL ANAESTHETICS

1. Calculate the maximum dose based on the patient's ideal weight. Administer the required amount and disregard the rest.
2. They can be mixed with adrenaline to increase the duration of action (0.1 ml of adrenaline for every 20 ml of local anaesthetic).
3. Always aspirate before injecting local anaesthetics, with or without adrenaline. Many are cardiotoxic.
4. Local anaesthetics should not be coadministered with vasoconstrictors in the limbs, tail, or other appendices.
5. To avoid pain when injecting local anaesthetics, they can be mixed with bicarbonate (1 part bicarbonate with 9 parts anaesthetic). This gives a quicker onset of action, but it also reduces the overall duration.
6. Doubling the concentration of a local anaesthetic only increases its effect by around 30 %.

α_2-Agonists in epidural anaesthesia

There are only a handful of publications on the epidural use of these drugs and, while beneficial, the side effects were very similar to those observed when used by more traditional routes (IM or IV).[42]

Analgesic combinations for surgery and the postoperative period

In the last 5 years, the intensive care units of many hospitals have turned to the use of constant rate infusions with analgesic combinations. **Morphine–ketamine–lidocaine** (MKL) or **fentanyl–ketamine–lidocaine** (FKL) are two of the most used combinations. Both combinations produce excellent analgesia and are very well tolerated (Table 12).

Table 12. Doses of drugs for constant rate infusions in cats and dogs.

Drug	Dose	Loading dose
Butorphanol	0.1–0.2 mg/kg/h	0.1 mg/kg IM or IV
Methadone	0.05–0.2 mg/kg/h	0.1–0.2 mg/kg slow IV
Fentanyl	0.02–0.06 μg/kg/min (0.0012–0.0036 mg/kg/h)	0.003–0.005 mg/kg IM or IV
Ketamine	2–10 μg/kg/min (0.12–0.6 mg/kg/h)	0.50 mg/kg IV
Morphine	2–6 μg/kg/min (0.12–0.36 mg/kg/h)	0.1–0.5 mg/kg IM
Lidocaine	10–50 μg/kg/min (0.6–3.0 mg/kg/h)	0.5–1 mg/kg slow IV
Medetomidine	1–5 μg/kg/h (0.001–0.005 mg/kg/h)	2.4 μg/kg
Dexmedetomidine	0.5–2.5 μg/kg/h (0.0005–0.0025 mg/kg/h)	1–2 μg/kg IV
Propofol	0.05–0.2 mg/kg/min	1–5 mg/kg IV
Alfaxalone	0.1 mg/kg/min	2 mg/kg IV
Etomidate	50 μg/kg/min	0.5–1 mg/kg IV

These doses can be used in cats with the exception of lidocaine and opiates in which case it is better to apply the lower dose given in the table.

HOW DO YOU PREPARE AN MKL OR FKL COMBINATION?[43]

Materials:

- One 500 ml bottle of Ringer's lactate solution, physiological saline or 5 % glucose solution.
- 40 mg of morphine sulphate or 0.75 mg of fentanyl.
- 500 mg of lidocaine.
- 100 mg of ketamine.

Preparation:

1 Calculate the total volume (ml) of all the drugs and remove the same amount from the 500 ml bottle of solution.
2 Add the drugs to the bottle.
3 As morphine and lidocaine are photosensitive, the bottle should be protected from light (e.g. with aluminium foil).
4 Inject an initial loading bolus of 3 ml/kg, then start to infuse the rest of the bottle at a constant rate of 1–3 ml/kg/h.
5 Bear in mind that this "analgesic" volume has already been administered when performing fluid management throughout the rest of the operation. According to guidelines published in 2013, the AAHA/AAFP Fluid Therapy Guidelines for Dogs and Cats, the infusion rate should be 2–3 ml/kg/h for cats and 2–6 ml/kg/h for dogs.
6 If using the solution as an intraoperative analgesic, ensure anaesthesia is maintained by administering an intravenous or inhaled hypnotic.

The final doses given to the patient are:

- Morphine: 0.24 mg/kg/h with a concentration of 80 mg/l in the bottle.
- Fentanyl: 0.005 mg/kg/h with a final concentration of 1.5 mg/l.
- Lidocaine: 3 mg/kg/h with a concentration of 1,000 mg/l in the bottle.
- Ketamine: 0.6 mg/kg/h with a final concentration of 200 mg/l.

Note: for cats, it is recommended to prepare the dilution without lidocaine because of its potential toxicity. If it is included, never exceed a dose of 10 µg/kg/min or 0.6 mg/kg/h. Author's note: personally, for cats, I use a combination of fentanyl–ketamine (FK) or morphine–ketamine (MK) at the following doses for a 500 ml solution: 60 mg of morphine or 0.6 mg of fentanyl plus 60 mg of ketamine. I apply an infusion rate of 1–3 ml/kg/h for MK and 1 ml/kg/h for FK. If the cat has received an intramuscular dose of ketamine combined with an opiate agonist, I do not administer the loading dose.

THE OWNER'S PERSPECTIVE

No one likes to see their pet undergo anaesthesia. **Be empathetic.**

Explain to the owner each and every **stage of the anaesthetic procedure** and how the patient will be **controlled and monitored** throughout. If possible, the procedure should be recorded on **paper** and, after the intervention, you can hand a **copy of the report** to the owner.

It is important to **remind the owner that there is no such thing as a perfect anaesthesia**. That said, if the patient is in a good state of health, **there will be minimal complications**. If, however, their health is less than perfect, then you need to stress the importance of **diagnosing** and even **treating** any conditions that could complicate the anaesthetic procedure.

Do not take anything for granted. One of the things owners like the least about surgery is discovering their pet has been shaved in several areas to insert catheters, take ultrasound images, and so on. **We need to explain everything and emphasise the reasons why**.

Remind the owner that each animal responds to anaesthesia differently, which is why your clinic always **personalises anaesthetic procedures to each individual**. Furthermore, remind them that their pet is unique to them and that **your patients are also unique to your clinic**.

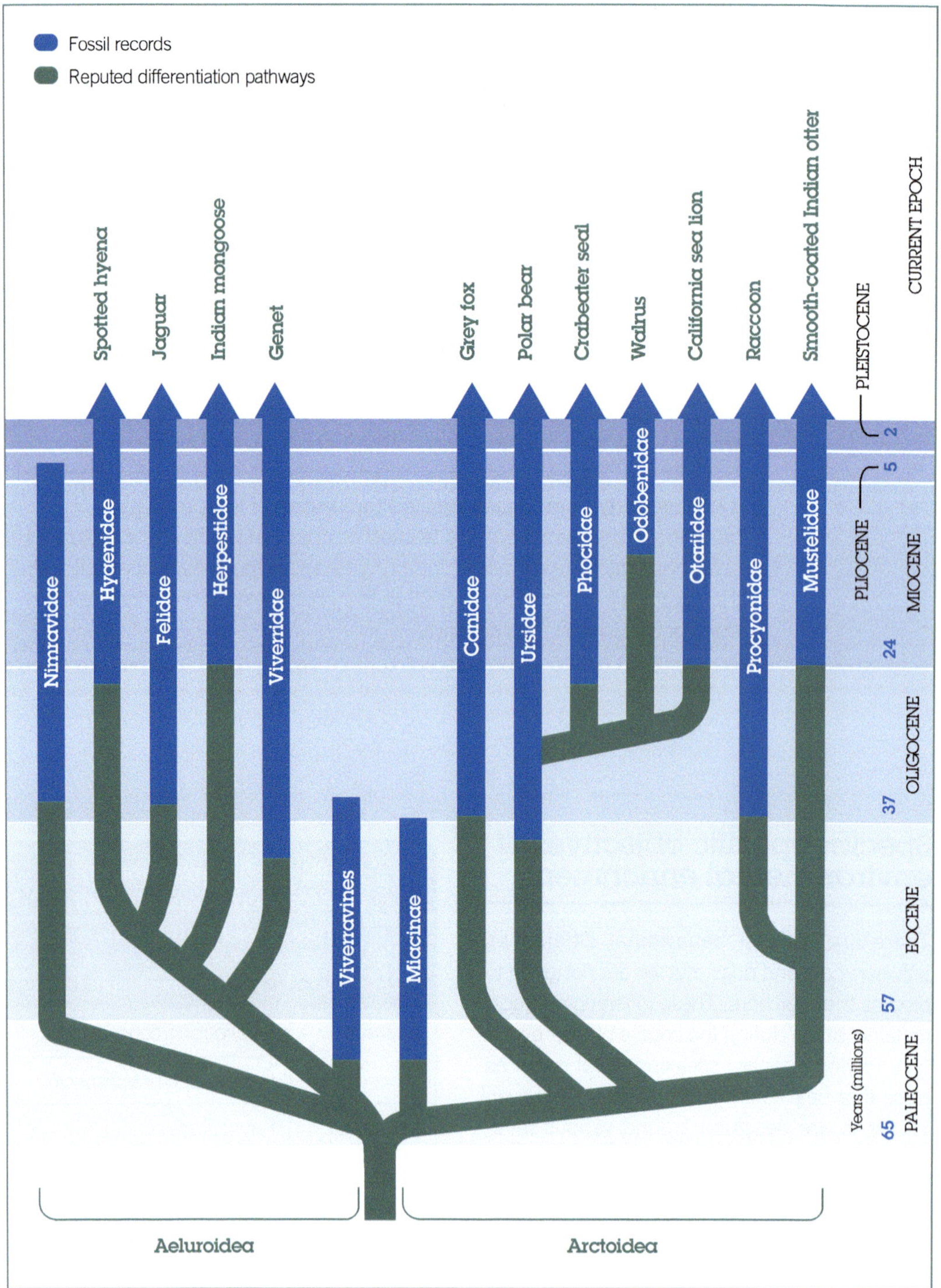

Figure 1. Phylogeny of carnivores.

EE plans have various objectives, but we can say that the overall aim is to improve the patient's physical and mental health by modifying the environment, that is, without using drugs (Box 1).[1–3] Adopting these measures will not only improve our patients' quality of life, but we can also resolve organic problems, such as feline idiopathic cystitis, which forms part of the recently discovered condition called Pandora syndrome.[4]

Animate enrichment

Animate EE refers to an animal's interactions with other beings, whether from the same or a different species. This enrichment is **conspecific** when the interaction is with an individual from the same species or **heterospecific** when it is between species. In animate enrichment, the quality of socialisation with the species the patient interacts with is key to obtaining a positive outcome and avoiding worse problems or injuries.

Box 1. AIMS OF ENVIRONMENTAL ENRICHMENT.

To increase behavioural repertoire.

To reduce the frequency of behavioural alterations.

To increase the range of species-appropriate behaviour.

To improve the ability to exploit the environment.

To increase the capacity to overcome difficulties naturally.

Conspecific social contact

It has been shown that **dogs** need contact with members of their own species, particularly in situations of isolation. Otherwise, they can develop undesired conducts.[5–8] The closer this contact, the better it is for the dogs; however, it may also introduce a greater health risk (infections) and chance of injuries (bites).[6] When dealing with a dog that has barely socialised with other dogs, it is better to start with just visual contact before allowing more intimate contact, since simply being able to smell, hear, or see another member of their species can be a sufficiently enriching experience for the patient.[9]

Given their solitary and strongly territorial origins, conspecific contact in **cats** has not been received much research attention. However, some recent articles and studies assessed intraspecific relationships and concluded that this type of contact may also be beneficial for cats.

A few premises have to be satisfied so that cats may live together peacefully and beneficially for all, namely: an abundance of food and other essential resources (litter trays, sleeping areas, drinking bowls) and certainly some degree of kinship.[10–12] Free-roaming cats tend to create groups formed by females and their offspring, which suggests that cats will coexist in a single home more smoothly if they are related.[13,14] Unfortunately, due to a lack of data, we cannot say whether this facility to create and maintain relationships with family members is merely because of shared genetics, their socialisation together from an early age, or a combination of both (Fig. 2).[15]

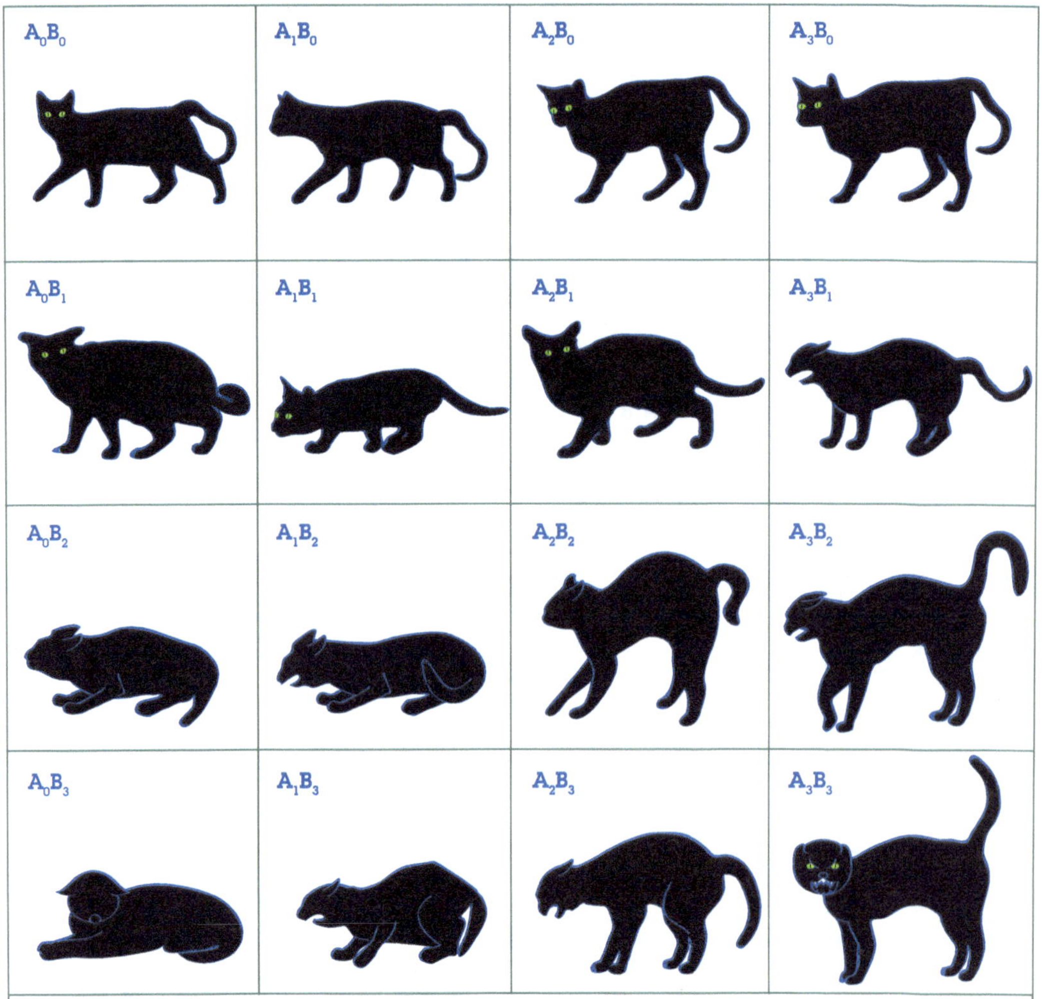

Figure 10. Bodily postures in cats. The series $A_0B_0 \rightarrow A_3B_0$ shows an ever more offensive cat, whereas the progression $A_0B_0 \rightarrow A_0B_3$ depicts a cat growing more defensive. A_3B_3 is a typical posture of a cat displaying defensive and offensive behaviour, while A_0B_0 is that of a relaxed cat. A_3B_0 shows an aggressive attitude in an offensive sense. The owners of such cats tend to report situations of extreme intraspecific aggression or unprovoked attacks on humans.
Adapted by Karen Overall from Paul Leyhausen's *Cat Behavior: The Predatory and Social Behavior of Domestic and Wild Cats.* New York, Garland STPM Press, 1979.

QUESTIONNAIRE ON ENVIRONMENTAL ENRICHMENT FOR CATS

Please read this form carefully. There are no correct or incorrect answers, we would just like to know more about your cat's living conditions. After reading it, fill out the requested background information and for the rest of the questions, place an X next to the applicable response. Please answer all the questions.

DK/NR: don't know/no response.

N/A: not applicable.

Thanks for your cooperation.

Background information

Owner's name and surname(s): ____________________
Cat's name and age: ____________________
Names and ages of other cats in the home: ____________________
Name of the cat's dry or wet diet: ____________________
Name or type of litter tray material: ____________________
Problem and date it started: ____________________

Questions

1. **Does each cat have its own food bowl?** Yes ☐ No ☐ DK/NR ☐ N/A ☐
2. **Does each cat have its own water bowl?** Yes ☐ No ☐ DK/NR ☐ N/A ☐
3. **Are the food/water bowls located so the cats can use them without being bothered?**
   Yes ☐ No ☐ DK/NR ☐ N/A ☐
4. **Are the food/water bowls cleaned regularly?**
   Yes ☐ No ☐ DK/NR ☐ N/A ☐
5. **Are the food/water bowls close to any appliances that can turn on automatically?**
   Yes ☐ No ☐ DK/NR ☐ N/A ☐
6. **Does each cat have a litter tray in a well-ventilated location where it can use it without being bothered?** Yes ☐ No ☐ DK/NR ☐ N/A ☐
7. **Are the litter trays close to any appliances that can turn on automatically?**
   Yes ☐ No ☐ DK/NR ☐ N/A ☐
8. **Is the tray scooped clean of any litter at least daily?**
   Yes ☐ No ☐ DK/NR ☐ N/A ☐
9. **Is the litter tray cleaned with soap and water at least weekly?**
   Yes ☐ No ☐ DK/NR ☐ N/A ☐
10. **Does each cat have a resting area in a location that provides some privacy?**
    Yes ☐ No ☐ DK/NR ☐ N/A ☐

Continued on the next page.

QUESTIONNAIRE ON ENVIRONMENTAL ENRICHMENT FOR CATS

11. **Can other animals bother the patient while in its resting area?**
Yes ☐ No ☐ DK/NR ☐ N/A ☐

12. **Is the resting area close to any appliances that can turn on automatically?**
Yes ☐ No ☐ DK/NR ☐ N/A ☐

13. **Does each cat have a platform or shelves from where it can monitor the rest of the home's inhabitants?** Yes ☐ No ☐ DK/NR ☐ N/A ☐

14. **Can each cat move about the home freely?** Yes ☐ No ☐ DK/NR ☐ N/A ☐

15. **Can each cat jump, play, scratch, and climb as much as it wants?**
Yes ☐ No ☐ DK/NR ☐ N/A ☐

16. **Does each cat have access to warm or cool areas?** Yes ☐ No ☐ DK/NR ☐ N/A ☐

17. **Do you leave the radio or television on when there is nobody home?**
Yes ☐ No ☐ DK/NR ☐ N/A ☐

18. **Does the patient get a chance to play with other animals or humans at least once a day?**
Yes ☐ No ☐ DK/NR ☐ N/A ☐

19. **Can each cat hide from other animals or humans throughout the entire day?**
Yes ☐ No ☐ DK/NR ☐ N/A ☐

20. **Does the patient get a chance to see cats from outside the home, even if only through the window?** Yes ☐ No ☐ DK/NR ☐ N/A ☐

21. **How much time do you spend at home where the cat can see you?** ____________ hours/day.

22. **How long do you play with your cat each day?** ______________ minutes/day.

23. **How long do you spend stroking your cat each day?** ______________ minutes/day.

24. **Does the patient have toys?** Yes ☐ No ☐ DK/NR ☐ N/A ☐

25. **Do any of the toys move?** Yes ☐ No ☐ DK/NR ☐ N/A ☐

26. **Can the toys be grabbed, lifted, tossed around, etc.?**
Yes ☐ No ☐ DK/NR ☐ N/A ☐

27. **Do you rotate the toys regularly?** Yes ☐ No ☐ DK/NR ☐ N/A ☐

28. **Does the cat have vertical scratchers at home?** Yes ☐ No ☐ DK/NR ☐ N/A ☐

29. **And horizontal scratchers?** Yes ☐ No ☐ DK/NR ☐ N/A ☐

Please use this space to add any comments you feel relevant:

____

____

____

____

Again, thank you for your collaboration and placing your trust in our team.

THE OWNER'S PERSPECTIVE

Owners are often surprised to discover that their pet might not feel completely happy or "fulfilled" in their home. Others **refuse to acknowledge** the **signs of stress** displayed by their pet. From our experience, in most cases this is due to one of two scenarios: a sense of **guilt** because they did not do more for their pet or **because they do not want to do more**. Evidently, there are other possible causes, but these two are the most common. For example, cat owners are often reluctant to switch from a silica litter to an unperfumed agglomerated litter whether because of the price, weight, or convenience of not having to change the litter for several weeks. It is easy to imagine that this type of owner would also be averse to adding more litter trays.

When the reason for consultation is **something that troubles the owner** (urine or faeces in inappropriate places, barking, destructive or even aggressive behaviour), then in our experience they are **more likely to cooperate** with the vet. However, if the vet recommends an EE plan to treat obesity due to frustration or boredom or a series of changes to **improve the quality of life** of a patient with osteoarthritis, then we find **owners are less likely to heed our advice**.

Even when the **owner is engaged in the EE plan**, the measures often **become diluted over time**. It is important to underline that EE not only **helps make pets "happier"** (mental health), but it also **improves their physical health**, which equates to fewer visits to the veterinary clinic.

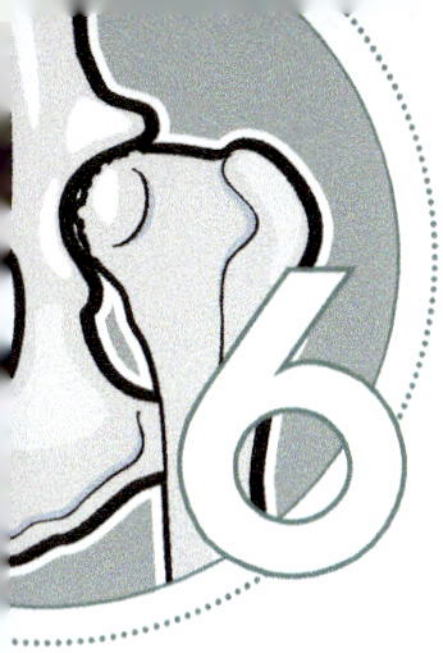

Chronic pain Arthrosis

The main problem veterinary surgeons have to overcome when treating patients in pain is that they cannot tell us what hurts or how much; we have to assess it and make a judgement. This means the pain in itself, even in the same patient, is treated with different strength drugs and at different dosages depending on the clinician they visit.

In light of this problem, which is inherent to the patient, the vet must train themselves to detect and treat chronic pain so that neither the pet nor its owner suffers unduly because of the situation.

Introduction. Definitions and basic concepts

Before starting, it helps to clarify some concepts so we can move forward with a strong foundation. Many aspects of chronic pain differ from those of acute pain. Merely defining chronic pain is no easy feat, as it encompasses a range of distinct types, such as musculoskeletal, neuropathic, or oncological pain, among others. Therefore, the International Association for the Study of Pain (IASP) defines acute pain as: "an unpleasant sensory and emotional experience associated with actual or potential tissue damage ... Pain is always subjective, and each individual learns to apply the concept based on experiences related to injuries in early life."[1] And their definition of chronic pain is: "pain without apparent biological value, lasting longer than the typical healing time" (Table 1). Obviously, the second definition is open to interpretation. When does pain have or lack biological value? What is the typical healing time? We could go even further and ask ourselves; how do we decide when a patient has healed if they express pain differently from us?

However, it is not all bad news. Owners are keenly sensitised to their pet's pain and, in most cases, show support for investigating and treating the cause in order to alleviate the patient's suffering. This is largely because humans also suffer both acute and chronic pain. After all, 76.2 million people in the United States suffer from chronic musculoskeletal pain, which is over 25 % of the country's population and more than those with heart disease, diabetes, and cancer combined.[3] Furthermore, in a US

Table 1. Basic differences between acute and chronic pain.

Acute pain	Chronic pain
Refers to initial tissue damage	No identifiable tissue damage
Has protective value	No protective value
Relatively easy to treat	Hard to treat and sometimes treatment refractory[4]
These features give it a "physiological" component	These features give it a "pathological" component

survey conducted to discover whether humans with pain would prefer to reduce the pain or the degree of associated disability, they found more respondents would prefer less pain than less disability.[6] So we can reasonably expect that when owners notice their cat or dog is in pain, they will bring them to the clinic and empathise with their pet's need for analgesic treatment.

Our patients' pain must be treated and not just because owners want us to treat it, but because pain causes alterations in the individual that may eventually result in severe consequences. In humans, cardiovascular disease, metabolic syndrome, kidney disease, depression, and anxiety are some of the consequences associated with the presence of chronic pain.[5]

TAKE NOTE!

Any acute pain that is not treated correctly can become chronic, and the resulting chronic pain will become increasingly hard to manage due to both central and peripheral sensitisation.[2,4]

Pathophysiology of pain

This section briefly reviews the pathophysiology of acute and chronic pain to help refresh the veterinary surgeon's knowledge of the physiological basis of pain so they may treat it through a reasoned, scientific approach.

The perception of pain is the culmination of the spatial or temporal transduction of stimuli from peripheral nociceptors. There are specific nociceptors that sense pain, as well as others for other types of stimuli (mechanical, thermal, chemical, and electrical).[8]

The painful stimulus ascends to the central nervous system via both **myelinated** (A-delta fibres) and **unmyelinated pathways** (C fibres). Various neurotransmitters are involved in these pathways, including substance P, neurokinin, neurotensin, glutamate, and N-methyl-D-aspartate. Once the fibres reach the dorsal horn of the spinal cord they synapse. At this point, the signal passes through different modulation systems then the information is decussated and ascends to the upper spinal segments before finally reaching the neural centres in the brainstem and midbrain. There are other tracts that carry the signal through the thalamus before projection in the cortex (Fig. 1).

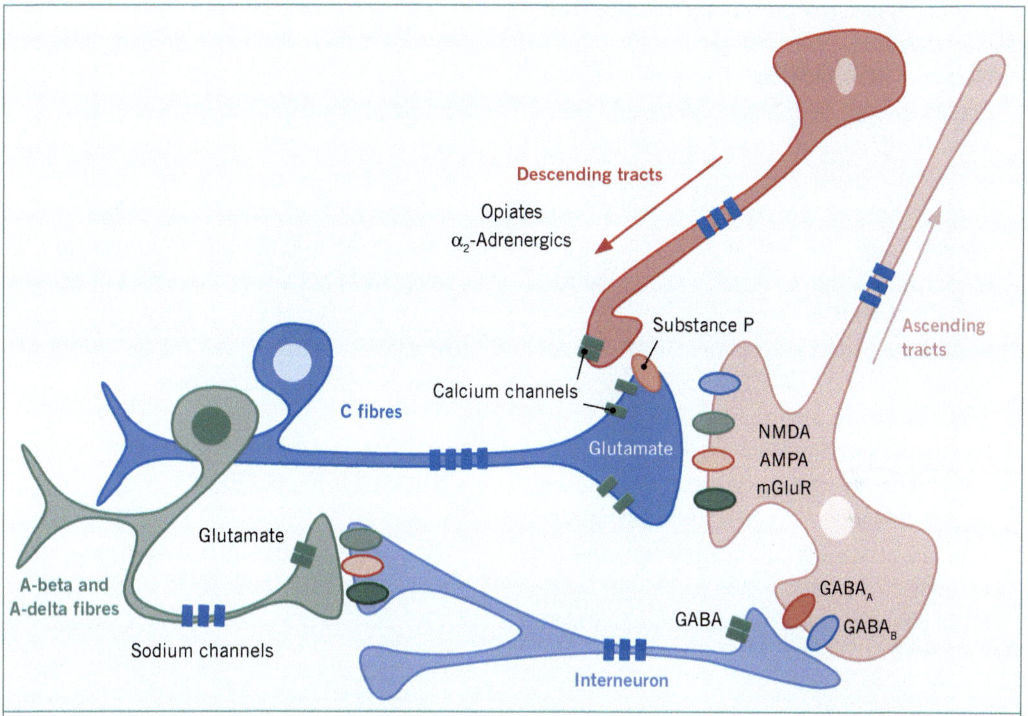

Figure 1. Anatomy of pain. Taken from Vinik et al., 2006.

ALTERATIONS KNOWN TO OCCUR IN ANIMALS WITH CHRONIC PAIN[7]

- Central and peripheral sensitisation
- Increase in sympathetic innervation of the dorsal root ganglions
- Inhibition of inhibitory modulation
- Redistribution of nociceptors in the lamina of the spinal cord
- Alterations in the phenotype of the sensory fibres in the damaged nerve and neuroreceptors
- Changes to interneuronal communication patterns in the spinal cord
- Changes in the grey matter

The pathophysiology of chronic pain involves two differentiating processes, namely:

- **Neuronal sensitisation.**[8] This phenomenon occurs in both peripheral and central neurons. Peripheral neurons are sensitised to chemicals released during cell destruction. These chemicals form what is called a "**sensitising soup**". Central sensitisation, on the other hand, is due to the activation of **glutamate** and **NMDA** receptors.[9] This process creates the perfect environment for the development of chronic pain syndrome in a mechanism known as wind-up (Fig. 2).
- **Neuronal plasticity.**[8] Prolonged activation of pain pathways, due to sensitisation, causes synaptic degeneration and remodelling with side branches sprouting between nearby neurons. This phenomenon can trigger functional changes in the neurons, and they start releasing a new neurotransmitter for the first time.[a] If there is also nerve damage, there will be increased activation of the cholecystokinin (CCK) system in the afferent neurons.[10] CCK is known to possess antiopioid activity and suppresses the analgesic effect of both endogenous and exogenous opiates. Studies have shown that the administration of CCK antagonists enhances the effect of opiates. Which could go at least some way to explaining why opiate derivatives are less effective in patients with neuropathic pain.

TAKE NOTE!

Neuropathic pain includes some degree of neural injury.

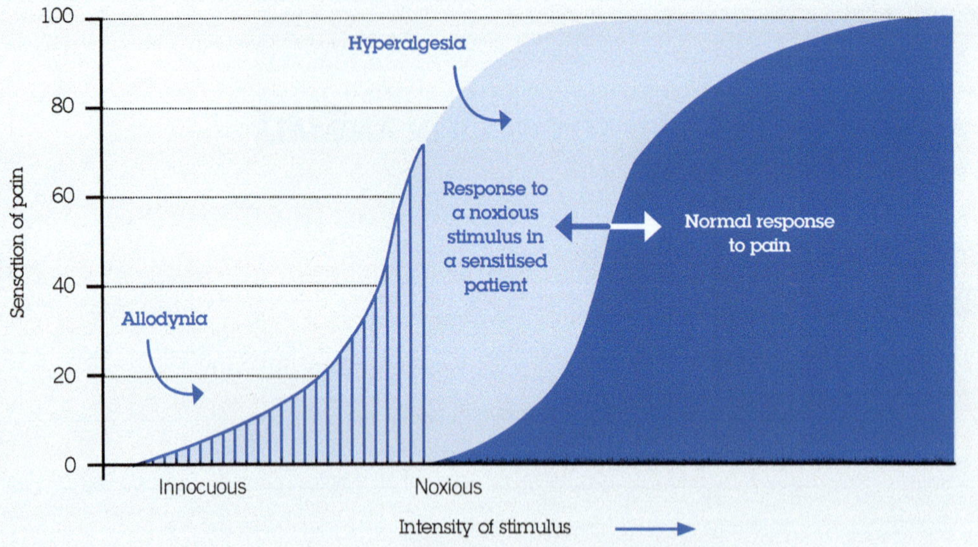

Figure 2. Chronic pain syndrome or wind-up.

[a] For example, a nerve fibre (A-beta) may start to produce substance P for proprioception and convert previously innocuous signals into painful ones.

To summarise, all these morphological and functional changes lower the pain threshold, cause overactivation of pain pathways, ectopic discharges, and a decline in normal inhibitory processes.

Identifying pain

The identification of pain forms the central linchpin of this chapter. You must be able to recognise a clinical sign or disease in order to treat it. Although we may have patients in pain, sympathetic owners, and a spectrum of medical technologies at our fingertips, it is all worthless if we cannot recognise pain. Our patients, like human newborns or people with severe mental health problems, cannot verbalise their pain, which means its detection is entirely in the clinician's hands. Which is why the IASP declared: "the inability to verbalise is no excuse for neglecting to treat a patient's pain."[1] Evidently the IASP was not thinking about vets, or their patients, when they stated this perspective. However, the concept is very befitting for veterinary medicine. Table 2 and Figure 3 together provide a helpful guide to identifying pain in our patients.

TIP

In the case of chronic pain, as the changes may have occurred weeks or months earlier, the owner can find it hard to understand the situation. If the vet suspects but is not certain the patient is in pain, it is worth applying a therapeutic test and assessing their response to treatment.

Treatment of chronic pain

The clinician needs to bear various premises in mind when treating chronic pain:

1. **The patient's age and metabolism.** Although not always, patients with chronic pain are usually mature or elderly.
2. Monotherapies do not tend to work well in the case of chronic pain. A **multimodal approach** is usually required and often not just pharmacological.

Table 2. Signs of pain (modified from AAHA/AAFP Pain Management Guidelines 2007).

General signs	Specific signs
Variation from normal behaviour	Reduction in activity and/or loss of appetite, lethargy. Hard to assess at the clinic.
Expression of abnormal behaviours	Inappropriate elimination or vocalisation, reduced interaction with the family or other pets, altered facial expression, altered posture, restlessness.
Reaction to touch	Body is notably tenser or animal withdraws from gentle contact in the area(s) of suspected pain.
Changes in physiological parameters	Increased blood pressure, body temperature, and heart and respiratory rates. Dilated pupils.

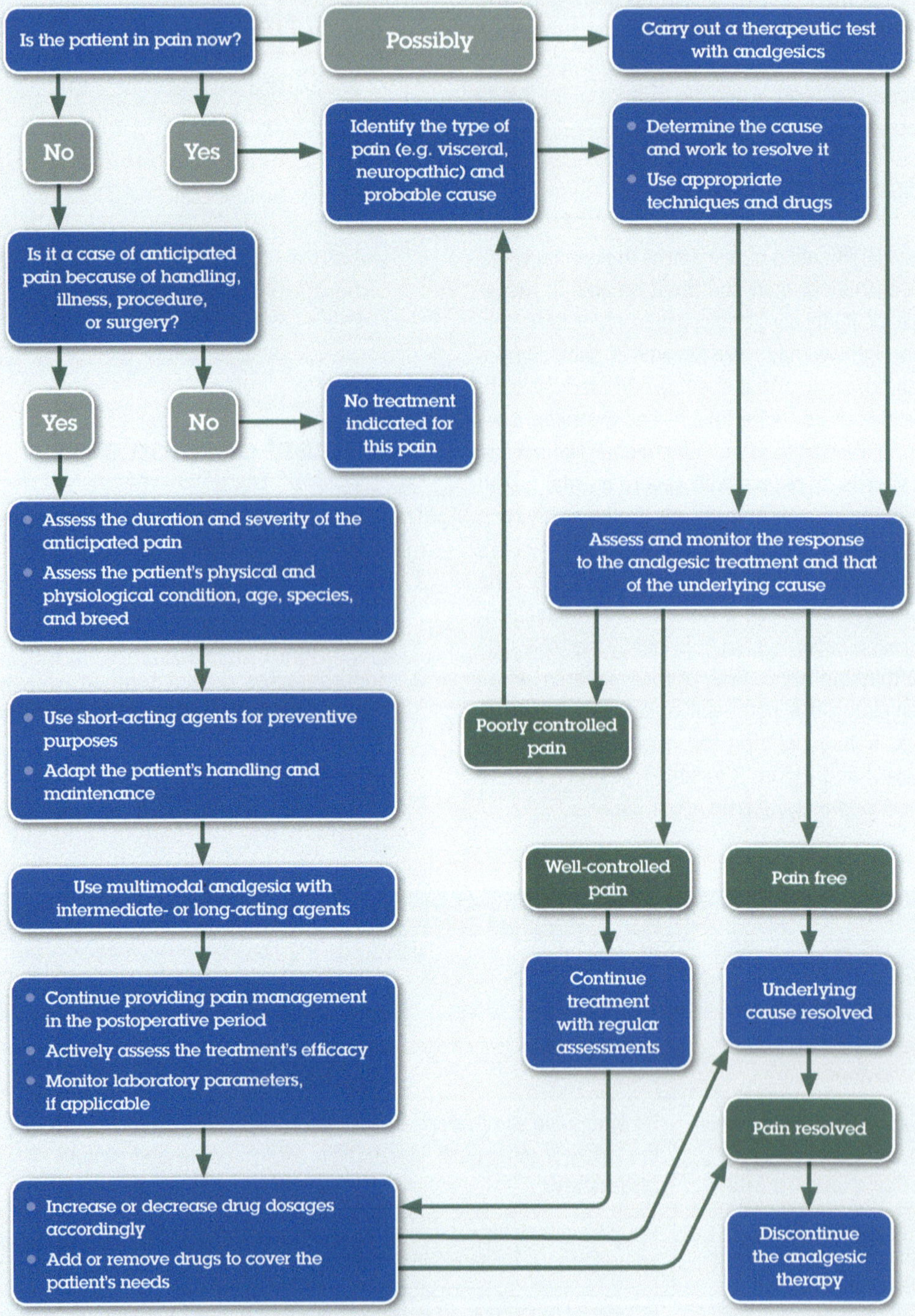

Figure 3. Diagnostic algorithm for pain.

3. **Communication with the owner** is essential. These treatments are typically permanent and palliative, as the problem is rarely fully resolved. It is important to explain the treatment goals very clearly and ensure they are attainable.
4. The perception of pain is very **dynamic**, so the medication regimen must be adapted accordingly (e.g. osteoarthritis pain is more intense when the weather changes).

In 1984, the World Health Organization (WHO) elaborated some recommendations for treating patients with cancer pain depending on the intensity and need for drugs. It was called the "**WHO analgesic ladder**" (Fig. 4). A patient in pain climbs this ladder as it is observed that their pain does not go away and requires more medication. This involves a lot of time and, in the meantime, pain for the patient. Which is why, in 2002, Dr Luis M. Torres Morera, the Head of Anaesthesia and Reanimation at the Puerta del Mar Hospital, Cadiz, Spain, proposed the "**analgesic elevator**", in which the patient is treated for the patient-reported and/or directly suspected pain. If the treatment proves effective, the number and dose of the drugs are gradually reduced. So it is like pressing the button to take the elevator directly to the required analgesic level without waiting. We can take inspiration from these approaches to treating pain. However, as mentioned in Chapter 4 on anaesthesia, there are no standardised protocols with a full guarantee of success. Thus, we can use and adapt the ladder and elevator according to the patient, their type of pain, previous treatments, associated diseases, owner, and need for results.

Lastly, remember pain is a dynamic sensation in constant change and its management may require fine-tuning or even "**rescue**" medications.

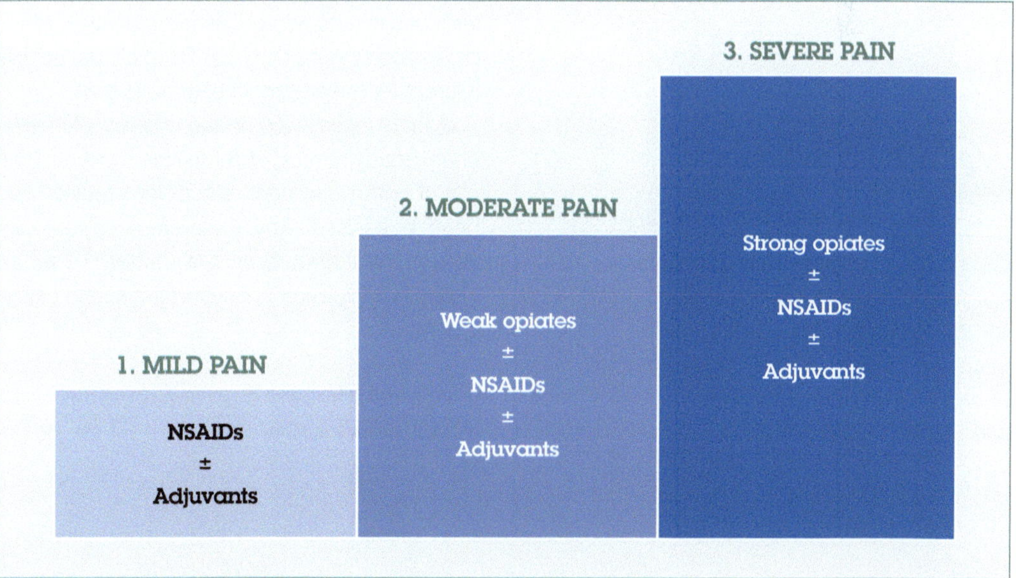

Figure 4. WHO analgesic ladder.

FACTORS TO CONSIDER WHEN TREATING CHRONIC PAIN

There is no such thing as just a little pain.

Chronic pain is hard to assess.

The time available is variable. The owner may decide that euthanasia is best for the patient at any moment. While sometimes it is necessary, it should not be because the vet advanced too slowly.

The time scales for discontinuing or adding drugs to the regimen depend on the vet's judgement.

Each case is unique and individualisation is the key to success.

TIP

It is important to plan these medications in advance and, where necessary, the owner could keep them at home so there is no delay in the patient's treatment if the pain appears to worsen.[b]

Analgesic agents

When a vet comes across a patient suffering from chronic pain, their first instinct is how are they going to alleviate this pain. However, within seconds a barrage of questions come to mind, such as: can I give this drug to a cat or dog with this underlying disease? At what dosage? How often? For how long? And if we opt for multimodal drug therapy, the number of questions grows exponentially. To help simplify this period of uncertainty, the following sections briefly summarise each drug or group of drugs, so the reader is armed with the basic information to help them select the most appropriate drug or drugs for each patient and set of circumstances.

Nonsteroidal anti-inflammatory drugs

In recent years, this group of drugs has developed into the most frequently used to treat chronic pain in small animal veterinary practice. Even in feline medicine, where there has been a lot of reluctance to use NSAIDs, they have gained acceptance and a guide to their long-term use in cats was published recently.[11] Many professionals consider NSAIDs to be the central fulcrum for the treatment of chronic pain.

A lot of information on the pharmacokinetics, pharmacodynamics, and multiple reviews of the use of NSAIDs in dogs and other species have been published. Any interested readers can peruse the literature on the matter,[12–15] as an in-depth discussion is beyond the scope of this chapter.

It is widely known that **nonsteroidal anti-inflammatory drugs** (NSAIDs) act by, at the

[b] The author normally uses tramadol at 2–5 mg/kg every 8–12 hours as rescue medication.

least, inhibiting cyclooxygenase 1 and 2 (COX-1 and COX-2). These enzymes break down arachidonic acid into prostaglandins and thromboxanes (Fig. 5).

- **COX-1** is called "**constitutive**" because it is a key component in various organs and tissues and is necessary to maintain homeostasis.
- **COX-2** is known as an "**inducible**" enzyme as it was originally thought to be induced or overexpressed by inflammatory processes. However, we now know that COX-2 is also constitutive of several organs and tissues including the kidneys, gastrointestinal tract, and parts of the central nervous system.

All NSAIDs available for veterinary use are designed to block COX-2 without inhibiting COX-1. This can be achieved through two strategies:

1. **Depending on the dose:** this applies to NSAIDs with a low selectivity for COX-2, which means that at the correct dose they will inhibit COX-2 but not COX-1. Always try to use the lowest effective dose.
2. **COX-2 selectivity:** NSAIDs with a high COX-2 selectivity inhibit COX-2 much better than COX-1. However, they are not without side effects.

It is very hard to reach a scientific decision as to which NSAID is better for the treatment of chronic pain in our canine patients, as every drug on the market has proven efficacy, but this is also coupled with side effects. The situation in cats is more straightforward because only two drugs are authorised for long-term use, namely meloxicam and robenacoxib. What is more, the assessment of chronic pain is highly subjective, and it is not always easy to design an experiment or assessment scale. So, in 2008, M. G. Papich suggested:[12]

- All NSAIDs, regardless of their COX-1/COX-2 selectivity, can cause gastrointestinal lesions, particularly at high dosages.
- All NSAIDs, selective or nonselective, can cause other gastrointestinal signs, including vomiting, diarrhoea, and loss of appetite, without producing ulceration.

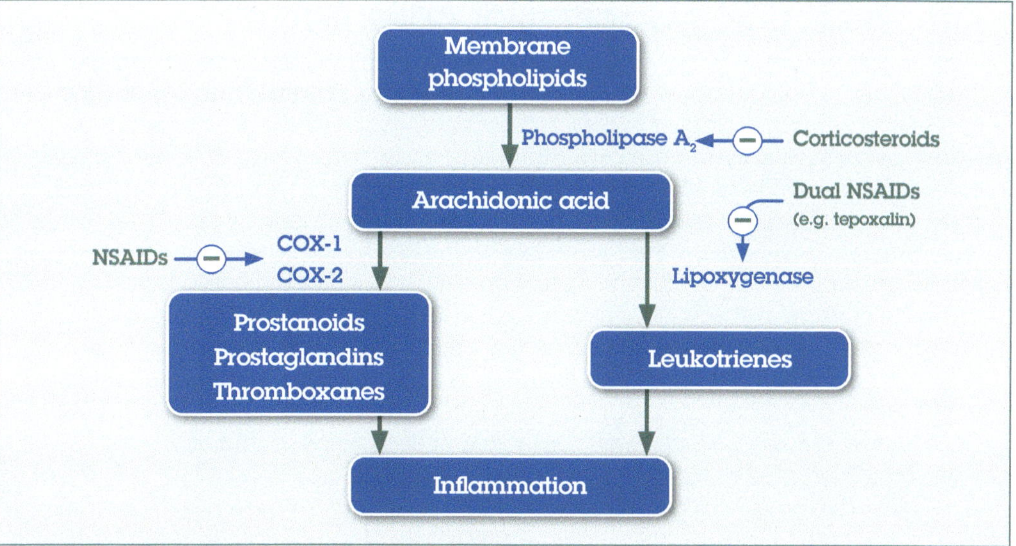

Figure 5. Action of nonsteroidal anti-inflammatory drugs (NSAIDs).

- All NSAIDs have the potential to cause liver damage. The susceptibility seems to be idiosyncratic and unpredictable.
- All NSAIDs have the potential to cause kidney damage. Prior kidney injury, low levels of certain electrolytes, and dehydration increase this risk.
- There is no definitive difference between NSAIDs in terms of their clinical efficacy.

Opiates

Historically, opiates have scarcely been used to manage chronic pain in pets. The need to use opiates has declined because of the availability of a growing range of NSAIDs and because drugs in the opiate family are hard to administer orally. Notwithstanding, they play an important role in veterinary analgesia and their use should not be disregarded (Table 3).

Morphine

First isolated from opium extract in 1805, morphine is an analgesic subject to controlled distribution. Unlike in human medicine, oral morphine is rarely prescribed for cats or dogs because its absorption is unpredictable and it has a low bioavailability (<20 %).[17,18] Morphine is metabolised rapidly in the liver and even the use of delayed-release drug formulations is not enough to maintain blood levels over long periods. A delayed-release formulation was approved recently, but while it provides better longevity of morphine blood levels, its bioavailability is still too low.[19] Despite this, morphine offers good efficacy when adhering to the recommended dosages, and the range of pharmaceutical forms available (capsules, tablets, oral solutions, etc.) makes it a good option for treating chronic pain in dogs. The most common side effects are constipation and sedation. Following oral administration, vomiting and nausea are less frequent side effects. Any undesirable effects tend to subside after 1 week of administration. A high-fibre diet or laxatives can be prescribed as a prophylactic measure for animals treated with oral morphine.

AND WHERE DOES PARACETAMOL COME INTO IT?

Traditionally, small animal vets have avoided the use of paracetamol due its toxicity. However, this only applies to cats, but not dogs. In fact, there are no reports of kidney or gastric lesions at normal doses. In one study, there were no signs of toxicity even at doses as high as 100 mg/kg.[16] Nevertheless, the references found are merely anecdotal and from cases where there was no alternative medication.

Many clinicians no longer classify paracetamol as a NSAID, because it does not affect the aforementioned COX enzymes in the same way. On the other hand, recent studies have shown that paracetamol inhibits COXs but in cells where the concentration of arachidonic acid is low. Hence it seems its inhibition of COXs occurs in situ. Paracetamol has also been shown to inhibit the COX-1 variant called COX-3. COX-3 is found in the CNS and was discovered in dogs before humans; it is also believed to hold greater significance in dogs.

Table 3. Dosages and notes on opiates in cats and dogs.			
Drug	**Dosage in dogs**	**Dosage in cats**	**Notes**
Tramadol	2–5 mg/kg PO every 8–12 h	1–4 mg/kg PO every 8–12 h	Possesses opiate effects. Its effect is mainly acute.
Oral morphine	0.5–2 mg/kg PO every 6–8 h (or even every 2–4 h)	0.25–0.5 mg/kg PO every 6–8 h (or even every 3–4 h)	High doses can produce dysphoria, sedation, nausea, and vomiting, which last for a week.
Oral, long-acting morphine	2–5 mg/kg PO every 6–12 h	Hard to administer in cats	For chronic use, increase the frequency before increasing the dose.
Codeine	1–2 mg/kg PO every 6–8 h	0.1–1 mg/kg PO every 4–8 h	
Codeine–paracetamol	1–2 mg/kg (codeine) PO every 8–12 h	Toxic in cats	
Transdermal fentanyl	3–5 μg/kg/h	Same as for dogs	Patches last 2 to 3 days.
Methadone	0.1–0.5 mg/kg SC or IM every 2–4 h	0.1–0.5 mg/kg SC or IM every 2–4 h	There are only doses for injectable forms. Has a certain degree of NMDA receptor antagonism.
Buprenorphine	0.01–0.03 mg/kg SC, IV, or IM	0.01–0.03 mg/kg SC, IV, IM, or transmucosal PO	

Codeine

It was first synthesised in France in 1832 and can be isolated from opium or morphine. Not much information has been published regarding its use in small animals, but its pharmacokinetics have been well studied.[20,21] Codeine is rapidly metabolised by the liver and, like morphine, eliminated in the urine. In humans, 10 % is metabolised into morphine which is believed to be why it has an analgesic action. Yet this differs in cats and dogs as less than 1.5 % of codeine is converted into morphine. Therefore, it is reasonable to conclude that codeine has a mild analgesic effect.

Methadone

Methadone is a purely synthetic opiate that was first synthesised in Germany in 1937. It is a controlled prescription drug that has attracted a lot of interest recently. This is because besides being a pure antagonist of mu (μ) or OP_3 opioid receptors, it also has a certain degree of antagonism with **NMDA receptors**, which is especially important in patients with neuropathic and chronic pain.

As with the other opiates we have discussed so far, after its oral administration to dogs, methadone has a short half-life, rapid clearance, and low bioavailability.[22] The side effects of methadone are similar to those described for morphine.

If we compare the cardiovascular effects of morphine against those of methadone in conscious dogs, the latter has a stronger impact. It causes a bigger and more prolonged reduction in heart rate and cardiac index[c] than the decreases induced by morphine. Methadone also provokes a greater increase in systemic vascular resistance and bigger decline in the partial pressure of oxygen.[23] Indeed, in humans, methadone often triggers a prolonged QT interval and can cause fatal arrhythmias; however, these effects have not been observed in cats or dogs.

Tramadol

Tramadol is a centrally acting analgesic that was first synthesised in Germany in 1962. It is structurally related to morphine and codeine, which is probably where it derives its mu opioid receptor agonist activity. However, its analgesic effect is also accompanied by inhibition of **serotonin** and **norepinephrine** reuptake. Tramadol is a racemic mixture in which the (+)-enantiomer has opiate-like activity and acts on serotonin metabolism, whereas the (–)-enantiomer affects norepinephrine uptake. These different actions are complementary and apparently synergistic in so far as tramadol's analgesic activity. The pharmacokinetics of tramadol have been extensively studied in both cats and dogs.[24–26] While tramadol's bioavailability following oral administration is similar in dogs and humans, its half-life, on the other hand, is very short in dogs. Furthermore, dogs eliminate unaltered tramadol in the urine, yet this does not occur in humans or cats where tramadol undergoes hepatic demethylation into O-desmethyltramadol, which also has mu agonist effects. This metabolism produces an extended analgesic effect.

TAKE NOTE!

There are no reports in veterinary medicine of tramadol-induced serotonin syndrome, but it should be taken into account whenever tramadol is coadministered with drugs that also increase serotonin concentration.

Drugs used for neuropathic pain (Table 4)

Gabapentin and pregabalin

These two drugs are structural analogues of the inhibitory neurotransmitter known as GABA (γ-aminobutyric acid), yet their effect does not stem from this similarity and their mechanism of action is not fully understood. Current thinking is that they block presynaptic, high-voltage calcium channels, the number of which is known to increase in situations of chronic pain. This diminishes the presynaptic release of neurotransmitters and attenuates postsynaptic excitability. Some patients need to take gabapentin for the rest of their lives; however, in many patients its use can be discontinued once the pain has subsided. It is important to note that gabapentin withdrawal must follow a stepwise schedule (from days to weeks) to avoid a rebound effect.[27] The most common side effect of gabapentin administration is sedation. It will disappear if the dose is reduced, but interestingly it will not develop again if the dose is then slowly increased back to the original concentration. The level of sedation is greater in animals who are also receiving opiates.

[c] The cardiac index (CI) is a haemodynamic parameter that relates cardiac output (CO) to the body surface area (BSA), in other words, it relates heart performance to the size of the individual. It is measured in l/minute/m².
CI = CO/BSA = Vsyst × HR/BSA, where Vsyst: systolic volume and HR: heart rate.

Table 4. Dosages and notes on drugs used for chronic and/or neuropathic pain in cats and dogs.

Drug	Dosage	Notes
Amantadine	2–5 mg/kg every 24 h, for at least 21 days.	As part of multimodal treatment. NMDA receptor antagonist.
Ketamine	0.5–2 mg/kg PO every 6–8 h (or even every 2–4 h) 8–12 mg/kg PO every 6 h 2 µg/kg/min IV (CRI)	NMDA receptor antagonist.
Gabapentin	1–10 mg/kg PO every 8–24 h	Ca^{2+} channel blocker.
Pregabalin	1–2 mg/kg PO every 8–12 h	Ca^{2+} channel blocker.

Amantadine

Amantadine is an FDA-approved antiviral drug for the treatment of influenza virus infections in humans. Its value in the treatment of chronic pain is due to its antagonism of NMDA receptors. Some pharmacokinetic data on amantadine use in cats and dogs have been published.[28,29] In human medicine, it is used to relieve both acute and chronic pain (including when it is neuropathic). Studies suggest that it should be coadministered with an NSAID for at least 21 days to achieve effective pain management. No side effects or interactions with other drugs have been reported to date.[30]

Osteoarthritis

Osteoarthritis (OA) is not just part of "normal ageing", it is a specific problem that affects some very specific locations and has identifiable predisposing factors. As such, we can and should react to any clinical signs of OA observed in our feline or canine patients.

OA is defined as the final outcome of a slowly advancing disease, or group of diseases, that affects mobile joints and which is clinically characterised by the gradual onset of pain, stiffness, and limited mobility in affected joints. It can affect any joint, even the metacarpo- and metatarsophalangeal joints (Fig. 6) or vertebral facet joints.

TAKE NOTE!

Despite its high prevalence among elderly dogs, osteoarthritis is still a commonly underdiagnosed and undertreated condition.

As vets, we all perform a thorough examination of the musculoskeletal system when visiting a large- or giant-breed dog, but all breeds and species can suffer from OA. Joint instability and incongruence (Fig. 7), irregular weight distribution, and injuries all subject the cartilage to chronic stress and inflammation. Consequently, the body tries to stabilise the area leading to the growth of bone spurs or OA (Fig. 8).

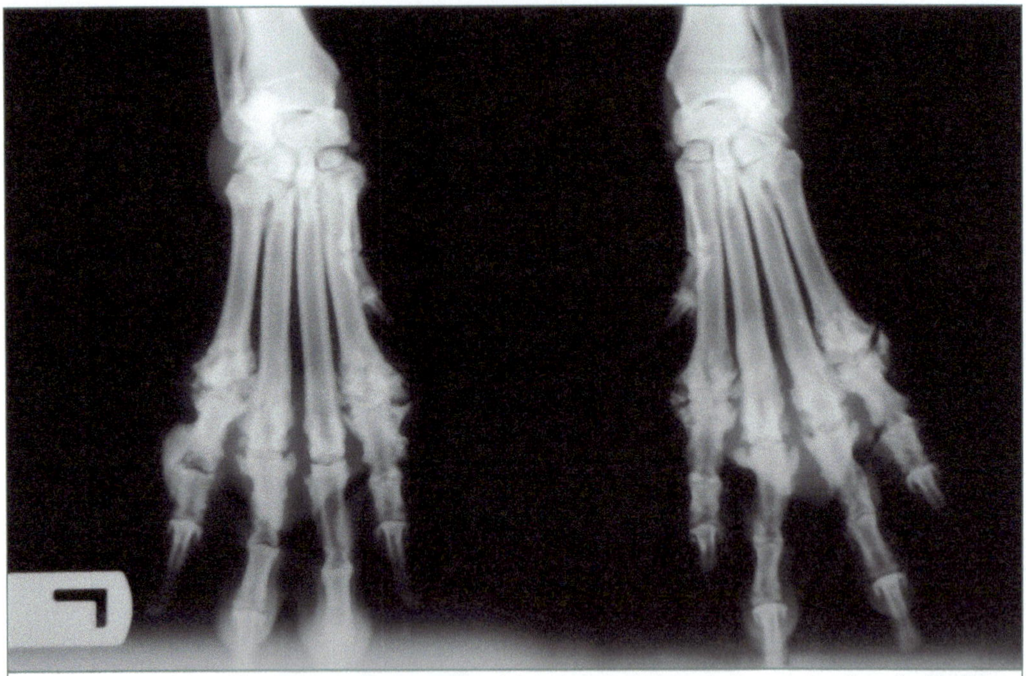

Figure 6. Osteoarthritis of the phalanges. Image courtesy of Antonio Peña, Lisboa veterinary centre, Alcorcón (Madrid).

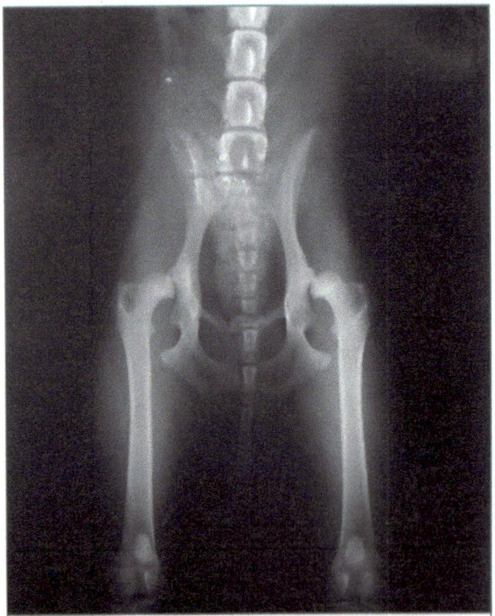

Figure 7. Joint dysplasia of the hip, with no arthrosis yet, in a female dog aged 10–12 months. Image courtesy of Antonio Peña, Lisboa veterinary centre, Alcorcón (Madrid).

The diagnose or identification of OA during annual checkups, by incorporating joint pain assessment protocols, is generally well received by dog owners, who often attribute their pet's decline in mobility and lack of vitality to its advanced age. Systematic muscle palpation, including of the masticatory, cervical, paraspinal muscles, and major muscle groups in each limb, makes an excellent place to start an OA pain assessment protocol. If muscle palpation reveals any painful areas or contractures, it should be complemented with, at the least, a neuro-orthopaedic exam of the affected area.

Before coming to a diagnosis of OA, it is important to rule out other potential causes of musculoskeletal pain, such as:

- Osteosarcoma
- Osteomyelitis
- Septic arthritis
- Soft tissue injuries

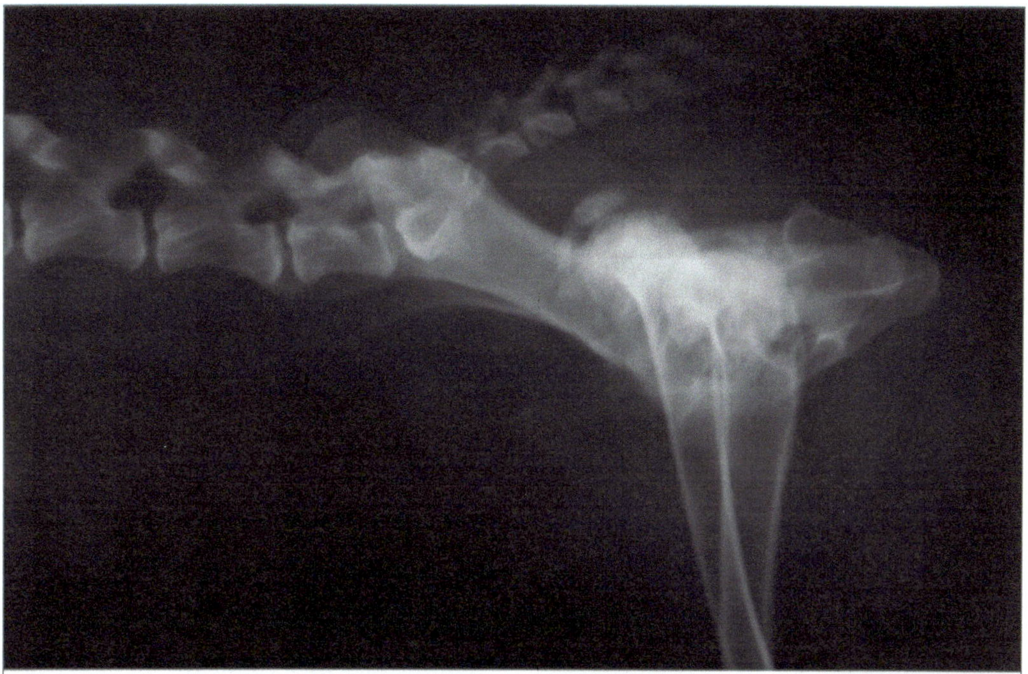

Figure 8. Hip dysplasia with terminal arthrosis and luxation.

To this end, besides a complete medical history and thorough clinical exam, X-rays of the painful regions detected in the exam are also required. X-rays will help highlight changes in bone tissue in the painful joint and surrounding tissue (Figs. 9–11) and can be used to rule out osteolysis, bone spurs, and other abnormalities unrelated to OA.

RADIOGRAPHIC SIGNS OF OA

- Irregular loss of joint space
- Osteophyte formation
- Subchondral sclerosis
- Irregular joint surfaces

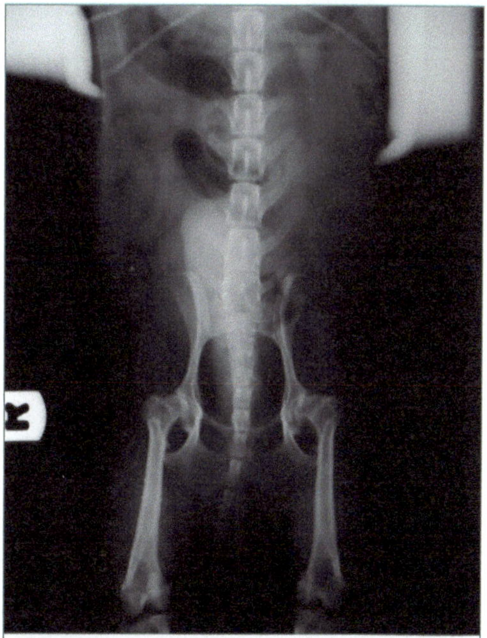

Figure 9. Arthrosis of the hip. Image courtesy of Antonio Peña, Lisboa veterinary centre, Alcorcón (Madrid).

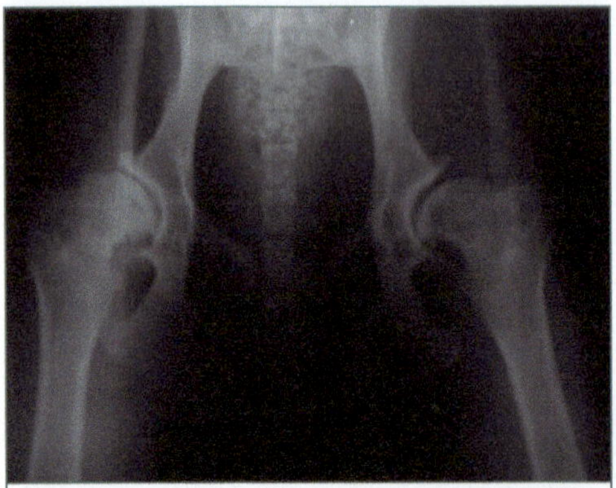
Figure 10. Arthrosis of the hip.

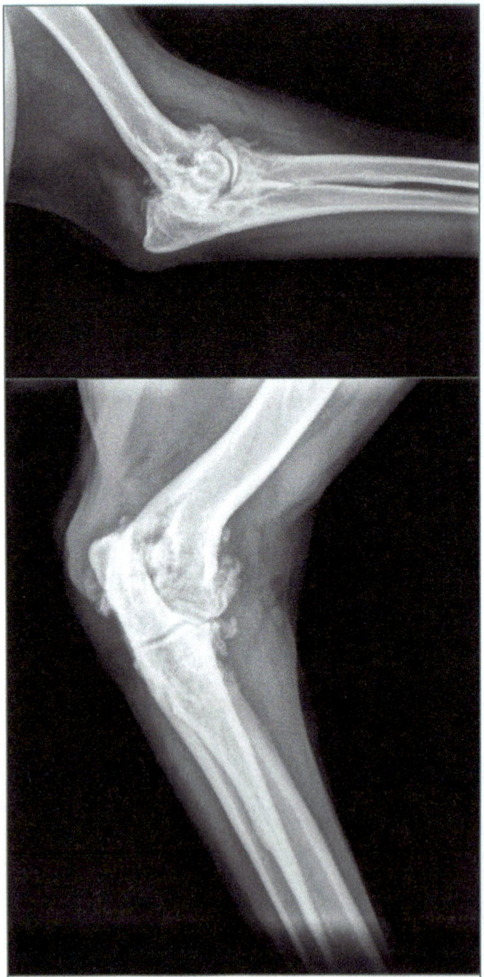
Figure 11. Arthrosis of the elbow.

Treatment of osteoarthritis

The chronic pain caused by OA should be treated by means of a multimodal approach. In addition to the various combinations of analgesics (discussed earlier), we should not forget the nonpharmacological measures that can mark the difference between success and failure (Fig. 12).

Nonpharmacological measures include:

- Weight loss and control programmes
- Nutraceuticals
- Unconventional analgesic measures (acupuncture, thermotherapy, transcutaneous electrical nerve stimulation, and laser therapy)
- Rehabilitation techniques
- Environmental enrichment

Weight loss and control

Studies have shown that just by reducing a patient's weight it improves their clinical signs of OA and mobility. Obesity is one of the most prevalent factors predisposing animals to OA, since it places extra strain on joints. It also contributes to a state of chronic systemic inflammation, because adipose tissue can synthesise metabolically active cytokines.[31,32]

Nutraceuticals

The nutraceuticals used for OA can be placed in four groups:

1. **Glycosaminoglycans:** products with glucosamine and low-molecular-weight chondroitin are the most prescribed nutraceuticals for cats and dogs with OA. Scientific evidence of their efficacy is variable and depends on the product used.[33,34] Some studies found a reduction in the degree of pain, while others reported counterproductive effects.[35] However, the evidence derived from these studies is not totally convincing.

> **TIP**
>
> It is essential our clients are given sound advice on the quality and bioavailability of the products used,[36] as well as their expected effects.

2. **Undenatured type II collagen (UC-II):** this product has gained a place among the nutraceuticals used to treat arthrosis in both cats and dogs, as well as in horses and humans. It has excellent oral bioavailability, which means that even at very low doses (a few milligrams are enough) it brings about improvements in patients affected by OA. However, its strong market entrance among the range of nutraceuticals for OA is thanks to its novel mode of action. Undenatured type II collagen is not digested in the stomach like denatured collagen, but rather it crosses the intestinal mucosa and is recognised by intestinal dendritic cells. This activates a cascade of molecular reactions culminating in the increased synthesis of interleukin-4, interleukin-10, and transforming growth factor β (TGF-β) by regulatory T cells. These substances appear to contribute to the repair and reconstruction of damaged cartilage thanks to the oral tolerance phenomenon that starts in the gut-associated lymphoid tissue.[37–39]

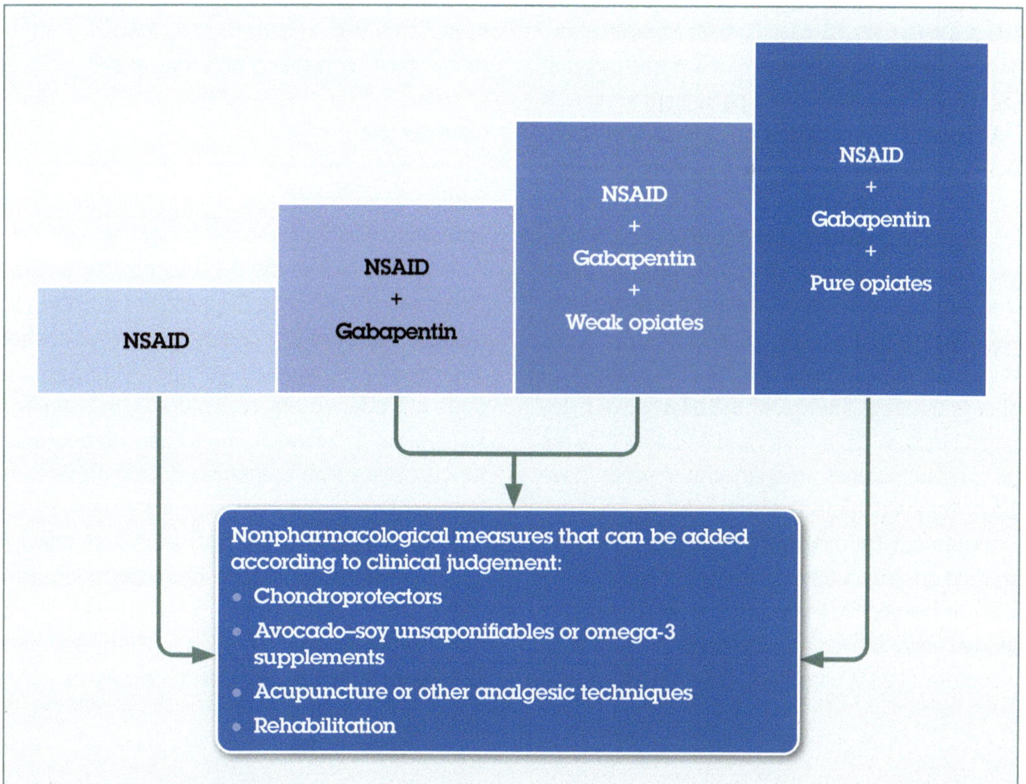

Figure 12. Treatment ladder suggested for patients with OA.

3. **Omega-3 unsaturated fatty acids:** fish oils rich in eicosapentaenoic acid (EPA) and docosahexaenoic acid (DHA) are well known for their "anti-inflammatory" effects in both humans and animals. They are also known to improve heart, kidney, and dermatological health, as well as reducing the rate and recurrence of neoplasms.[40–43] At present, they are the nutraceuticals backed by the most scientific evidence in terms of treating OA.
4. **Avocado–soy unsaponifiables:** these products could be the latest advance in nutraceuticals that improve the signs of OA. Several promising studies have already been conducted in cats and dogs.[44,45] However, we still need further, more in-depth studies before making recommendations on dosage and the correct avocado:soy ratio.

Unconventional analgesic measures

This section sets out some of the measures that can be recommended for a patient suffering with OA. These techniques are quickly gaining popularity in the treatment of chronic pain in veterinary patients. This manual does not set out to list and explain all of these techniques or specialties, although we must stress that this does not mean they are any less important or useful; actually, we will probably refer more and more patients to receive some of these therapies. Acupuncture stands out from the rest of the alternative measures because it provides good results. While not all of acupuncture's mechanisms of action have been fully elucidated, some of them are fully understood, for example, endorphin release, muscle spasm relaxation, and reduced nociceptive transmission to the spinal cord.[27] A myriad of studies have proven the analgesic utility of acupuncture, yet it is hard to manage OA pain using only acupuncture without any other measures, whether pharmacological or not.[46] It should be noted that owners have enthusiastically welcomed the improvement in their pets after acupuncture sessions.

Rehabilitation techniques

Rehabilitation forms part of many techniques, all of them intended to increase the functionality of the affected joint or joints. The exercises and techniques applied depend on the patient's degree of pain or reduction in functionality. Aerobic exercises that help strengthen muscle have proven useful in people with OA.[47]

New treatments

Just in recent months, various new products have been launched in Spain and added to our arsenal of drugs for the treatment of chronic pain in patients with osteoarthritis. Here we summarise their names and how they work.

Grapiprant

Grapiprant is the first member of the piprant family to be marketed as an analgesic and anti-inflammatory for dogs struggling with OA. It selectively blocks the EP_4 receptor for prostaglandin E_2 (PGE_2). The EP_4 receptor is known to regulate inflammatory nociception in the central and peripheral nervous systems. As grapiprant does not affect other receptors or the synthesis of other prostanoids, then their homeostatic functions are also preserved during grapiprant treatment.

Several inflammatory mediators that activate or sensitise neurons have been discovered in patients with inflammatory pain. These include not only prostaglandins, such as PGE_2, but also nerve growth factor (NGF) and bradykinin.

Based on current data and commercial registers, OA in dogs should be treated at grapiprant dosages of 2 mg/kg/day. For cats, although plasma concentrations are known to vary greatly, grapiprant did not accumulate after 27 days of administration. However, we do not have enough data at this time to support recommending grapiprant for cats.

Anti-NGF monoclonal antibodies: frunevetmab and bedinvetmab

NGF is an essential signalling protein for the survival of sensory and sympathetic neurons during the body's development. In adults, NGF and its interaction with tropomyosin receptor kinase A (TrkA) has been associated with various actions. Possibly the most interesting of these actions, from a therapeutic perspective, is its function in nociception and the role it plays in neural plasticity during painful processes. Studies have concluded that NGF is a key factor in the transmission of OA pain in humans, cats, and dogs as it has been found in higher concentrations in the synovial joints of OA sufferers. In adults, nerve growth factor fulfils an important function in pain signalling and is a key component in central sensitisation (wind-up), spinal cord plasticity, and unadapted pain signalling.

NGF is a neuropeptide secreted in large amounts by mast cells close to the nociceptive neurons whenever there is chronic inflammation in synovial joints. When NGF binds with TrkA on the surface of neurons, it is internalised before retrograde neuronal transport takes it to the dorsal root ganglion of the spinal cord (pain modulation area) where it modulates or increases the activity of the nerve cells. These changes in peripheral nerve function induced by NGF cause the release of mediators, such as calcitonin gene-related peptide (CGRP) and substance P, near the nerve endings, which results in neurogenic inflammation. Neurogenic inflammation and NGF contribute to the development of new blood vessels and neuronal sprouts, which can increase the joint's overall sensitivity. So, a vicious circle has been set in motion leading to greater joint degeneration and more pain.

It should be added that NGF also binds to TrkA in inflammatory cells. This stimulates more NGF synthesis, which further contributes to the vicious circle of inflammation and pain occurring in the chronic processes.

Monoclonal antibodies that neutralise NGF (anti-NGF mAbs) have been developed for use in both cats and dogs. In fact, bedinvetmab was first made available on the European market for the treatment of OA pain in dogs in early 2021. Then in September 2021, frunevetmab, the felinised active substance, was launched for the same indication in cats.

When these monoclonal antibodies bind to NGF, it reduces the amount of NGF available to bind with the TrkA receptors in the patient's OA affected joints, thereby limiting the activation of receptors in neurons, the immune system, and other cells in the joint. In turn, the limited activation of these receptors means the pain signal travelling through the peripheral and central nervous system to the brain is weaker and, what is more, it allows the nerve to return to a "more normal" shape and level of function. The monthly, subcutaneous administration of monoclonal antibodies is a new treatment option for chronic pain in patients with OA.

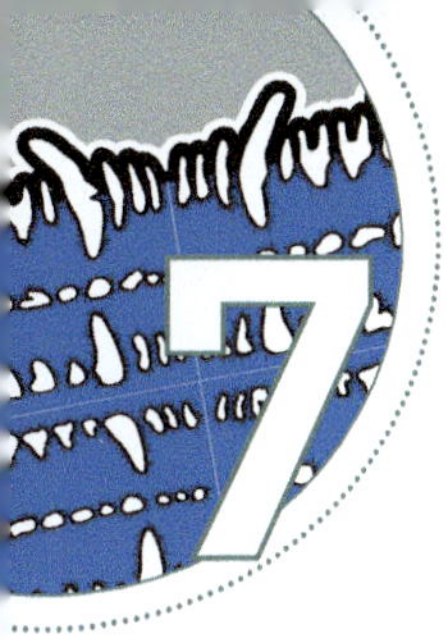

7 Orodental problems in elderly animals

The mouth and teeth of geriatric cats and dogs frequently require extra care and attention. According to Veterinary Pet Insurance (VPI), dental treatments were the tenth most requested services by their clients in 2010, with over 17,000 claims. Owners, however, are often reluctant to approve anaesthesia for their pets for something they consider merely an "aesthetic" problem.

Prevention is the key, and as tends to be the case, it is cheaper than curative treatment, so it helps the owner save money. This chapter provides a detailed description of the stages of an orodental consultation.

Considerations before starting

The first thing we should ask ourselves as veterinary practitioners when a "lifelong client" (over 10 years) brings their pet to our clinic for an orodental consultation is: have we done everything possible to help maintain the animal's oral health? In other words, have we kept the owner fully informed about how to look after their pet's dental health over the last 10 years? Have we shown owners how to train their pet to allow them to clean its teeth? Have we recommended a full dental health plan? And going even further, what do we mean by a dental health plan? Have we developed one for our clinic? If so, do we promote it correctly? We should be honest with ourselves when answering these questions and act accordingly. Unfortunately, it is not one of the aims of this chapter, but there are several publications that can help anyone interested in creating and developing their own **dental health plan**.

However, the last chapter of this manual does contain information about general health plans for geriatric patients. Another good source of information is the American Animal Hospital Association's 2005 Dental Care Guidelines for Dogs and Cats.[1]

TAKE NOTE!

If lesions are observed during the conscious exam, it is a clear indication that more may be found on further inspection and the owner should be informed of this possibility.

The orodental exam

An orodental consultation in veterinary medicine consists of two different and complementary examinations: a conscious and an unconscious or anaesthetised exam (Fig. 1).

- The **conscious exam** is helpful, but it is often limited to a rather superficial visual or tactile exploration. Besides looking inside the oral cavity, this stage should also include an examination of the facial bones, temporomandibular joints, salivary glands, and submandibular lymph nodes. For the final step of the initial exploration, inspect the patient's dental occlusion by gently lifting the lips and make a preliminary assessment of the teeth.
- An **anaesthetised exam** is essential for a complete assessment of orodental health. First inspect inside the mouth and check its nondental structures (oropharynx, tongue, palate, lips, and cheeks) (Figs. 2 and 3). The next step is the actual dental examination. The anaesthetised exam is often combined with dental prophylaxis; in fact, in many cases it would not make sense to do one without the other. Therefore, there is a step-by-step description of both procedures later in this chapter.

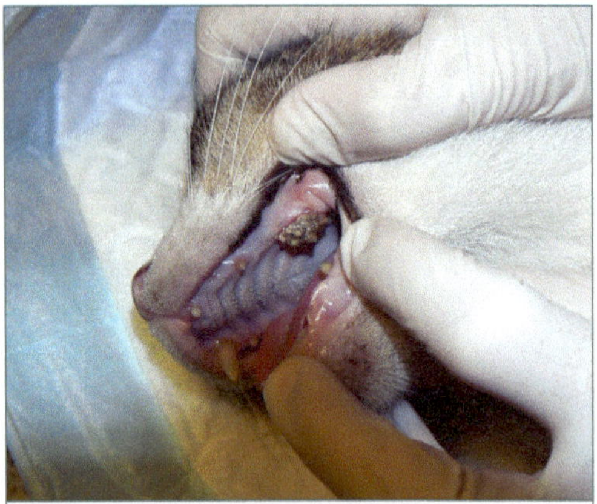

Figure 1. Dental exam and assessment.

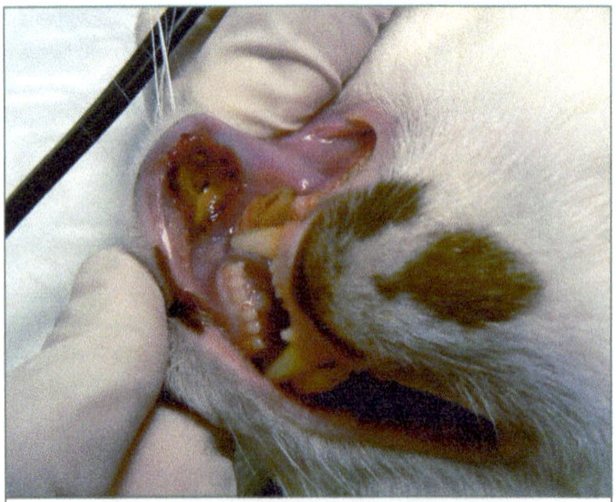

Figure 2. Gingival ulcers in a cat examined under anaesthesia.

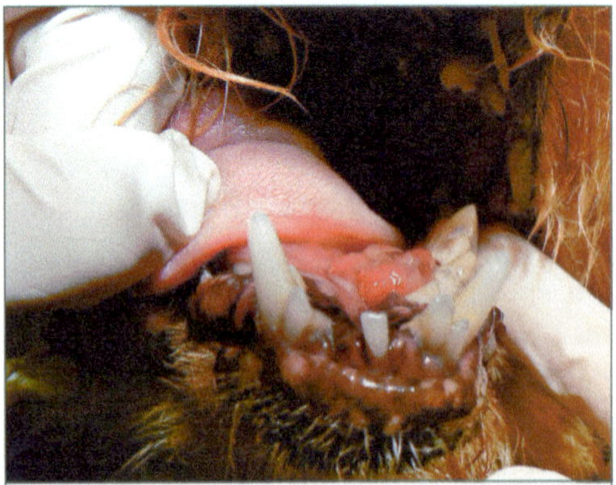

Figure 3. Squamous cell carcinoma in a Yorkshire Terrier detected during an anaesthetised exam of the oral cavity.

TIP

Always bear in mind that many patients admitted for dental procedures may be suffering from chronic pain. It is hard to treat chronic pain, and NSAIDs and opiates alone may not be enough. Never underestimate dental pain.

It can be hard to earn the full trust of some owners. Dedicate as much time as is needed to discover any reservations the owner may have and clear up all their doubts about the process. Many owners, however, will trust their pet's treatment to a vet who demonstrates empathy, sound knowledge, and professionalism.

Preparing patients for anaesthesia

On the day the patient is brought to the clinic for their anaesthetised dental procedure, they should be assessed again, and all their vital signs recorded before administering any drugs. If the owner is overly nervous, they often feel calmer after watching the vet check their pet again before sedation, even if it is for the umpteenth time. An anaesthesia protocol sheet, where you can note down the drugs administered, their doses, and the patient's vital signs, not only provides a record of some crucial information, but it can also help boost the owner's confidence after somewhat reluctantly agreeing to the proposed treatment.

It is good practice to administer the first sedatives with the owner still in the room, particularly when treating cats and dogs that are relaxed by their owner's presence.

Before administering any sedative, insert an intravenous catheter, if possible, to ensure quick access to the patient's circulation. Once inserted, and depending to some extent on each patient, start fluid therapy with Ringer's lactate solution or an isotonic glucose saline solution. In healthy animals, the administration rate can range between 2 and 3 ml/kg/hour for cats and between 2 and 6 ml/kg/hour for dogs. Lower rates may be more suitable for patients with kidney or heart disease or high blood pressure. If antibiotics are required, they should be administered at least 1 hour before the procedure.

The antibiotics we currently use the most at our clinics are ampicillin (20 mg/kg slow IV) and clindamycin (5.5–11 mg/kg slow IV). However, if there is patent pyorrhoea (Fig. 4) or an abscess is suspected, we would recommend starting antibiotic therapy 3 to 7 days prior to the dental procedure.

Dental prophylaxis

Prophylaxis is basically preventive treatment before any **irreversible disease** develops in the teeth or gums. It is what is commonly known as "**mouth cleaning**". Logically, any patient

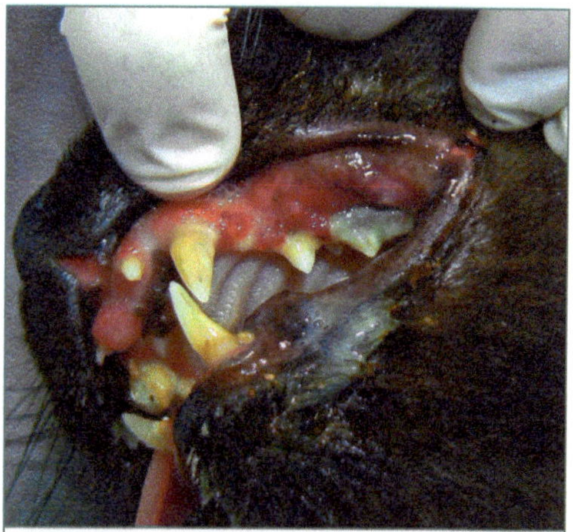

Figure 4. Pyorrhoea in a cat.

undergoing a dental procedure who also has an orodental condition that needs curing must receive more than just prophylaxis; consequently, in this case, the vet should not call it prophylaxis treatment.

TIP

Vets often give patients curative treatments under the concept of "mouth cleaning". However, this means that many clients fail to appreciate the high cost of their pet's actual treatment. So we advise giving clear definitions of the concepts and procedures to help avoid misunderstandings.

Similarly, the interpretation of dental prophylaxis tends to vary between clinics or depending on the veterinary professional. A full dental prophylaxis treatment should include the following eight steps (including the steps in the anaesthetised exam):

Step 1: removal of supragingival calculi and assessing gum health

Supragingival calculus (Figs. 5–7) is normally removed using manual tools and according to the vet's needs or preferences. These instruments should never be introduced beneath the gum line. In our experience, **tartar forceps** (Figs. 8 and 9) give the best results, and it is a rapid, inexpensive technique. After removing the larger calculi, the next step is to clean with an ultrasonic scaler (Fig. 10).

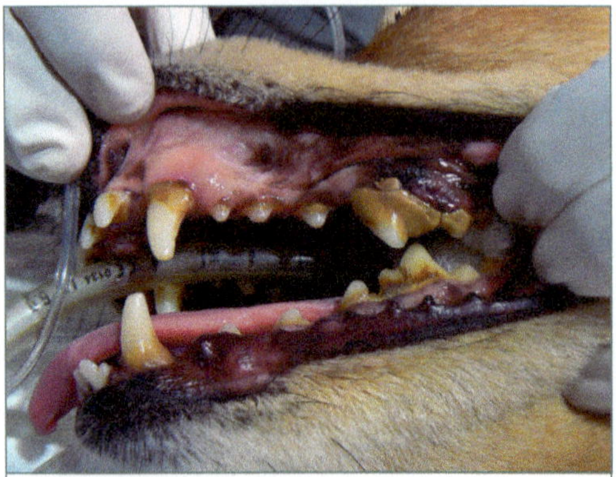

Figure 5. Supragingival calculus in an 11-year-old male dog.

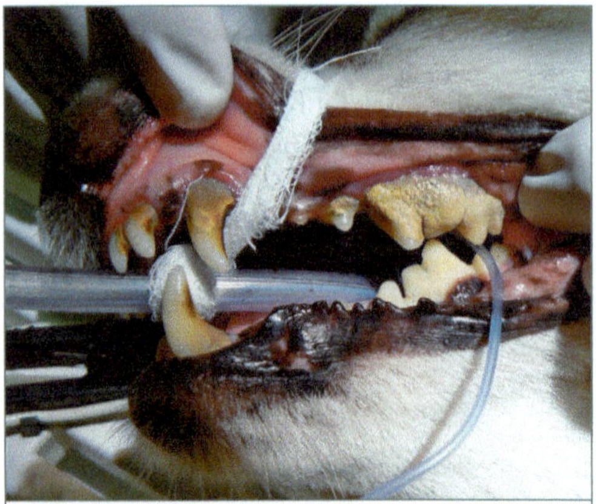

Figure 6. Supragingival calculus in a 10-year-old female dog.

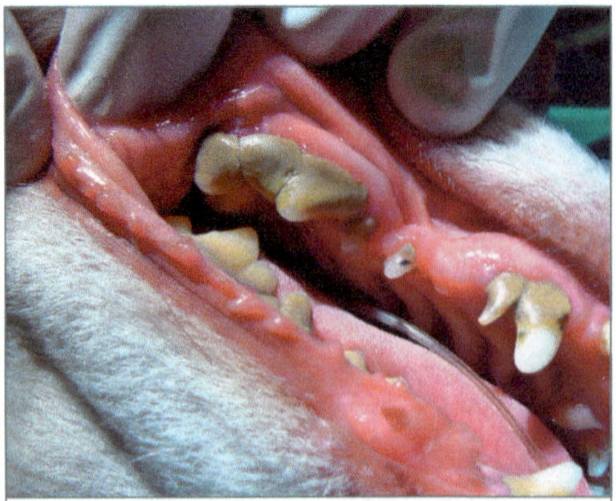

Figure 7. Supragingival calculi and severe gingivitis in a 10-year-old male dog.

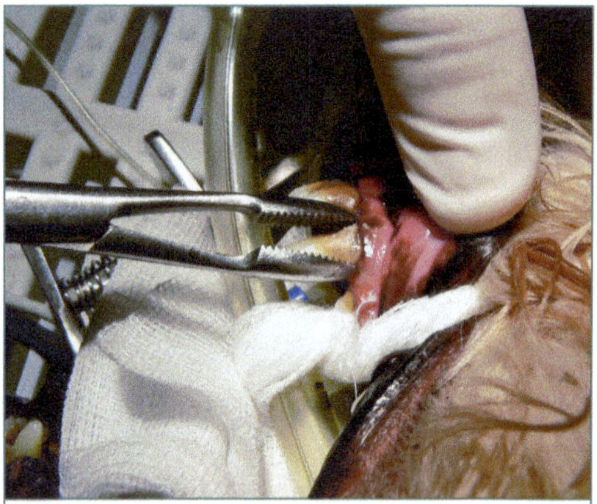

Figure 8. Tartar forceps.

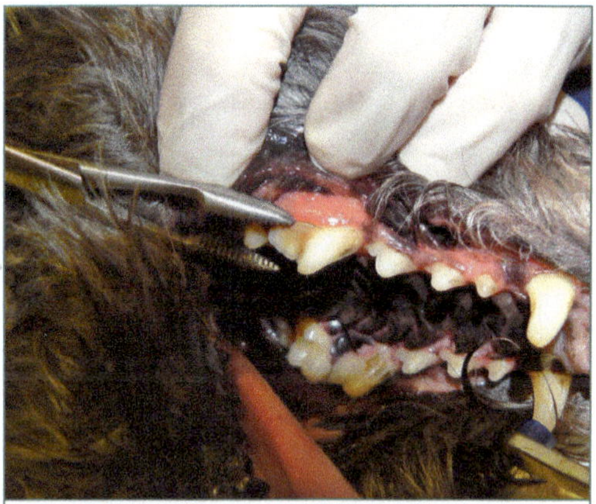

Figure 9. Using tartar forceps to eliminate supragingival calculi.

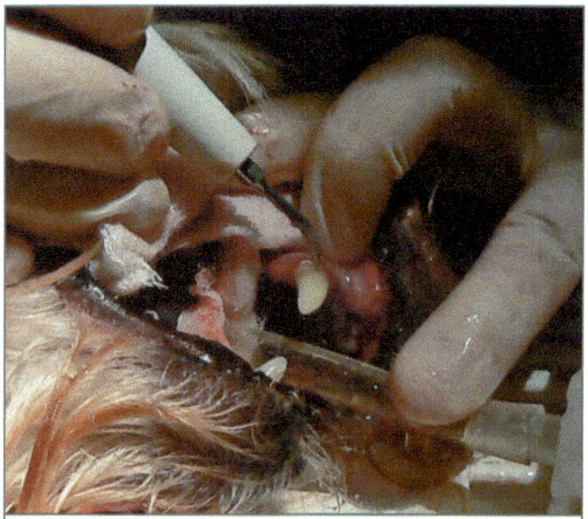

Figure 10. Application of an ultrasonic scaler.

TIP

Be sure to read the manufacturer's instructions carefully and replace the scaler's tip as soon as it becomes necessary.

These tools quickly eliminate any small remains of plaque still adhering to the teeth. It works by generating a high-speed vibration that breaks up the plaque. Apply the tip of the scaler correctly and without too much force; let the vibration do the work to avoid damaging the enamel and to keep the instrument in good working order. After cleaning the external surfaces of the teeth (supragingival), the next step is to clean the subgingival areas. There are many different tips available, so the professional can use whichever best suits their needs in each situation, but it is practically impossible to do everything with just one. This step is essential to the future health of our patient's mouth. If the subgingival space is not cleaned properly, bacterial plaque will continue destroying the periosteum unabated and eventually result in tooth loss.

Step 2: probing subgingival pockets

It is relatively easy to probe the subgingival pockets (Figs. 11–13), yet there are still some points to bear in mind to avoid mistakes. First of all, you must determine whether the height and shape of the gingival margin are physiologically correct. If so, the margin should coincide exactly with the cementoenamel junction. If, on the other hand, the gum line has receded, the pockets may be only shallow but of greater clinical significance. Similarly, in the case of **gingival hyperplasia**, the pocket may be much deeper than the actual loss of tooth attachment. During this step, it is essential to record the depths measured in the patient's dental file for reference in subsequent checkups (see boxes). These files will provide justification for future checkups and follow-up visits. The observation of any **furcation defects** should also be noted.

GINGIVAL INDEX

0: normal, healthy gums.

1: slight inflammation or erythema, no bleeding on probing. There may be oedema or changes at the free gingival margin.

2: moderate inflammation and moderate-to-severe erythema. Oedema and bleeding upon probing the subgingival pockets (Fig. 14).

3: severe inflammation or erythema. Oedema, ulceration, and spontaneous bleeding.

BONE SUPPORT INDEX

0: no loss of bone support.

1: horizontal loss of periodontal support tissue not exceeding one-third of the tooth's width.

2: horizontal loss of periodontal support tissue exceeding one-third of the tooth's width but not encompassing the total width of the furcation area.

3: complete horizontal loss of periodontal support tissue.

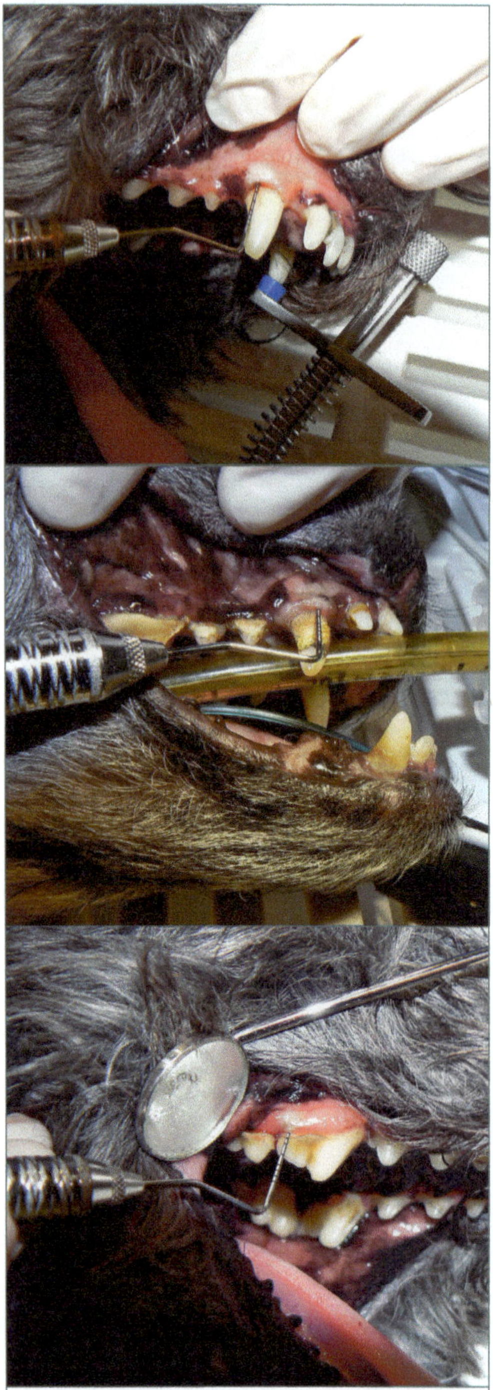

Figures 11, 12, and 13. Probing of the subgingival pockets.

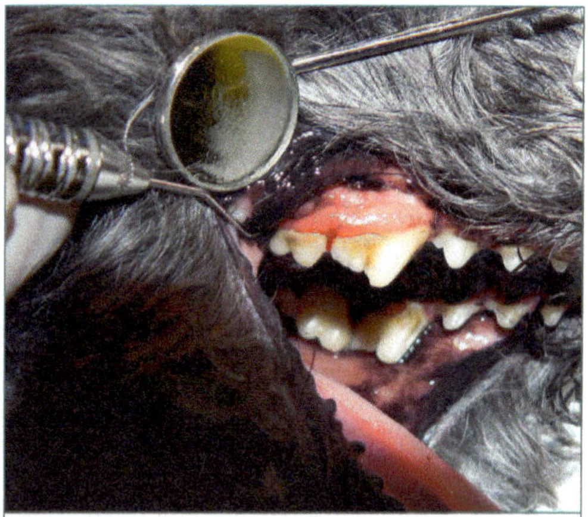

Figure 14. Bleeding on probing of the subgingival pockets.

TOOTH MOBILITY INDEX

0: no apparent mobility.

1: perceptible mobility, but less than 1 mm buccolingually.

2: mobility of between 1 and 2 mm.

3: clear mobility exceeding 2 mm buccolingually or vertically.

Step 3: detecting hidden calculi and plaque

There are various techniques for detecting any calculi or plaque that escaped the first cleaning. You can use a sickle probe to help feel where any calculi are still adhering to the tooth. Air flow or drying is another commonly used method. These instruments dry the surface of the tooth, thus highlighting any calculi which take on a whitish colour similar to chalk. Lastly, but not because it is the least used technique, are calculi disclosing solutions. Disclosing solutions can be applied with the aid of a cotton swab. After irrigating with water to remove the excess dye, calculi are visible as red/pink or blue stains depending on the brand of product used. Having detected the remains of tartar, they can easily be removed to leave a totally clean tooth.

PERIODONTAL DISEASE STAGING

Stage 0: no gingivitis, healthy gums.

Stage 1: only gingivitis, no loss of periodontal support tissue.

Stage 2: loss of <25 % of support tissue.

Stage 3: loss of 25–50 %.

Stage 4: loss of >50 %.

Note: add one stage for multiroot teeth with a furcation defect (e.g. a multiroot tooth with stage 2 periodontal disease and a furcation defect should be upgraded to stage 3 to account for the presence of the lesion).

Step 4: polishing

Polishing has two basic objectives. The first and more apparent aim is to smooth or soften the enamel surface as it may be damaged after cleaning. The second is to eliminate any plaque that remains bound to the teeth. Polishing is important because it helps prolong the benefit of the dental prophylaxis. Correct polishing depends heavily on the tools used for the task (Fig. 15). Teeth should be polished at a relatively low speed (3,000 to 8,000 rpm) with a rubber cup or nylon brush. The use of electric brushes is not recommendable at this stage.

Step 5: pocket irrigation and topical fluoride

Subgingival pocket irrigation also has two goals: to remove remains of calculi that have been dislodged but not expelled from the pocket, and to oxygenate the area. Irrigation can be done with a saline, fluoride, or 0.12 % chlorhexidine solution. However, for pockets with periodontal disease, perhaps the best option is 0.05 % saline solution. Pockets can be irrigated using a syringe fitted with a 25-gauge blunt needle (Fig. 16). This is a convenient moment to apply a fluoride gel or foam. The application of this type of products will delay the appearance of new plaque. They are generally left in contact with the teeth for 3 to 5 minutes, but of course the manufacturer's instructions should be followed for each product. After the allotted time, the product can be removed with gauze, it should not be rinsed off.

Step 6: periodontal diagnostic tests

At this stage, if not completed earlier, it is now time to measure and probe the subgingival pockets. After that, the next step is to take intraoral X-rays.

TAKE NOTE!

Intraoral radiography has earned its place as the most valuable diagnostic tool for periodontal disease, and there is growing support for the use of full-mouth radiography.[3,4]

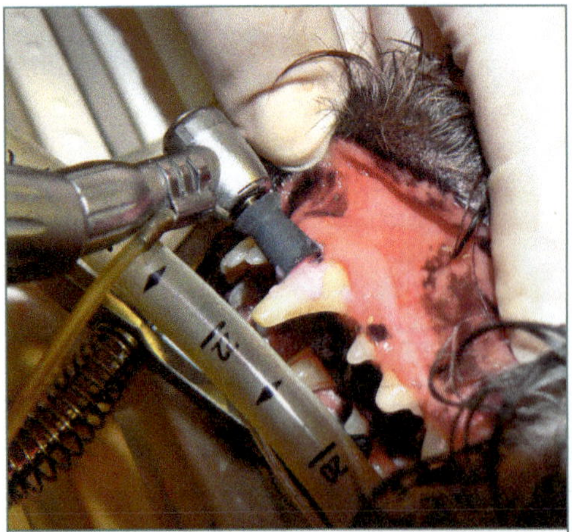

Figure 15. Polishing dental enamel with a cream.

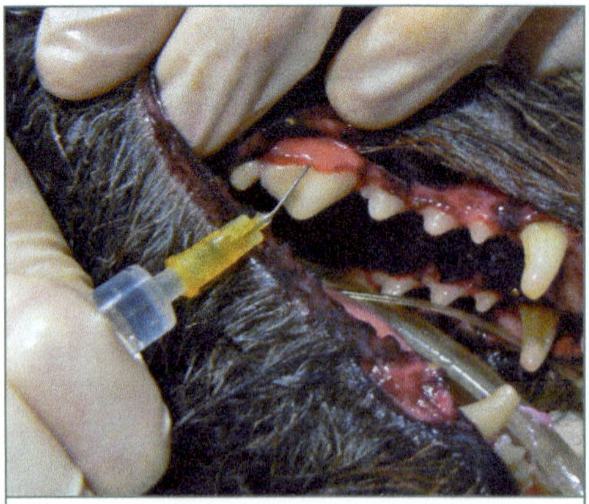

Figure 16. Irrigation of subgingival space with saline solution.

Step 7: recording data in the patient's dental file

It is important to record all the changes and procedures applied to each tooth and the scores for any indices assessed. Also make a note of any follow-up treatment required after the prophylaxis, if necessary. Shorthand codes come in handy when quickly jotting down all this information.

Step 8: home care measures

Remind the owner that without their collaboration the prophylactic effect of the procedure may last for far less than expected. Explain that a layer of glycoproteins forms within 20 minutes of cleaning, which helps bacteria adhere to the tooth surface, and the first bacterial colonies will develop within just 6–8 hours unless a fluoride or chlorhexidine solution is applied. These colonies are the root cause of bacterial plaque. The bacterial plaque dies after 3–5 days, which is when calcium in saliva binds to the plaque to form tartar.

Home care and maintenance of oral hygiene prevents or at least slows the formation of plaque and therefore tartar. Although oral hygiene ideally involves daily brushing, this is often unpractical, so home care measures can and should be adapted to each pet and each owner's means. The daily use of a chlorhexidine solution diluted in the pet's drinking water is one option, but this might not be enough. Some chlorhexidine solutions contain xylitol, and even though xylitol has been shown to be toxic to cats, one manufacturer has registered such a solution for daily use in cats. We prefer to use xylitol-free chlorhexidine solutions at our clinics.

CONSEQUENCES OF DEEP SUBGINGIVAL POCKETS (>4 mm)

Contain more pathogens and often anaerobic ones.

Deep pockets cannot be assessed without anaesthesia.

Deep pockets and furcation defects must be cleaned every 3–4 months.

Deep pockets are more difficult and take longer to clean.

How to complete a patient's dental file

Keeping an individual dental file for each pet where you can record all the problems detected really helps the vet conduct a full orodental consultation correctly. Dental files also help ensure the patient is followed up correctly and mean any other vet at the clinic or an external service can assess them and advise us on the best treatment for the given case. The owner should also be given a copy of their pet's dental file.

Every orodental examination should include an assessment of all the structures of the mouth and throat, as well as an in-depth dental exam that includes measuring the gingival pockets with a probe and recording any supernumerary or absent teeth, caries or feline odontoclastic resorptive lesions (FORL) (Fig. 17), the presence of tartar and/or pus, the state of the gingival mucosa and its degree of inflammation, any gingival recession or hyperplasia, and the level of tooth attachment, among others.

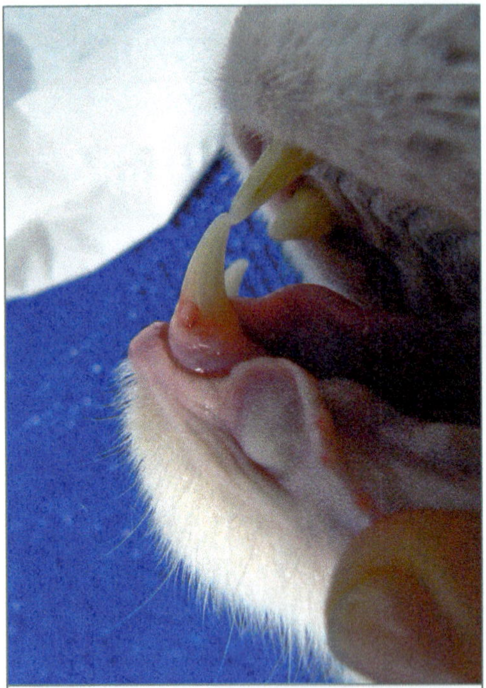

Figure 17. Feline odontoclastic resorptive lesion, or FORL, in a male cat.

All of these points have almost certainly been checked already, but is the information being written down? Besides its utility in the follow-up, recording the information in the dental file helps when justifying to the patient's owner the cost of treating any problems identified in the exam.

You can choose from several tooth numbering systems to identify pieces in the dental file; however, the most popular is the **modified Triadan system**,[2] which divides the mouth into four quadrants and numbers the teeth from 1 to 10. Once you know which tooth is problematic, you need a code to save time and ensure nothing is omitted when recording the data. In many cases, you should also note down the severity of these lesions and alterations.

The next page shows a copy of the dental file we use at our clinics.

DENTAL EXAM SHEET

ANIMAL HEALTH FILES No. 001

EXAMINATION

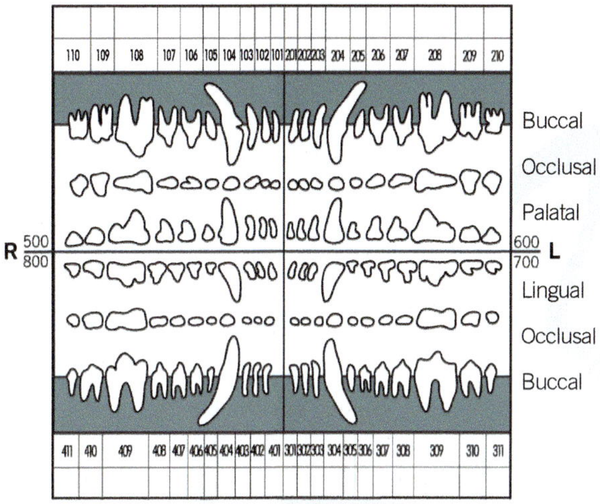

TREATMENT

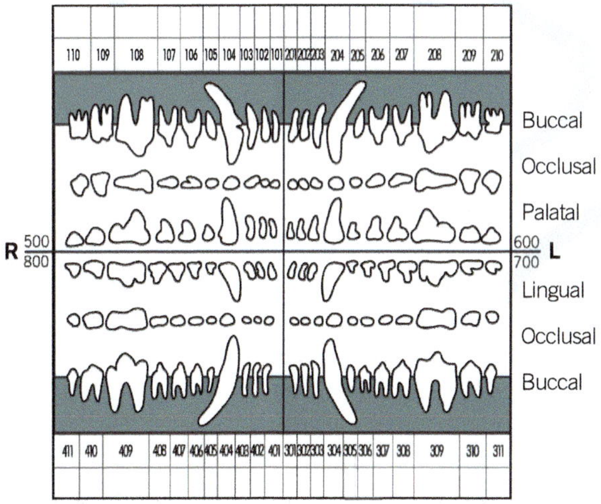

Clinical evaluation	Circle the correct option N = normal A = abnormal
Extraoral facial symmetry	N A
Lymph nodes	N A
Oral mucosa	N A
Tongue	N A
Palate	N A
Tonsils	N A
Pharynx	N A
Salivary flow	N A

Last dental prophylaxis (months)	
Home treatment	
Brushing: Yes ☐ No ☐	Materials:
Dental rinse: Yes ☐ No ☐	Materials:
Diet: Dry ☐ Wet ☐ Other ☐	
Oral habits: Chews hard objects ☐ No chewing ☐	

Treatment	
Home treatment	
Cleaning	
Extraction	
Comments:	

ABBREVIATIONS

BE Biopsy, excisional
BI Biopsy, incisional
CA Caries
CI Calculus index (1 to 3)
CR Crown restoration
FI Furcation index (1 to 3)
FX Fractured jaw or tooth
G Granuloma
GI Gingival index (1 to 3)
GH Gingival hyperplasia
GR Gingival recession
MI Mobility index (1 to 3)
OM Oral mass
PC Pulp capping
PE Pulp exposed
PI Plaque index (1 to 3)
PP Periodontal pocket
PRO Dental prophylaxis
R/C Composite filling
RD Retained deciduous
RRT Retained root tip
ST Stomatitis
T/A Tooth avulsed
T/I Tooth impacted
TR Tooth resorption (1 to 5)
X Simple closed extraction
XS Nonsurgical extraction with tooth sectioning
XSS Surgical extraction

THE OWNER'S PERSPECTIVE

After the conscious exam, **explain to the owner what is wrong with the patient** and the treatment options. Be sure to **address any doubts** the owner may have while explaining their pet's situation.

It is worth spending the time to fully clarify three points where most owners are generally wary of orodental procedures in pets. The **three issues that must be addressed** are:

- **Cost:** the price is a vital factor when deciding whether a patient will undergo an orodental treatment. The procedures in themselves are not particularly expensive. However, the final cost is often elevated by the need for anaesthesia and complementary tests. Whenever a geriatric patient has to be anaesthetised it involves a series of relatively extensive preoperative tests (see Chapter 4), in addition to dental X-rays and often complex medical treatments. It is always important to quote a price as close as possible to the final bill, but this is even truer of veterinary dentistry. However, this is particularly difficult given the lack of a full examination when estimating the price. At our clinics, we always ask for a contact number so we can call the owner after completing the full oral exploration during their pet's dental procedure to explain any new findings and discuss possible treatment options and their cost. If this is not possible, we suggest obtaining the owner's advance authorisation for the worst-case scenario or, if on the other hand permission is not granted, request approval to finish the intervention and wake the patient without performing all the required procedures. Any agreement should be recorded in writing and signed by the vet responsible for the treatment and the owner. Both parties should then keep a copy.
- **Anaesthesia:** this is clearly the point that scares owners the most. It is hard to work out how much information each client is willing to receive. Regardless of this, they must be given at least a minimum of information even if only in writing.[5] If any members of the clinic specialise in anaesthesia, this is a good moment for them to meet the owner and clear up any doubts they may have. The anaesthetic procedure should be explained using plain, straightforward language, including the stages, use

of anaesthetics, analgesics, anti-inflammatories, etc., and the monitoring equipment used to minimise the risks associated with anaesthesia. Although discussing the possibility of perianaesthetic death[a] is not very popular with most veterinary surgeons, we believe it helps convince a lot of owners that it is better to carry out the intervention before their pet's situation declines.

- **Dental extraction:** one of the main issues at our clinic when a patient is brought in for orodental treatment is that clients are unaware of the difference between veterinary and human dentistry, especially with respect to extractions. Many owners want to preserve their pet's teeth. If possible, all attempts should be made to preserve pieces; however, it should be made patently clear that if extraction is the appropriate treatment and it is not performed, then the patient's orodental and overall health may be at risk in a relatively short time. Owners should also be reminded that it often costs more to save a tooth than extract it.

It is good practice to **record the conversation** when dealing with a **difficult client**. If so, the owner must be informed and their consent to the recording registered in writing. Some mobile telephones have features or apps that can record conversations in a digital file.

Other issues that must also be addressed are the need to **shave one or more areas** to **insert catheters** and obtain **blood samples**. Similarly, you should obtain **permission to photograph** the patient's mouth before and after the dental treatment and conduct the **treatments needed before and after** the actual dental procedure.

[a] Around 0.1 to 0.2 % of healthy cats and dogs die during the perianaesthetic period. This rate is 10 times higher for patients with a suboptimal state of health. Remember that over 60 % of perianaesthetic deaths occur during recovery. Hypothermia, hypoxia, and hypotension are among the main causes.

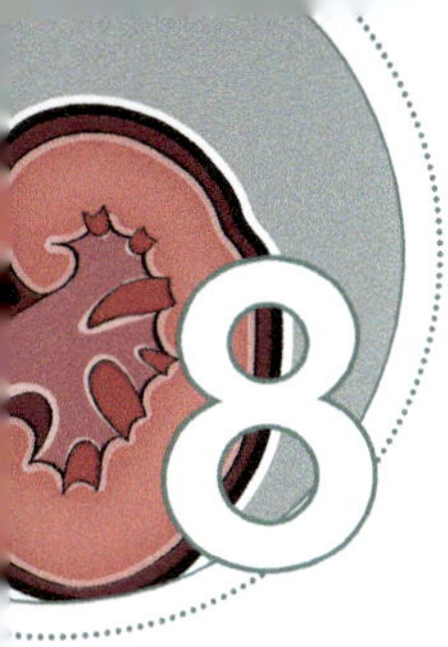

Chronic kidney disease

We could dedicate an entire book, or even several volumes, to describing the physiology, pathophysiology, and myriad of techniques available for the diagnosis of kidney disease in small animals. Kidney injury or damage has a lot of potential causes; nevertheless, we are generally unable to reach an aetiological diagnosis and have to make do with a clinical diagnosis, which tends to be enough to treat the patient in question.

This chapter starts by reviewing basic renal physiology, before providing more detailed information on the most useful diagnostic tests. Lastly, and accompanied by the scientific evidence, we shall explore the world of kidney disease and its treatment.

Definition and prevalence

The kidneys perform various functions to help maintain homeostasis, and to do so they receive around 25 % of cardiac output. Due to their complex architecture and multifunctional role, they are always subject to ongoing research. A brief account of their functions and anatomical location are given later in the chapter.

Chronic kidney disease (CKD) is defined as the progressive loss of normal kidney function over a period of more than 3 months (Fig. 1). The term encompasses a group of diseases that affect kidney function and which eventually follow a similar clinical course. As such, do not be fooled into thinking this is an aetiological diagnosis, as it is in fact a clinical diagnosis. Although, as mentioned above, it is often hard to reach an aetiological diagnosis; but if one can be reached, it would benefit the patient because it opens the door to a more specific treatment and, in theory, possibly even stopping the damage produced by the causal agent or lesion.

The prevalence of CKD in animals increases with age. Accordingly, the prevalence in geriatric dogs may be up to 10 %, while as many as 35 % of elderly cats have CKD. Expressed from a more practical perspective; 1 in 10 dogs aged over 8–10 years and 1 in 3 cats over 10 will suffer from "kidney problems".[1] Given its high prevalence, vets really need to be well informed about CKD.

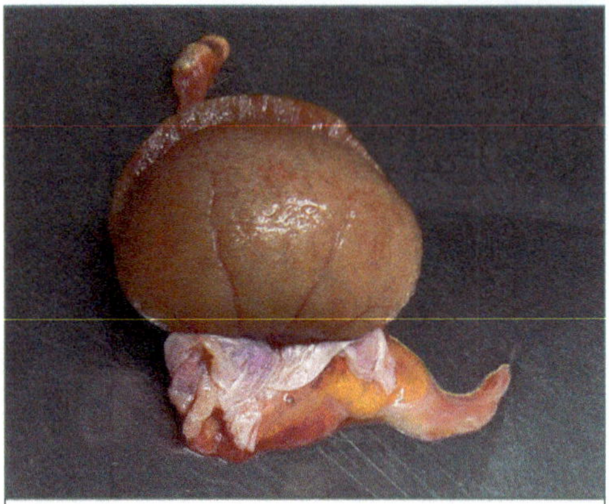

Figure 1. A kidney with interstitial nephritis; a common cause of CKD in cats. Note the fibrotic and pleated surface. The ipsilateral adrenal gland visible at the top is calcified, which is a clinically insignificant finding in a geriatric cat.

Renal physiology

Given the complex nature of renal physiology, and in line with the adage that a picture paints a thousand words, Figure 2 shows a diagram summarising all the kidneys' functions according to the anatomical location in nephrons.

Diagnostic techniques and early diagnosis

When nephrons are affected by any of the causes that can lead to CKD, the consequent damage and functional impairment is practically irreversible, so vets must learn to use quick, reliable diagnostic techniques to minimise the kidney injury and maximise the patient's life expectancy.

If you ask another vet which is the best technique or test in the diagnosis of CKD, you will receive a lot of different answers. In light of this and the elevated prevalence among our geriatric patients, when an elderly cat or dog is brought to the clinic for whatever reason, you should always pay attention to several details that could be key indicators of CKD that has just started but which may not yet develop any clinical manifestations for weeks or months. Box 1 presents the clinical findings and reasons for consultation most commonly encountered in patients with CKD.

Do not underestimate the value of measures such as body condition score, weight, water intake, and food intake. For example, in a retrospective study of 258 cats, weight loss preceded death for various reasons, one of them being CKD. The subjects started to lose weight 2.5 years before their demise. In the first year, they lost around 6 % of their weight, and over the second year, before death, they lost over 10 % of their initial weight.[3]

TIP

It helps if owners of elderly cats or dogs can try to estimate their pet's daily water intake before each visit and bring a urine sample with them. A urine specific gravity test gives quick results that can indicate whether further, more specific tests are required. Healthy cats and dogs drink around 20–70 ml/kg/day and urinate 20–45 ml/kg/day.

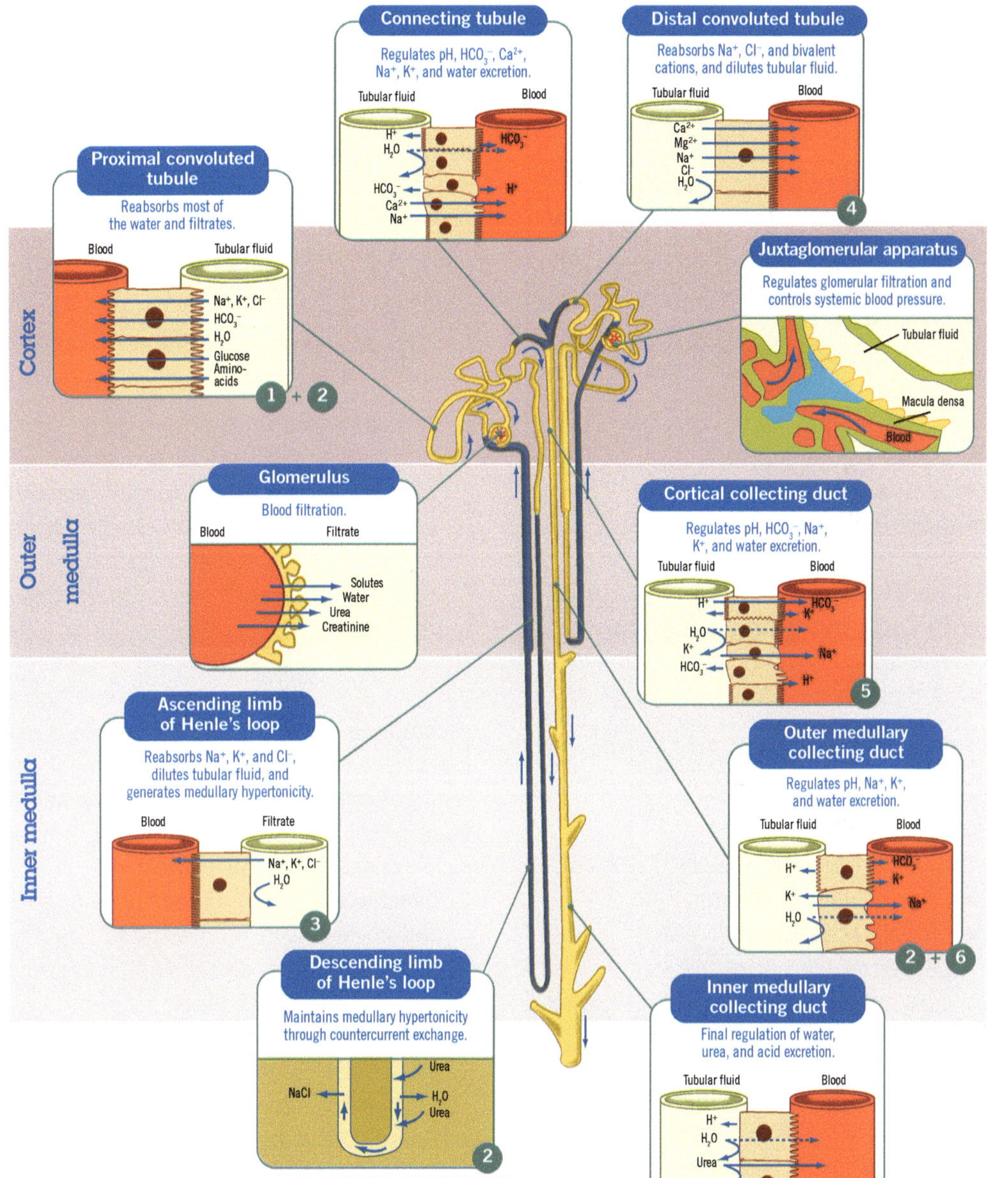

Diuretics key:
1. Carbonic anhydrase inhibitors (e.g. acetazolamide)
2. Osmotic diuretics (e.g. mannitol)
3. Loop diuretics (e.g. furosemide)
4. Thiazides
5. Aldosterone antagonists (e.g. spironolactone)
6. Antidiuretic hormone receptor antagonists (e.g. demeclocyclin)

This diagram does not include erythropoietin (Epo) synthesis. Epo-producing cells are an uncommon type of cell located in the cortex, in the interstitial space surrounding the renal tubules. Their morphology is characteristic of endothelial cells, so they are most probably peritubular capillary endothelial cells, especially given the space between the renal tubules is essentially occupied by peritubular capillaries.[2]

Figure 2. Schematic diagram of a renal nephron and the juxtaglomerular apparatus organised by segments and their functions. The arrows indicate the flow of tubular fluid. The circuit starts in the glomerulus. The numbers represent the principal site of action for the various diuretic agents used in routine clinical practice.

Box 1. CLUES THAT SHOULD AROUSE SUSPICIONS OF CKD.

Reasons for consultation in patients with CKD, including early stages:

- Reduced appetite
- Weight loss
- Increased water intake
- Increased urine output
- Vomiting
- Lethargy
- Exercise intolerance
- Sudden blindness

Clinical signs observed in patients with CKD, including early stages:

- Pale mucous membranes
- Dehydration
- Oral alterations (halitosis, ulcers)
- Abnormal renal palpation
- Hypertension
- Eye fundus alterations (hypertensive retinopathy)
- Loss of body condition
- Osteodystrophy (bone pain, pathological fractures).
- Oedema

Urinalysis

A urinalysis is a rapid, simple, and even cheap test. Maybe this is why the information it can provide is often underestimated or undervalued. However, a complete urine test can offer an array of information that helps with the diagnosis and prognosis of kidney disease. It is important to standardise the test in order to get reliable, reproducible results.

There are many different brands of urine test strip, but only some of them have been validated for use in cats and dogs. Bear in mind that test strips also have certain limitations; for instance, as they are based on a colorimetric method, high levels of pigments (bilirubin, biliverdin, urobilin, haemoglobin, or myoglobin, among others) can produce false results.

TAKE NOTE!

Test strips for human urine give unreliable results for nitrites, white blood cells, and urine specific gravity when used on samples collected from cats or dogs. Likewise, some urine glucose strips produce unpredictable reactions.

A **complete urine test** should include a reactive strip, a specific gravity measurement using a refractometer, a microscopic study, and the urine protein:creatinine ratio (UPC). A microscopic urinalysis consists of two parts:

1. **Direct exam:** place a drop of urine on a slide and cover it with a cover glass. Then use the microscope to search for and assess the nature of any crystalluria.
2. **Sediment exam:** centrifuge part of the sample (at least 3 ml) and place the resulting sediment on a slide and view it without stain. Finally, spread the sediment, dry it, and stain with a differential, Romanowsky-type stain. The UPC can only be measured if the end product is an inactive urine sediment (with no haematuria or inflammation). Any signs of infection (pyuria with/without bacteriuria) should be studied further through a urine culture and bacterial sensitivity analysis. You can use the data in Table 1 for guidance whenever a culture cannot be obtained.

TAKE NOTE!

All rapid panoptic staining kits are similar to one another; they comprise three bottles containing a fixative, a red acidophilic stain, and a blue basophilic stain. However, each brand works with different staining times, so pay attention to the instructions as one set of stains may require 10 seconds for each product while another brand may need a full minute.

With respect to the **urine protein:creatinine** ratio (UPC), the gold standard for calculating proteinuria is based on the measurement of protein contained in a 24-hour urine sample. Yet this sampling period has clear disadvantages in veterinary medicine, so vets started assessing the UPC ratio. This measurement links the amount of protein in urine to the amount of creatinine excreted. Several studies have shown that it correlates well with measurements based on 24-hour samples.[4]

Table 1. Diagnosis and treatment of principal bacterial infections.

Urinary pH	Bacteria characteristics	Probable organism	1st choice antibiotic	2nd choice antibiotic
Acidic	Bacilliform	*E. coli*	Sulphonamides/ trimethoprim	Cephalexin
		Klebsiella	Cephalexin	Sulphonamides/ trimethoprim
		Pseudomonas	According to the culture	-
		Enterobacter	Sulphonamides/ trimethoprim	Fluoroquinolones
Acidic	Coccus	Enterococci	Aminopenicillins	Fluoroquinolones
		Streptococci	Aminopenicillins	Cephalexin
Alkaline	Bacilliform	*Proteus*	Aminopenicillins	Cephalexin
Alkaline	Coccus	Staphylococci	Aminopenicillins	Cephalexin

Note: *E. coli* is by far the most common aetiological agent of bacillary infections in acidic urine. Potentiated fluoroquinolones and aminopenicillins should be saved for invasive infections. The drugs recommended in this table are supposed to have an efficacy of over 80 % against the given bacteria.

ASSESSING PROTEINURIA: STRIPS AND TURBIDITY TEST OR UPC RATIO?

First it is important to emphasise that each test is designed to meet different objectives. Both urine strips and the turbidity test with sulphosalicylic acid (SSA) are designed for the semiquantitative detection of protein in urine. The former detects urine protein when above 30 mg/dl, while the test with SSA can identify levels above 5 mg/dl. However, neither of these measures provides objective data and in fact they often give different results depending on the technician or laboratory carrying out the tests. Thus, we need a quick, reproducible, and numerically precise measurement so we can assess and quantify the proteinuria and response to treatment. What is more, as shown in Figure 3, we must not forget that urine test strips can show negative or trace results when the UPC is >0.4, which is a clinically relevant value and indicator that treatment should be initiated for the proteinuria.[5]

Therefore, the answer to our initial question should be: both, one is used to detect proteinuria, the other is used to quantify it. Proteinuria is a negative prognostic factor in both cats and dogs, and we must do everything possible to keep it under control. We can also use the UPC to classify the substages of CKD according to the protocol published by the International Renal Interest Society (IRIS).

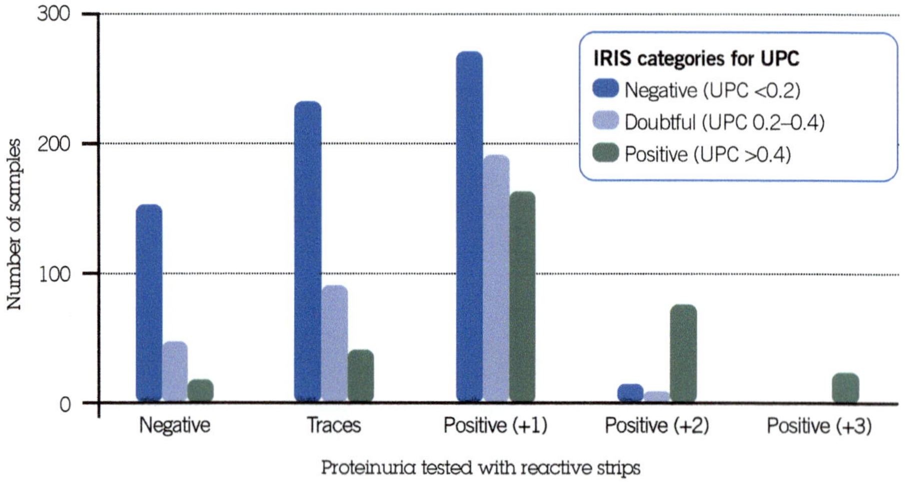

Figure 3. Correlation between proteinuria measured with strips and UPC ratio.[5]

Blood test

Numerous alterations can be observed in the blood count and blood chemistry of patients with CKD. The most frequently affected and well-known parameters are urea (blood urea nitrogen or BUN), creatinine, and phosphorus. However, many other parameters are influenced by the reduction in glomerular filtration (amylase, specific pancreatic lipase, etc.), while yet more imbalances can develop because of secondary alterations (hypercalcaemia due to renal hyperparathyroidism, hypoalbuminaemia secondary to proteinuria, etc.). Box 2 lists the minimum laboratory tests that should be conducted in patients with nephropathy, and Table 2 shows the changes in certain blood parameters over the course of CKD.

Before concluding this section, let us have a more detailed look at the latest lab parameter to receive attention, that is, **symmetric dimethylarginine** (SDMA). As with creatinine, SDMA is eliminated exclusively via the kidneys and also follows a close correlation with the glomerular filtration rate (GFR). SDMA holds certain advantages over creatinine, as it is not influenced by changes in the patient's muscle mass and can be used to detect altered renal function in the earliest stages of CKD. The International Renal Interest Society (IRIS) has now incorporated SDMA in its panel of recommended tests, and the same group of experts also advises vets to always assess SDMA along with the other indicators and pay attention to studies reporting information on its diagnostic efficacy.

Diagnostic imaging

Imaging techniques can be used to assess the degree of kidney compromise, bilateralism, structural alterations, and ureteral permeability, among others. Nowadays, CKD is never diagnosed without confirmation from imaging tests. Ultrasound is the method of choice for CKD.

Box 2. BASIC LABORATORY TESTS IN PATIENTS WITH SUSPECTED NEPHROPATHY.

Blood count

Albumin

Creatinine

Urea

Phosphorus

Calcium*

Symmetric dimethylarginine (SDMA)

Bicarbonate

Potassium

In cats, total T_4 and ALT

Complete urinalysis:
- Urine test strips
- Sediment
- UPC**

* Calcium measured in cats must be ionised calcium and it is also advisable for dogs.

** Only determine UPC if the sediment is inactive.

Table 2. Changes in blood parameters over the course of CKD.

Parameter	Type of change or reason	Pathophysiological cause	Treatment or care
Anaemia	Nonregenerative	• Reduction in red blood cell half-life • Decreased protein intake due to anorexia or hyporexia • Decreased levels of group B vitamins due to polyuria • Release of inflammatory cytokines that cause iron chelation in the liver, provoking anaemia due to chronic inflammation • Reduction in erythropoietin (Epo)	• Correct the patient's hydration status and uraemia • Prescribe a renal diet • Administer Epo
Urea and creatinine	Elevated	Reduced glomerular filtration rate (GFR)	• Fluid therapy • Renal diet
Phosphorus	Elevated	Reduced GFR	• Fluid therapy • Renal diet • Chelating agents
Potassium	Decreased	• Reduced intake • Urinary loss	• Renal diet • Potassium supplements
Blood pressure	Increased	Multiple causes: activation of the renin–angiotensin system, sodium retention, extracellular volume expansion, etc.	• Ca^{2+} channel blockers • Angiotensin II receptor antagonists (AIIRAs) • Angiotensin converting enzyme inhibitors (ACEIs) (mainly in dogs)
Proteinuria	Present	Glomerular hypertension or glomerulonephritis	• AIIRAs • ACEIs • Ca^{2+} channel blockers
Blood pH	Reduced or acidosis	Multiple causes	• Renal diet • Alkalising agents (sodium bicarbonate, potassium citrate)

Renal X-rays

A plain film X-ray is sufficient to assess the size and shape of both kidneys. The observation of smaller than normal kidneys may be a sign of CKD. For example, one study found that 33 % of cats with CKD had small kidneys, 40 % were of normal size, and 27 % were larger than usual.[6] Evidently, besides their size, important information can be obtained by comparing their shape and size relative to each other. Renal atrophy tends to be associated with scarring and/or chronic fibrosis and often compensatory renal hypertrophy in the contralateral kidney if it is not directly affected by CKD. An irregular margin is common in cases that course with renal cysts, infarcts, or masses (Fig. 4).

Lastly, do not forget to assess bone density when looking at X-rays for renal patients. Although subjective, this measure can help in the diagnosis of secondary cases of renal osteodystrophy or renal hyperparathyroidism.

Nevertheless, it should be noted that while plain X-rays have a specificity of 100 % for kidney and ureteral stones, the sensitivity is only 60 %. Ultrasound, on the other hand, has a sensitivity of 77–100 % and a specificity of just 33 %. The use of both techniques to identify lithiasis reaches a sensitivity of 90 %.[7–10]

You can use the second lumbar vertebra (L2) as a reference for estimating kidney size in ventrodorsal X-rays (Fig. 5).

TAKE NOTE!

In dogs, a normal sized kidney is 2.5 to 3.5 times the length of L2. In females and entire male cats, it is 2.1 to 3.2 times the length of L2, and in castrated males a little smaller, i.e. 1.9 to 2.6 times L2.[11]

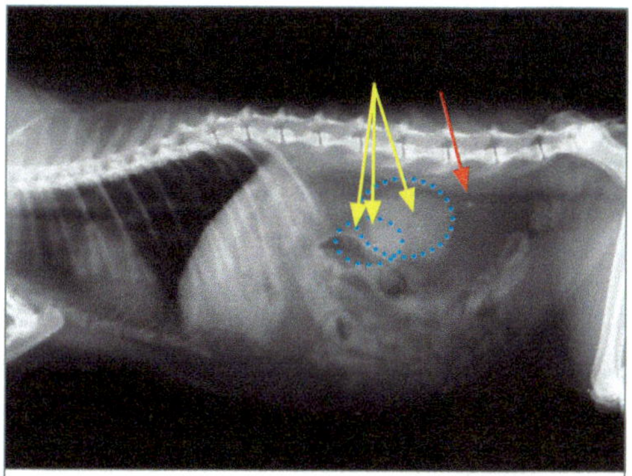

Figure 4. Laterolateral X-ray of a 5-year-old male cat. The blue circles highlight irregular margins and a smaller kidney with compensatory hypertrophy in the other. There are also kidney stones (yellow arrows) and a ureteral stone (red arrow).

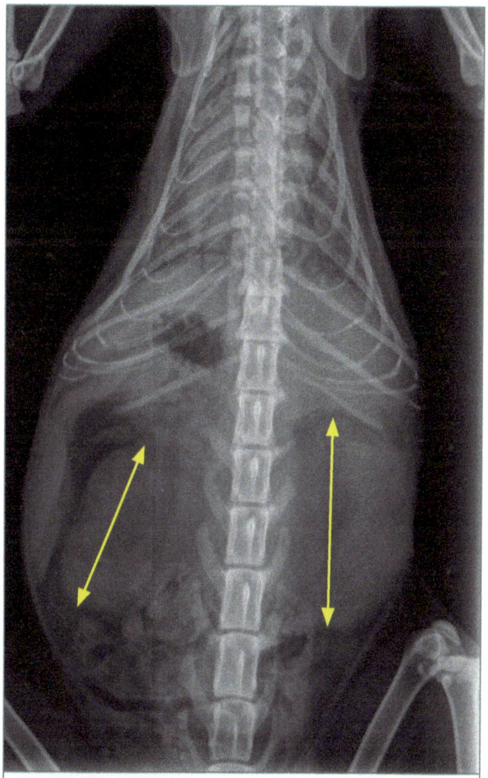

Figure 5. Dorsoventral X-ray of an 11-year-old female cat with pulmonary and renal metastasis of a mammary carcinoma. Both kidneys are between 3.5 and 4 times the size of the second lumbar vertebra.

Renal ultrasound

An abdominal ultrasound can be used to examine not just the size and shape of the kidneys, but also their architecture (Fig. 6). A normal feline kidney should measure 3.8–4.4 cm on an ultrasound image, provided there is no renal pelvic dilatation. Various parameters have been used as yardsticks in dogs, such as renal volume and the ratio between kidney length and aortic diameter, but with limited success due to the large range of sizes in different breeds of dog.

Renal ultrasounds of patients with CKD tend to display a loss of corticomedullary differentiation, hyperechoic cortices, and irregular margins. You may also identify renal cysts, which are often a sign the process is becoming chronic (Fig. 7).[12] Unfortunately, renal ultrasound scans of patients with CKD can also appear totally normal.

To finish off, you could try to obtain images of the parathyroid glands. The technique is not difficult, but it does require some practice and you often need to shave the ventral region of the neck. If there is hyperplasia in the glands, the patient probably has renal hyperparathyroidism. One study found that dogs with CKD had larger parathyroid glands (3.9–8.1 mm) than those with acute kidney disease or healthy subjects (2.0–4.6 mm).[13]

TIP

Although it seems obvious, it is important to remember that the size of the kidneys and parathyroid glands is proportional to the size of the dog.

Renal biopsy

Biopsy is not typically used as a means of diagnosis. This is because it is a relatively invasive method that may entail complications for the patient. In spite of this, when absolutely necessary, the collection of biopsy samples can be particularly useful as their examination usually leads to an aetiological diagnosis. A renal biopsy should be performed in the case of:

- nephromegaly (with suspicion of neoplasm),
- proteinuria that is hard to diagnose by other means, or
- CKD in young animals.

The owner should be given a clear explanation of the difficulties and risks involved with the technique before carrying out a renal biopsy on a patient. Do not proceed if the patient is very small (<5 kg), has disrupted homeostasis, or

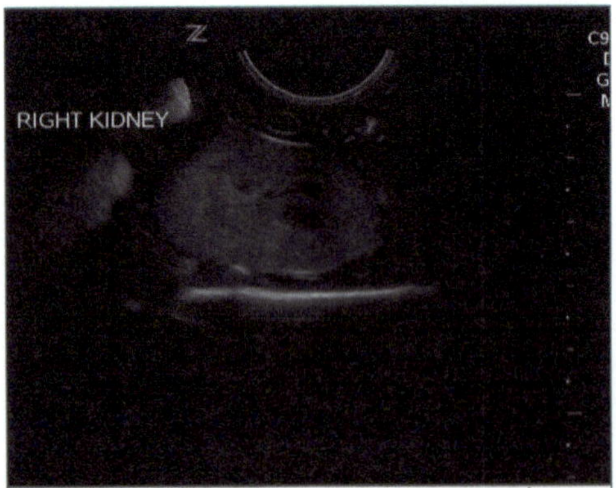

Figure 6. Renal ultrasound.

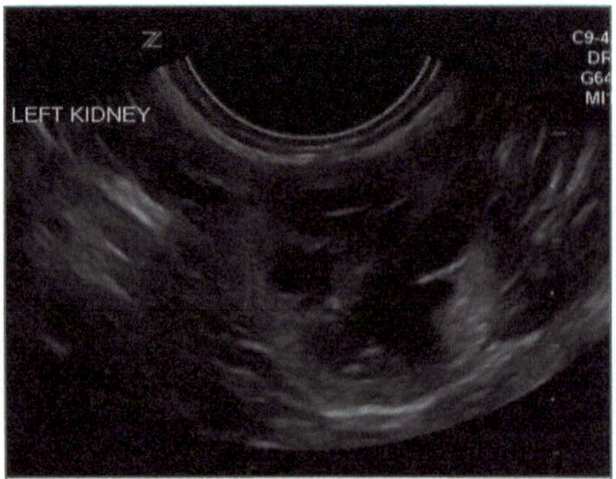

Figure 7. Ultrasound of a polycystic kidney.

hypertension that cannot be controlled with medication.[14,15] Indeed, one retrospective study found that the group with most complications were animals over 4 years old, weighing under 5 kg, and with a blood creatinine level of over 5 mg/dl.[16]

Box 3 lists the main complications that can arise after a renal biopsy, ordered as per their frequency of presentation.

Box 3. LEADING COMPLICATIONS FOLLOWING RENAL BIOPSY.

- Arteriovenous fistula formation
- Biopsy of nonrenal tissue
- Renal cyst formation
- Death
- Haemorrhage
- Micro- or macroscopic haematuria
- Peri- or intrarenal haematoma
- Renal vessel laceration
- Intra-abdominal haemorrhage due to laceration of organs or vessels
- Hydronephrosis
- Infarct and thrombosis
- Infection
- Formation of scar tissue and fibrosis

Fine-needle puncture can be used to try and obtain samples from small patients.

IRIS classification

The IRIS designed a simple system for the clinical staging of CKD in cats and dogs. Basically, the method involves determining the blood creatinine concentration, assessing proteinuria by calculating the UPC, and measuring systolic blood pressure. The IRIS system classifies patients as having stage 1 to 4 CKD, with or without proteinuria and/or hypertension.

Once the patient's CKD has been staged, their treatment becomes more standardised and therefore straightforward. Table 3 shows the parameters and ranges that define each stage, as well as the corresponding clinical signs most often manifested by patients.

Evidence-based treatment of CKD

Given the wide range of treatment options available for patients diagnosed with CKD, veterinary clinicians often find themselves a little unsure as to which are the most effective and safest treatments, and ultimately which of them will mark the difference.

TAKE NOTE!

The objective of evidence-based medicine is to facilitate the application of current standards of medical care based on the best data available regarding the benefits, limits, and risks of the therapeutic measures.

Table 3. IRIS staging and substaging of CKD.

Stage	Blood creatinine and SDMA levels
Stage 1 100 % renal function	Dogs: creatinine <1.4 mg/dl; SDMA <18 µg/dl Cats: creatinine <1.6 mg/dl; SDMA <18 µg/dl
Stage 2 33 % renal function	Dogs: creatinine 1.4–2.8 mg/dl; SDMA 18–35 µg/dl Cats: creatinine 1.6–2.8 mg/dl; SDMA 18–25 µg/dl
Stage 3 25 % renal function	Dogs: creatinine 2.9–5.0 mg/dl; SDMA 36–54 µg/dl Cats: creatinine 2.9–5.0 mg/dl; SDMA 26–38 µg/dl
Stage 4 <10 % renal function	Dogs: creatinine >5 mg/dl; SDMA >54 µg/dl Cats: creatinine >5 mg/dl; SDMA >38 µg/dl
Interpretation of UPC	
Dogs <0.2: no proteinuria 0.2–0.5: incipient proteinuria >0.5: clinical proteinuria	**Cats** <0.2: no proteinuria 0.2–0.4: incipient proteinuria >0.4: clinical proteinuria
Interpretation of systolic blood pressure	
<140 mmHg: normotension. Minimal risk of target organ damage. 140–159 mmHg: prehypertension. Low risk of target organ damage. 160–179 mmHg: prehypertension. Moderate risk of target organ damage. ≥180 mmHg: severe hypertension. High risk of target organ damage.	
Note: whenever there is a discrepancy in the staging between a patient's creatinine and symmetric dimethylarginine (SDMA) blood levels, the vet should consider the potential loss of muscle mass and reassess both parameters after 2–4 weeks. If there is still disagreement between the values, the patient should be graded at one stage higher than that marked by the blood creatinine level.	

An ideal treatment would increase the patient's life expectancy, improve their quality of life, minimise any side effects or adverse reactions, and always strive to accommodate any reasonable demands from the owner regarding treatment duration and cost while causing the least possible impact on the patient–owner relationship. As a given treatment achieves less and less of these objectives, then the chance of failure, lack of follow-up, and even patient euthanasia all increase.[17]

Any attempts to determine which are the safest and most effective therapeutic measures should be based on scientific evidence. This evidence has been graded on a 4-point scale, where grade 1 is the most reliable evidence and grade 4 only provides weak support for the recommendation (Table 4).

At present, and in line with both the IRIS guidelines and scientific evidence, as vets we must apply a logical approach to assessing and justifying the various therapies at each stage. Table 5 summarises the treatment recommendations for cats and dogs and the level of their supporting evidence.

Table 4. Grades for evidence-based medicine and their significance.	
Scientific evidence	How it is attained
Grade 1	There is at least one properly conducted randomised controlled trial (RCT) or a meta-analysis of several RCTs. **Strong support for the recommendation.**
Grade 2	The data have been gathered from studies that use acceptable laboratory models or simulations in the target species. They estimate the efficacy in ideal conditions rather than real-life conditions. They may not coincide with the clinical working conditions of the case in hand. **Moderate support for the recommendation.**
Grade 3	Implies the existence of at least one well-designed, nonrandomised clinical trial, a cohort of controlled, analytical case studies, or a group of uncontrolled studies that have returned spectacular outcomes. **Moderate support for the recommendation.**
Grade 4	Implies recommendations from experts based on their experience, descriptive studies, studies in other species, pathophysiological reasoning, and reports from panels of experts. **Weak support for the recommendation.**

Main therapeutic measures for CKD

Renal diet

As far back as 1939, Mark Morris designed the first renal diet for dogs. The type of food was the first variable found to play a crucial role in improving the quality of life of patients with kidney disease. Nowadays, the nutrient composition of these diets has been greatly modified, but there are four key changes common to all commercially available renal diets.

1. **Reduced protein:** protein metabolism is responsible for the concentration of nitrogenous waste products in the blood. The level of nitrogenous waste in blood can be reduced by decreasing the total protein intake and increasing its biological value. It should be stressed that the amount of nitrogenous metabolites produced not only depends on the amount ingested but also on its biological value. The biological value is determined by the source of the protein; for example, protein derived from eggs and milk has a greater biological value.
2. **Reduced phosphorus:** in an effort to reduce the level of phosphates in blood, the first step is to prescribe a low-phosphorus diet. A high blood phosphate level leads to renal hyperparathyroidism with the subsequent risk of soft tissue calcification. If a renal diet does not bring blood phosphate levels under control, it should be supplemented with phosphate binders.
3. **Increased potassium:** a lot of patients with CKD, particularly cats, develop hypokalaemia during the course of the disease. Potassium deficiency causes myopathies that manifest clinically as a loss of muscle mass and the development of lameness. Furthermore, hypokalaemic nephropathy is one of the

Table 5. Scientific evidence for therapeutic measures applied in CKD.

Type of treatment	Examples	Indicated IRIS stage	Evidence	Treatment benefits
Renal diet	Commercial renal diet	Dogs in stage 3 or 4 Cats in stage 2, 3, or 4 Creatinine ≥2 mg/dl	Grade 1 in both cats and dogs (RCTs)	Improves blood urea, phosphate, and potassium levels
ACEIs and AIIRAs	Enalapril, benazepril, captopril Telmisartan at antiproteinuric doses	In stage 1 if UPC ≥2 Dogs in stages 2–4 if UPC >0.5 Cats in stages 2–4 if UPC >0.4	Grade 1 in cats and dogs for the reduction of proteinuria (RCTs) Grade 4 in cats and dogs for slowing disease progression	Reduces proteinuria
Calcitriol	Calcitriol	In stages 3 and 4	Grade 1 in dogs (RCTs) Grade 4 in cats (RCTs do not endorse its use)	Reduces degree of renal hyperparathyroidism
↓ Phosphataemia	Calcium carbonate, lanthanum carbonate, etc.	In stages 2–4	Grade 2 in dogs Grade 4 in cats	In stage 2 or 3, maintains phosphorus at ≤4.5 mg/dl or ≤5 mg/dl, respectively In stage 4: ≤6 mg/dl
↓ Hypertension	Amlodipine, telmisartan at antihypertensive doses, ACEIs (in dogs), etc.	In stages 2–4 to keep systolic blood pressure <140 mmHg	Grade 2 in cats (amlodipine) Grade 4 in dogs	Reduces the risk in target organs: kidneys, heart, retina, and CNS
Omega-3 fatty acids	Fish oils rich in omega-3 fatty acids	In stages 2–4 Stage 1 with proteinuria	Grade 2 in dogs Grade 4 in cats	Slows the progression of CKD

Table 5. Scientific evidence for therapeutic measures applied in CKD (continued).				
Type of treatment	**Examples**	**Indicated IRIS stage**	**Evidence**	**Treatment benefits**
Control of anaemia	Avoiding haemorrhages and administering Epo	In stages 3 and 4	Grade 3 in cats and dogs	Maintains haematocrit levels: • Dogs: 38–48 % • Cats: 30–40 %
Management of gastrointestinal (GI) signs	Gastroprotectants and antiemetics	In stages 3 and 4	Grade 4 in cats and dogs	Improves GI signs to increase food intake
Improve food intake	Feeding tubes and administration of orexigenic agents (e.g. mirtazapine)	In stages 3 and 4 with deficient food intake	Grade 4 in cats and dogs	Maintains body condition
↑ Blood potassium	Potassium gluconate or chloride	In stages 3 and 4	Grade 4 in cats and dogs	Keeps potassium at levels >4 mEq/l to prevent myopathy and hypokalaemic nephropathy
Correction of acidosis	Diet, sodium bicarbonate, potassium citrate	In stages 1–4	Grade 4 in cats and dogs	Keeps blood bicarbonate levels between 18 and 24 mEq/l Minimises catabolism
Maintain hydration status	Long-term subcutaneous fluid therapy	In stages 3 and 4	Grade 4 in cats and dogs	Reduces azotaemia and progression of CKD

causes of CKD that we have the greatest capacity to address. If the potassium obtained from the diet is not enough to maintain a sufficiently high concentration in the blood, it should be provided as a supplement.

4. **Increased energy density:** cats and dogs affected by a process involving CKD have a strong tendency to lose weight. This is partly due to the clinical course of their illness, as nutrients are lost in urine (albumin, B group vitamins, potassium), but it is also true that patients often lose their appetite because of alterations (anorexia and uraemic gastritis) caused by metabolites. Furthermore, and above all in cats, many patients are not interested in eating, and especially not a

low-protein diet. To overcome these problems, commercial diets incorporate an extra energy source, usually a kind of fat, which increases the calorie intake and improves the palatability. Of the fats added to diets, omega-3 (ω-3) fatty acids are the latest to be included for their anti-inflammatory and potential antifibrotic action, as well as their effects on the circulatory system (vasodilator action). Recent studies appear to demonstrate the effect of these polyunsaturated fatty acids,[18–20] but it depends heavily on the source of origin. Cats, for instance, seem to only benefit from animal sources of omega-3.

Treatment of proteinuria

There are two main groups of drugs for reducing proteinuria, namely, angiotensin converting enzyme inhibitors (ACEIs), such as enalapril, benazepril, captopril, etc., and angiotensin II receptor antagonists (AIIRAs), such as telmisartan. So, if a dog or cat has a UPC >0.5 or >0.4, respectively, then treatment with an antiproteinuric agent is strongly recommended. However, in light of recent studies into the use of antiproteinurics, there may not be sufficient grounds to administer them if proteinuria cannot be detected. Despite this, they are very popular drugs in the treatment of CKD. ACEIs can be used to lower blood pressure in dogs; but not in cats, however, as their antihypertensive effect is normally too weak. Finally, their use can be justified in some animals with CKD who do not have hypertension or proteinuria, as patients receiving ACEIs usually eat better, and their owners tell us that their pet seems to have improved.[21–26]

ACEIs lower the GFR through vasodilation of the efferent glomerular arterioles. Accordingly, creatinine levels in blood often increase at the start of treatment. But the dose only needs to be reduced or the use of ACEIs reconsidered if it is a substantial increase. AIIRAs, on the other hand, cause vasodilation of both afferent and efferent glomerular arterioles, so they should not produce a significant increase in blood creatinine.

WHEN SHOULD A RENAL DIET BE PRESCRIBED?

This question often comes up among veterinary clinicians. In response, a renal diet should be started when any of the following conditions are met: the patient has proteinuria, hyperphosphataemia, or a blood creatinine >2 mg/dl. However, it is important to pay close attention to the patient. In many animals, it will work to their detriment if they are changed to a very-low-protein diet too quickly. These animals should eat a diet with a physiologically moderate amount of protein and receive close monitoring. There is a saying in the treatment of CKD that any vet would do well to remember: "patients live longer and better if they eat a renal diet, while those who eat whatever they like live longer than those who eat nothing at all."

Phosphate binders

There is a wide range of products that act as chelating agents for dietary phosphorus. From aluminium hydroxide to lanthanum carbonate, they all work in the same way more or less. They bind to phosphorus in the intestinal lumen, thus blocking its absorption and therefore improving its elimination in the faeces. Chelating agents should be considered in two situations during the course of CKD:

- Whenever blood phosphate cannot be reduced adequately despite the patient following a renal diet. The maximum effect of a low-phosphorus diet is observed 2 to 6 weeks after starting the new regimen. If after waiting 6 weeks the diet has not brought the blood phosphate concentration down to the low end of the range, then it is time to prescribe phosphate binders.
- In animals given a nonrenal diet and who, consequently, have a blood phosphate level that tends to increase. Although it is not the ideal treatment for either hyperphosphataemia or CKD, it is the only practicable strategy in some patients.

Monitor blood pressure

As we all know, hypertension can be either a cause or a consequence of CKD. As such, blood pressure should be monitored in all animals diagnosed with CKD (Box 4). The initial aim is to keep the systolic blood pressure (SBP) below 160 mmHg, but whenever possible we should try to maintain the patient's SBP at less than 140 mmHg. Treatment should be started if the SBP remains above 160 mmHg, even when there are no observable lesions to target organs (heart, kidneys, retina, or CNS) or when there is damage to these organs and the SBP is over 140 mmHg. The final goal is to keep the patient's SBP beneath 140 mmHg and free from any signs of hypotension. Treatment for hypertension should be initiated with ACEIs in dogs, while amlodipine or telmisartan can be used in cats. Always bear in mind that telmisartan produces an antiproteinuric effect at a dosage of 1 mg/kg/day, while this must be increased to at least 2 mg/kg/day to obtain an antihypertensive effect. Antihypertensive drugs can be combined to treat refractory cases, but caution must be exercised as side effects are more likely to develop.

Box 4. POINTS TO CONSIDER WHEN ASSESSING SBP IN PATIENTS WITH CKD.

SBP should be assessed in all patients suspected of having CKD.

And it should be monitored regularly in all patients diagnosed with CKD, especially if they are a suffering a uraemic crisis.

When measuring the SBP, also note down the cuff used, the animal's weight, the time, and the staff member making the measurement.

The result is more accurate if you measure the SBP a few times and work out the average. Some people omit the highest and lowest values. If the result is abnormal, it is worth waiting a few minutes for patients to acclimatise to their surroundings before measuring it again.

Patients with hypertension normally need lifelong treatment with antihypertensives which should only be suspended if the SBP is <110 mmHg, if there are signs of hypotension, or if blood creatinine does not stabilise and gradually increases after their prescription.

Treating anaemia

Nonregenerative anaemia is a very common finding in patients with CKD. As mentioned earlier, there are a lot of distinct reasons for this anaemia. Therefore, we cannot simply rely on a single therapeutic measure to function in all cases. The rest of this section goes through each measure one by one and indicates some treatment options.

Strive to control azotaemia

Azotaemia reduces the half-life of red blood cells in patients with CKD. The azotaemia is undoubtedly a consequence of the CKD, but this does not mean that the only option is to prescribe a renal diet. Patients that are successfully encouraged to increase their water intake will obtain maximum benefit from their remaining level of renal function. Thus, the administration of soft diets or dry foods moistened with warm water or water with flavourings, the addition of a fountain or establishing a timetable for drinking from the tap, or even training owners in subcutaneous fluid administration are all options worth considering.

> **TIP**
>
> Learning how to administer subcutaneous fluids can be a traumatic experience for owners and patients alike. You must be patient and spend as long as necessary explaining everything in detail. Subcutaneous catheters can be helpful in certain cases.

Strive to control uraemic gastritis

Uraemic gastritis is a cause for concern because:

- It is hard to quantify.
- It implies gastric discomfort which will affect the patient's appetite.
- It increases the likelihood of vomiting.
- If it causes bleeding, blood tests would return false results for urea and creatinine due to partial digestion of the blood products.

There are three main types of drugs used to treat uraemic gastritis:

- **Antiemetics.** Nowadays, maropitant, an NK1 receptor antagonist and, therefore, substance P blocker with a potent antiemetic effect, is available for use in both cats and dogs. While it has been shown that maropitant does not increase the life expectancy of renal patients, in our experience, however, a lot of owners consider the possibility of euthanasia if the vet is unable to control the animal's vomiting. Although maropitant is not indicated for long-term use, evidence from several studies shows it can be administered to renal patients with vomiting for as long as necessary without cause for concern.

- **Acid secretion inhibitors.** This group consists of two families of drugs:
  - Histamine H_2-receptor antagonists (ranitidine, famotidine), moderate potency.
  - Proton pump inhibitors (omeprazole, pantoprazole), high potency.

  The choice depends on the vet, patient, and client.
- **Mirtazapine.** In human medicine, this active substance is classified as a noradrenergic and specific serotonergic antidepressant. It is known to stimulate appetite in cats more effectively than other drugs that were used until quite recently. Mirtazapine can be given orally or, alternatively, transcutaneous forms are also available. It has a mild antiemetic effect, which is of some benefit in this sort of patient. Given its serotonergic action, it should not be used in combination with serotonergic drugs due to the risk of serious side effects. Furthermore, it is recommendable to start on low doses in renal patients, because they are more susceptible to serotonergic agents.

Administration of erythropoietin

An Epo deficiency is another cause of nonregenerative anaemia secondary to CKD. There are currently various types of recombinant human Epo available, some of which (epoetin alfa and darbepoetin) have proven useful in the treatment of anaemia related to CKD in small animals. Unfortunately, they can provoke an antibody-mediated response, resulting in the rapid degradation of exogenous Epo. This is why cats and dogs often stop responding to exogenous Epo after a period of treatment with human Epo, during which the patient's red blood cell levels improve substantially. The resulting anaemia is worse than before treatment, which suggests that the antibodies generated have cross-reactivity with the patient's endogenous Epo.

TIP

Before starting treatment with human Epo, make sure the patient has sufficient reserves of iron and B group vitamins (especially B_9 and B_{12}). In their absence, the patient will only show a partial or insufficient response to the Epo.

TAKE NOTE!

Antibody-mediated anaemia can last for 2 to 12 months after withdrawing treatment. Hypertension is a common complication in patients treated with Epo.

THE OWNER'S PERSPECTIVE

Owners of pets with kidney disease often **find it hard to understand CKD**. Most of them realise that yellow urine is a bad sign compared to colourless urine. Make sure owners appreciate that **more is not necessarily better**, especially if it means the patient is dehydrated.

Graphic presentations in PowerPoint or Keynote can help get your message across. Remember that **a picture paints a thousand words**.

Also provide a clear explanation of the **follow-up schedule**, the **tests** that should be completed at each checkup, why they are needed, and how much they will **cost**. Similarly, the vet should point out that certain treatments or tests may sometimes cost more or less for various reasons. Explaining these things in advance avoids mistrust later on.

Tools such as **reminders via mobile phone text messages or emails** help owners adhere to their pet's appointments and checkups schedule; they also demonstrate just how much your clinic cares about their pet.

There are a lot of therapeutic measures for CKD, some with more scientific backing than others. Always **avoid "renal kits"**, in which case owners take home the same product for their renal pet regardless of their stage of CKD, and instead use whatever is necessary for each stage. Owners best understand the need for ongoing, regular monitoring when the rationale is to adjust their pet's medication regimen.

KEY POINTS VETERINARY PRACTITIONERS SHOULD BEAR IN MIND

Kidney patients can have a very long life expectancy. The vet should try to **make an early diagnosis** and provide the **most appropriate treatment** at each stage of the patient's CKD.

Patients with early stages of CKD should undergo **biannual checkups**, those with moderate CKD **quarterly**, and severe cases should be seen **monthly**.

Owners of animals with CKD can spend 3 to 25 times more than before their pet fell ill; this can seem like an unreasonable level of expenditure for some clients. It is therefore a good idea to **increase the added value of your actions** and **dedicate a little more time to these owners**.

Note that **owners of pets with CKD are often willing to do a lot of work at home to help the vet with the animal's care and treatment**. Weekly water intake tables, a log of the litter tray's weight before and after use, or a record of skinfold measurements are some of the things a collaborative owner can carry out at home. When **owners are involved** in their pet's disease, they demonstrate **better adherence** to both treatments and appointment schedules.

9

Liver problems in geriatric patients

Small animals do not tend to present with as many liver diseases as they do kidney conditions. What is more, most incidents of liver disease are secondary to an underlying primary condition, such as an endocrine disorder (hyperadrenocorticism, diabetes, hyperthyroidism), nearby alterations that can have a direct influence on the liver (e.g. inflammatory bowel disease, feline triaditis), metastatic liver cancer, or due to exposure to certain medications used to treat other diseases (e.g. barbiturates, chemotherapy). The liver's low incidence of primary disease but apparent susceptibility to secondary problems associated with the rest of the body is probably why vets tend to underdiagnose liver conditions, often overlooking the sequelae left by the primary cause once this has been diagnosed and is being treated.

This chapter describes some of the most common liver diseases encountered in elderly cats and dogs, as well as explaining their diagnosis and treatment.

Inflammatory liver diseases

Chronic inflammatory liver disease in dogs

Chronic hepatitis in dogs may be due to a range of causes including infections, drugs, abnormal copper accumulation, or immune mediated. Of these causes, hepatitis associated with infections, such as infectious canine hepatitis, canine acidophil cell hepatitis, or hepatic leptospirosis, initially appears in an acute form that will develop into chronic hepatitis unless it is diagnosed and treated correctly. The different types of chronic hepatitis generally follow a very similar pathophysiology; the process begins with cell necrosis and is followed by hepatic infiltration of lymphocytes, plasma cells, or macrophages. The infiltrates cause inflammation and eventually liver fibrosis and cirrhosis.

Box 1 lists the breeds of dog with the greatest predisposition to copper-associated hepatitis.

Diagnosis

Chronic liver disease initially courses with a very nonspecific clinical picture and, due to its slow progression, normally goes unnoticed. Weight loss, depression, anorexia, and polyuria/polydipsia (PU/PD) are some of the clinical signs that can appear in the early stages; evidently, none of these are particularly suggestive of a liver problem, unless the owner has noticed that their pet is drinking more water than usual.

Lab tests also give different results depending on the stage of the liver disease. For example, there is an initial increase in the serum activity of alanine aminotransferase (ALT) and aspartate aminotransferase (AST). Normally there are no signs of marked cholestasis at this point, so alkaline phosphatase (ALP) activity will remain unchanged, and there is no evidence of liver dysfunction. As the disease progresses, however, cholestasis does usually develop, which results in an increase in ALP and total bilirubin (TB) serum levels. Liver function also begins to decline gradually but very progressively. This initially translates into elevated concentrations of bile acids (BA), which is later followed by a drop in the serum levels of albumin (Alb), urea, and glucose (Gluc). It should be noted that by this stage a lot of dogs also show altered concentrations of blood coagulation factors. This is an extremely important point as many diagnostic techniques are based on punctures or biopsies that can cause potentially dangerous bleeding if the vet is caught unprepared.

X-rays do not usually provide any relevant information, unless the patient is in a very advanced stage of liver disease, which sometimes leads to ascites or microhepatia. Perhaps the most useful and quickest of all the modern imaging techniques is a liver ultrasound. Nevertheless, ultrasound also has its limitations, above all when dealing with a patient in the early stages of chronic hepatitis. Ultrasound images may be completely normal at the onset of hepatitis, or you may observe some nonspecific changes in echogenicity. However, in late-stage liver diseases, such as cirrhosis, ultrasound can reveal microhepatia, irregular lobe margins, focal lesions (corresponding to regenerative nodules),

Box 1. BREEDS OF DOG WITH THE GREATEST PREDISPOSITION TO COPPER-ASSOCIATED HEPATITIS.

- Airedale Terrier
- Bedlington Terrier*
- Boxer
- Bull Terrier
- Bulldog
- Cocker Spaniel (American and English)
- Collie
- Dachshund
- Dalmatian
- Dobermann*
- German Shepherd Dog
- Golden Retriever
- Keeshond
- Kerry Blue Terrier
- Labrador Retriever
- Norwich Terrier
- Old English Sheepdog
- Pekingese
- Poodle (standard)
- Samoyed
- Schnauzer
- Skye Terrier*
- West Highland White Terrier*
- Wire Fox Terrier

* Breeds known to have a hereditary predisposition to copper-associated hepatitis.

increased parenchymal echogenicity (due to fibrosis), splenomegaly, and ascites.

Ultimately, the definitive diagnosis of any liver disease can only be made after performing a histopathological study. The tissue samples can be stained to highlight copper accumulations. Either way, the most reliable means of determining the copper concentration in the liver is with a sample collected specifically for this purpose.

Treatment

The initial treatment should focus on eliminating the root cause of the lesion. This requires an aetiological diagnosis, which, unfortunately, is not always feasible. However, it can make a dramatic difference to the prognosis for the disease if the aetiological cause can be discovered. For instance, a patient with hepatitis who is being treated with phenobarbital or primidone as an anticonvulsant can be changed to gabapentin, potassium bromide, or imepitoin. If clinical signs compatible with leptospirosis are observed, antibiotic therapy with aminopenicillins may cure it; and if the patient has a very elevated hepatic copper level, D-penicillamine should be added to the regimen as a copper-chelating agent.

As mentioned earlier, given the difficulty of finding the primary aetiological agent, the therapeutic approach often revolves around a "generic" treatment. Table 1 shows the dosages and main indications of each agent administered generically to diminish or slow the advance of chronic hepatitis.

Purely symptomatic treatment should be applied if ascites or oedema develop. The pathophysiology of these fluid accumulations basically stems from two separate but interconnected mechanisms:

1. **Hypoalbuminaemia:** as the serum albumin concentration falls, so too does the oncotic pressure, which translates into a reduced

Table 1. Helpful drugs in the treatment of chronic inflammatory liver disease in dogs.

Drug	Dosage (oral)	Indications
D-penicillamine	10–15 mg/kg every 12 h	Copper-chelating agent and antifibrotic
Trientine	15–30 mg/kg every 12 h	Copper-chelating agent
Zinc (acetate)	1.5–4 mg/kg (elemental zinc) every 24 h	Reduces copper absorption
Prednisone	0.5–2.0 mg/kg every 24–48 h	Immunosuppressant, anti-inflammatory, and antifibrotic
Azathioprine	1.0 mg/kg every 24–48 h	Immunosuppressant
S-Adenosyl-L-methionine (SAMe)	18 mg/kg every 12–24 h	Increases glutathione levels (antioxidant)
Ursodeoxycholic acid	10–15 mg/kg every 24 h	Choleretic, cytoprotective, and immunomodulator
Vitamin E	10 IU/kg every 24 h	Antioxidant
Silymarin	4–8 mg/kg every 24 h	Antioxidant

capacity to maintain plasma water inside blood vessels.

2. **Changes in vascular hydrostatic pressure:** the liver experiences increased resistance to blood flow (i.e. portal hypertension), which can also lead to acquired portosystemic shunts, greater lymph formation, and an increase in the plasma volume.

Intravenous colloids can be given to reestablish the osmotic gradient in animals with hypoalbuminaemia and ascites, for example, dextrans and hydroxyethyl starch at a dose of 10–20 ml/kg over 1 or 2 hours. This dose can be repeated as required. Potassium-sparing diuretics (spironolactone: 2 mg/kg every 24 hours) and low-sodium diets can help in the treatment of both ascites and oedema.[1,2] If spironolactone proves ineffective, a second option is furosemide (2 mg/kg every 8–12 hours), but potassium levels must be monitored closely as these patients tend to develop hypokalaemia. Canine albumin is ideally suited for these cases; however, it is a fairly expensive therapy due to the large amounts required. Human albumin can be used as a temporary solution, but it comes with the risk of anaphylactic reactions (especially after repeated use), so it is rarely administered in daily practice.

Inflammatory liver diseases in geriatric cats

The inflammatory liver diseases usually encountered in elderly cats are known as **feline cholangitis syndrome** (FCS) or **cholangitis/cholangiohepatitis syndrome** (CCHS).[7] FCS can occur in neutrophilic, lymphocytic, and lymphoplasmacytic forms, with neutrophilic FCS being the most typical form in geriatric cats. These forms have acute and chronic presentations.[8] Neutrophilic

KEY POINTS REGARDING COPPER-ASSOCIATED HEPATITIS

Besides Bedlington Terriers, various other breeds are also predisposed to canine copper-associated hepatitis (Box 1).[3-5]

The disease progresses slowly and dogs usually die because of liver cirrhosis. Affected dogs normally have 3 to 5 times more copper in their liver than healthy dogs. The highest concentrations of hepatic copper are found in Bedlington Terriers. The condition is diagnosed through a biopsy in which copper granules will be found in larger quantities than to be expected given the degree of cholestasis or fibrosis.[3]

The treatment of copper-associated hepatitis includes reducing the amount of copper absorbed from the diet (with a low-copper diet and zinc supplement) and chelating the copper that has already accumulated in the liver. D-Penicillamine and trientine are used as copper-chelating agents. The latter is slightly quicker than the former and can be used if D-penicillamine causes vomiting. In the breeds mentioned above, even though copper-associated hepatitis is not suspected initially, some patients benefit from the addition of a copper-chelating agent or oral zinc to their treatment plan.[6]

An early diagnosis can be made in Bedlington Terriers by studying a DNA sample.

FCS is characterised by an inflammatory infiltrate consisting of predominantly neutrophils, whereas in the lymphocytic and lymphoplasmacytic forms the liver is infiltrated by mononuclear cells. In both cases, the nomenclature describes the main type of infiltrating cell, but there are also cases of mixed inflammatory reactions. Neutrophilic, lymphocytic, and lymphoplasmacytic FCS are the three most readily identifiable forms, each with their own clinical presentation and therefore requiring a distinct treatment.

Diagnosis

In cats, neutrophilic FCS tends to affect males and the typical signs at onset are vomiting and acute diarrhoea. The initial clinical presentation courses with jaundice, lethargy, fever, and dehydration. A lot of cats with the neutrophilic form experience moderate increases in ALT, AST, ALP, and GGT (γ-glutamyltransferase) activity.

A leukocyte count will normally reveal leukocytosis with a left shift. Less than 50 % of these cats have hepatomegaly. The bacteria most readily isolated in such cases are: *Escherichia coli*, *Staphylococcus*, α-haemolytic *Streptococcus*, *Bacillus*, *Actinomyces*, *Bacteroides*, *Enterococcus*, *Enterobacter*, and *Clostridium*.[9–11] Table 2 summarises the clinical data for cats with neutrophilic FCS and hepatic lipidosis.

Table 2. Clinical data for cats with acute and chronic neutrophilic FCS and hepatic lipidosis.

Parameter	Acute neutrophilic FCS	Chronic neutrophilic FCS	Hepatic lipidosis
Mean age (years)	5.7	9.7	6.2
Males:females ratio	86:17	56:44	55:45
Anorexia (%)	81	78	100
Weight loss (%)	56	33	84
Lethargy (%)	75	78	80
Vomiting (%)	43	67	70
Diarrhoea (%)	0	11	10
Fever (%)	71	11	6
Poikilocytosis (%)	28	44	85
Neutrophilia (%)	80	54	15
Left shift (%)	40	23	2
Elevated ALT (%)	71	78	95
Elevated ALP (%)	14	56	95
Elevated bilirubin (%)	57	78	85

Adapted from Weiss DJ, Armstrong PJ, Gagne J. Inflammatory liver disease. *Semin Vet Med Surg (Small Anim)*, 1997, 12(1):22–7.
Note: neutrophilic FCS is classed as chronic when it has been coursing for several weeks and cytology reveals predominantly neutrophilic but also mononuclear infiltrate.

Again, liver ultrasound is the most useful diagnostic imaging technique and may reveal marked cholangitis with thickening of the extrahepatic biliary tract and inflammation of the intrahepatic bile duct lumen. Other consequences are extrahepatic bile duct obstruction (observed as an increase in the size of the gallbladder, a dilated, tortuous common bile duct, and patent intrahepatic bile ducts), cholecystitis (laminar thickening of the gallbladder wall with adjacent fluid accumulation), and pancreatitis (patent, highly visible pancreas with hyperechoic peripancreatic fat). Cytology samples obtained via fine-needle puncture or biopsy reveal inflammation due to mainly neutrophilic infiltrates.

With the lymphocytic form of FCS most cats are ill for quite some time before diagnosis.[7] The clinical signs are much more subtle and can go unnoticed by the owner or they may report their cat suffered an episode of vomiting, diarrhoea, and anorexia a few weeks earlier. Many cats have hepatomegaly, jaundice, and perhaps even ascites. Lymphocytic FCS is often accompanied by inflammatory bowel disease, low-grade lymphocytic pancreatitis, and cholecystitis.

With respect to blood chemistry, cats with lymphoplasmacytic FCS tend to exhibit higher increases in ALT, AST, ALP, and GGT than cats with lymphocytic FCS. They may also develop severe lymphocytosis (>14,000 lymphocytes/l) with no other evidence of a lymphoproliferative disorder.

A multifocal hyperechoic pattern may be observed in ultrasound images due to peribiliary inflammation and fibrosis. However, in some cats the liver may appear totally normal under ultrasound. The cytological study of fine-needle puncture samples may not provide conclusive evidence of inflammation, or the degree observed may not correspond with the patient's actual level of inflammation. Therefore, in such cases a liver biopsy is more preferable than fine-needle puncture. Liver biopsy is more reliable, as it can demonstrate the presence of whole acinar units and portal triads.[7]

If the fine-needle puncture sample contains microorganisms, a Gram stain (Box 2) can help indicate the appropriate antibiotic, although samples should be sent for culture and sensitivity testing.

TAKE NOTE!

The occlusion should be treated in cats with extrahepatic bile duct obstruction. The retention of bile causes severe pain, and once the bile is drained, patients show an almost immediate clinical improvement.

Biliary drainage can be carried out during ultrasound (ultrasound-guided cholecystocentesis, Box 3) or by inserting a semipermanent drain. Other surgical options are not usually used to treat these conditions because of the high rate of associated mortality[12,13] and lengthy operating times they imply (>2.5 hours).

Treatment

Table 3 gives an overview of the most suitable drugs for routine use in feline inflammatory liver disease.

TIP

Before starting treatment for the liver disease as such, the vet must ensure that support therapy is in place.

Box 2. GRAM STAIN TESTING PROCEDURE.

Step 1: stain with methylrosaniline chloride (gentian violet).

Step 2: fix with an iodine solution. This stabilises the methylrosaniline chloride. All the bacteria in the solution remain purple or blue.

Step 3: extract with alcohol or another solvent. This discolours the gram-negative bacteria but not the gram-positive ones.

Step 4: stain with safranin. The gram-positive bacteria are already stained with methylrosaniline chloride and remain purple. The gram-negative bacteria will turn pink.

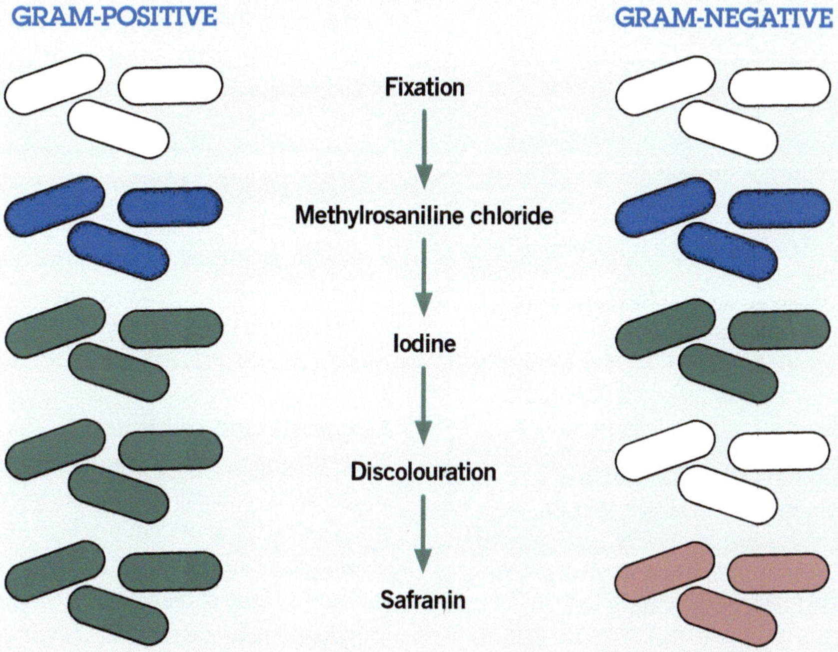

Box 3. ULTRASOUND-GUIDED CHOLECYSTOCENTESIS IN CATS.[14]

1 After fasting for 12 to 16 hours, patients are deeply sedated or lightly anaesthetised. Current recommendations are for combinations of alfaxalone (3–10 mg/kg IM, or 0.5–5 mg/kg slow IV) and methadone (0.1–0.5 mg/kg IM). If alfaxalone or methadone are unobtainable, they can be replaced with ketamine (2–5 mg/kg IV), butorphanol (0.1 mg/kg IV, or 0.2–0.4 mg/kg IM), or propofol (1–4 mg/kg IV).

2 Use a high-resolution ultrasound probe (7–13 MHz) to examine the liver and biliary tract.

3 Apply an aseptic skin preparation technique.

4 The gallbladder should be punctured with a 22-gauge needle that is at least 3.8 cm long and connected to 12 ml syringe.

5 The gallbladder should be approached through the right medial hepatic lobe, or from a right ventral location through the region of the falciform ligament.

6 Void the gallbladder completely. Make a note of the physical characteristics of the bile and always send a sample for microbiological study.

Be careful to avoid drugs that are known to cause hepatotoxicity or which are metabolised by the liver. The intake of the correct amount of calories and protein is of vital importance when treating inflammatory liver diseases. So whenever a cat goes more than 72 hours without eating, a feeding tube should be inserted without delay.

All cats suspected of having FCS should be assessed for extrahepatic biliary obstruction. If obstruction is detected, do not administer any choleretic agents (ursodeoxycholic acid). Besides ultrasound, which is irreplaceable in these cases, cats with complete biliary obstruction also lack any urobilinogen in the urinalysis. Furthermore, the presence of concurrent pancreatitis, inflammatory bowel disease, or lipidosis should also be ruled out in this group of patients.

TAKE NOTE!

Never give corticosteroids to patients with FCS and concurrent lipidosis or hepatic encephalopathy.

Prognosis and evolution

If the diagnosis was accurate and treatment administered according to the suggested guidelines, cats with acute neutrophilic FCS should show signs of improvement within 24–48 hours. In chronic cases of neutrophilic, lymphocytic, or lymphoplasmacytic forms of FCS, it may be days or weeks before any improvement emerges.

The lab results (neutrophil count, hepatic enzyme activity, serum bilirubin level) normally indicate improvement within a few days of starting treatment. Again, patients with acute cases improve more quickly than those with chronic FCS. Hepatic enzymes may require several months to return to normal values in all types of FCS.

Table 3. Recommended treatment for FCS arranged according to therapeutic priority.	
Treatment for neutrophilic FCS	**Treatment for lymphocytic/lymphoplasmacytic FCS**
Fluid therapy, as required	Fluid therapy, as required
Antibiotic therapy: ampicillin (20 mg/kg IV every 6–8 h), amoxicillin–clavulanic acid (22 mg/kg IV or PO), or marbofloxacin (2 mg/kg PO every 12–24 h)	Prednisolone (2–4 mg/kg every 24 h) or methylprednisolone
Potassium gluconate: 2–3 mEq/kg PO every 24 h; measure potassium levels weekly to avoid hyperkalaemia	Potassium gluconate: 2–3 mEq/kg PO every 24 h; measure potassium levels weekly to avoid hyperkalaemia
Vitamin E (100–200 IU/day) and/or SAMe (18 mg/kg every 24 h)	Vitamin E (100–200 IU/day) and/or SAMe (18 mg/kg every 24 h)
L-Carnitine (250 mg every 24 h), water-soluble vitamins (double maintenance levels), and vitamin K (0.5–1.5 mg/kg SC every 12 h for the first 3 doses, then weekly)	L-Carnitine (250 mg every 24 h), water-soluble vitamins (double maintenance levels), and vitamin K (0.5–1.5 mg/kg SC every 12 h for the first 3 doses, then weekly).
Palatable diet and, in some cases, pancreatic enzymes	Palatable diet and, in some cases, pancreatic enzymes
Lactulose for patients with mental compromise	Antibiotic therapy: ampicillin (20 mg/kg IV every 6–8 h), amoxicillin–clavulanic acid (22 mg/kg IV or PO), or marbofloxacin (2 mg/kg PO every 12–24 h)
Prednisolone (2–4 mg/kg every 24 h) or methylprednisolone	Lactulose for patients with mental compromise
Chlorambucil: 2 mg/animal PO every 72 h in cats <3 kg and every 48 h in cats >3 kg	Chlorambucil: 2 mg/m^2 PO every 24–48 h

Treatments vary between references. As such, in the case of neutrophilic FCS, corticosteroid treatment should be initiated if there is no clinical improvement after 3–4 days of aggressive antibiotic therapy. Similarly, if there is no significant improvement in patients with lymphocytic FCS after 4–5 days of corticosteroids, add ampicillin/amoxicillin (with/without sulbactam or clavulanic acid) to the regimen.[9,15]

Whatever the case may be, cats which eat, drink, and can maintain their body condition have a better prognosis than animals which do not. Patients that manage to reestablish normal levels in lab tests also have a better prognosis. Lastly, cats afflicted with acute neutrophilic FCS are more likely to survive than patients with chronic forms of FCS. On the other hand, patients that do not improve despite the medication have a poor prognosis. Nevertheless, they may live from months to years with the correct medication and veterinary monitoring. Progressive anorexia and multidrug-resistant bacteria in cultures are signs of a bad prognosis.

Infiltrative liver diseases

Liver disease is sometimes due to structural and functional changes that develop when hepatocytes are infiltrated by lipids, glycogen, amyloids, or other substances. Although hepatic lipidosis is a clinical entity that vets almost exclusively encounter in cats, it is actually a common histopathological finding in dogs with diabetes and can in itself develop into a significant clinical problem by causing liver dysfunction. Other less common infiltrative diseases are provoked by amyloid deposition in both dogs[16] and cats[17,18] and haemochromatosis.[19,20]

The excess of either exogenous or endogenous glucocorticoids can often lead to steroid hepatopathy in elderly cats and dogs alike, although it is perhaps more common in the latter.[21,22] Both species can develop severe liver dysfunction; dogs, however, seem to manifest less marked clinical signs. Lab test results in these dogs tend to reveal a sharp increase in ALP and GGT activity, sometimes reaching up to 60 times above the upper limit of the normal range.[23] Both cats and dogs usually have elevated levels of hepatocellular enzymes (ALT and AST), but not as high as those mentioned for ALP and GGT.

In some cases of iatrogenic hyperadrenocorticism in cats brought to our clinics, the patients had glycogen infiltrates in the liver, and they were all given slow-release glucocorticoids.

TAKE NOTE!

As cats do not possess the ALP isoenzyme induced by corticosteroids, it is not expected to increase in patients with hyperadrenocorticism. However, if hyperadrenocorticism is suspected, GGT levels should always be tested.

Dogs with hepatic glycogen infiltration generally have a normal total bilirubin concentration in serum, which suggests that the high ALP levels are induced by steroids and cholestasis.

Liver function tests may evidence slight increases in preprandial and postprandial bile acid concentrations.

The most typical and widely known type of infiltrative liver disease is **secondary hepatic lipidosis**. The most important feature of this clinical entity is the progressive infiltration of hepatocytes with fat, resulting in liver dysfunction (Figs. 1 and 2). Although it sometimes develops as a primary disease, it usually manifests as idiopathic hepatic lipidosis or hepatic lipidosis secondary to another underlying condition. In either case, it is always assumed that there is a primary cause, regardless of whether or not it can be identified. The classic clinical history is that of a somewhat overweight/obese cat that has stopped eating for a while (at least 3 days) and presents signs of muscle mass and weight loss, jaundice, and episodes of vomiting.[24] The onset of jaundice is a phenomenon indicative of a relatively advanced case (Figs. 3 and 4).

The blood chemistry basically shows evidence of cholestasis. There may be a relatively moderate, nonspecific increase in liver enzyme activities. ALP and GGT activities experience the largest variations compared to other diseases.

TAKE NOTE!

Patients with hepatic lipidosis tend to have a very high ALP activity, while GGT remains normal or only slightly elevated.

In liver ultrasound images it appears as a discrete and diffuse increase in echogenicity.[25] Unlike other liver diseases, the cytological study of a fine-needle biopsy sample tends to give a definitive diagnosis upon observing hepatocytes with marked vacuolar changes.[26]

The treatment comprises a two-pronged approach with the first aim being to remedy the primary cause and the second to restore any loss of nutritional status.

Feeding tubes are particularly helpful when treating hepatic lipidosis, as confirmed by higher recovery rates (see the box on the next page).

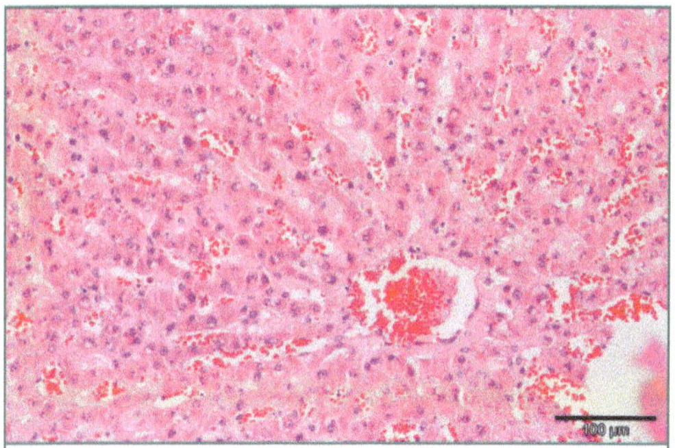

Figure 1. Histology image of a liver with congestion and diffuse fatty degeneration throughout the entire lobe (H&E, 20×). Image courtesy of Anapath laboratory, Granada (Spain).

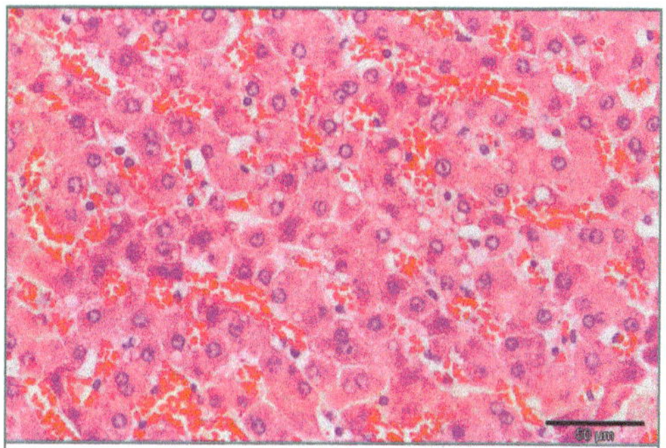

Figure 2. The drop-shaped vacuoles, unstained by haematoxylin and eosin, are clearly evident in the hepatocyte cytoplasm (40×). Image courtesy of Anapath laboratory, Granada (Spain).

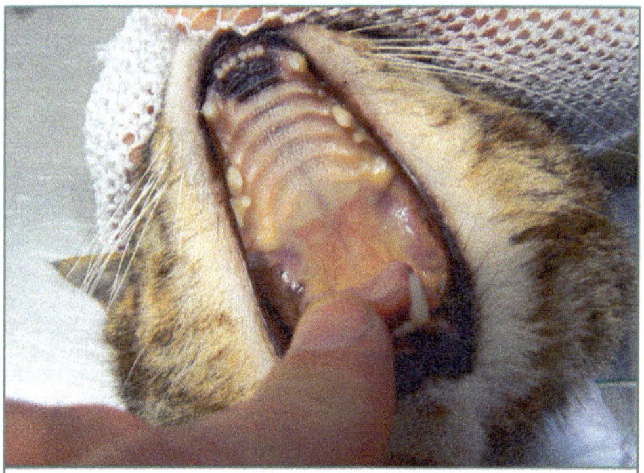

Figure 3. Ten-year-old female cat with jaundice due to hepatic lipidosis following the arrival of a new kitten in the home. Jaundice is sometimes more easily noted in the mucosa of the palate.

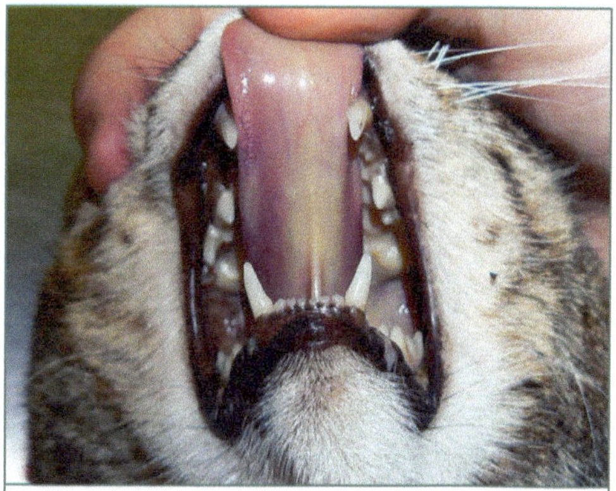

Figure 4. If the patient has a pigmented palate, the mucosa under the tongue is always another option.

STEP-BY-STEP INSERTION OF AN OESOPHAGOSTOMY TUBE

1. After anaesthetising the patient, tracheal intubation, and aseptic preparation of the area, measure the distance between the stoma placement site and base of the heart. The ipsilateral elbow can be retracted caudally to serve as a reference. Insert some mosquito or curved Kocher forceps into the oesophagus from the mouth, passing through the pharynx. When the forceps are in the desired location, press the tip forwards so the skin protrudes (1).

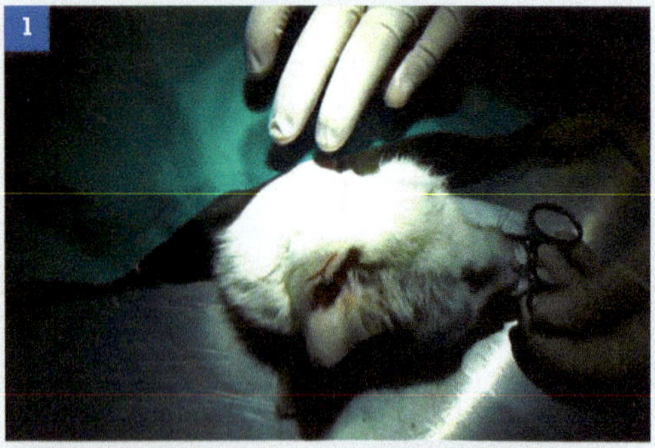

2. Use a scalpel to cut the skin and underlying layers until the forceps emerge from the stoma (2).

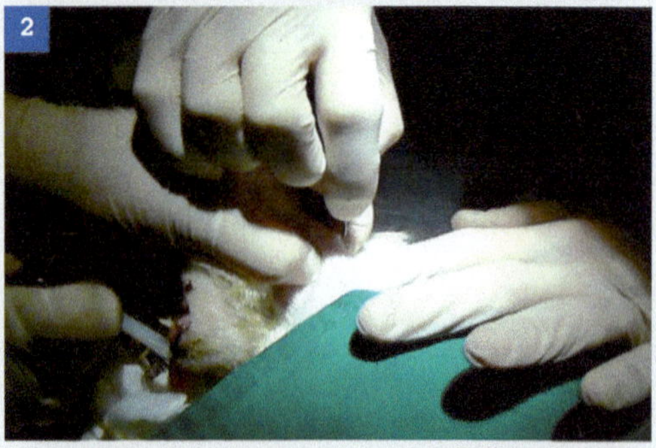

3. Open the forceps and grasp the end of the feeding tube (3).

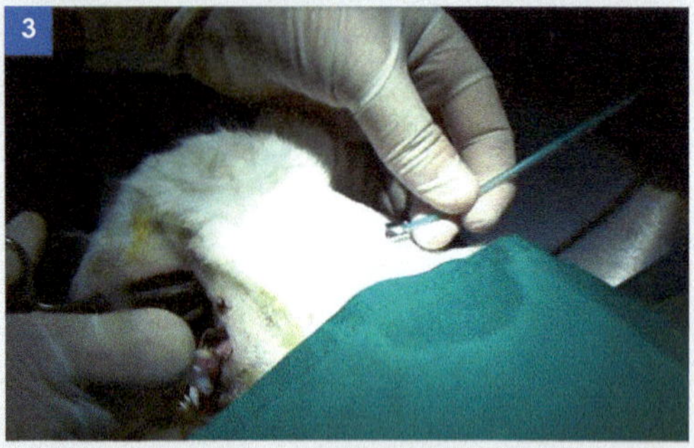

4. Withdraw the tube via the mouth and open the forceps (4).

5. Now feed the end that has just been withdrawn into the patient's oesophagus. If they are well intubated, there is no danger of entering the trachea (5).

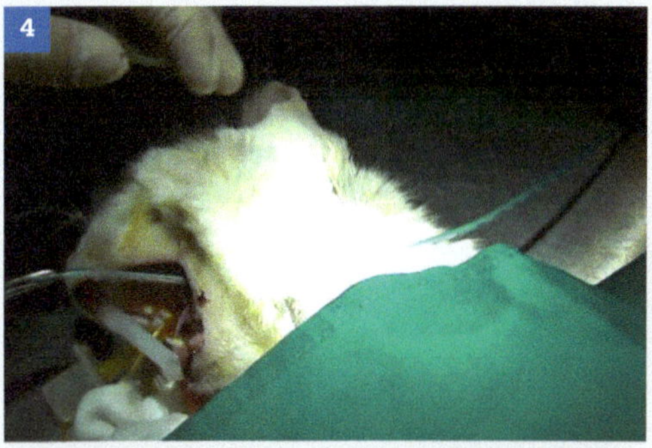

4

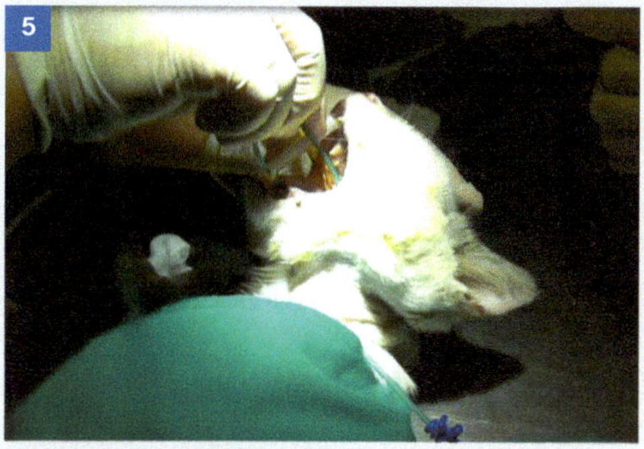

5

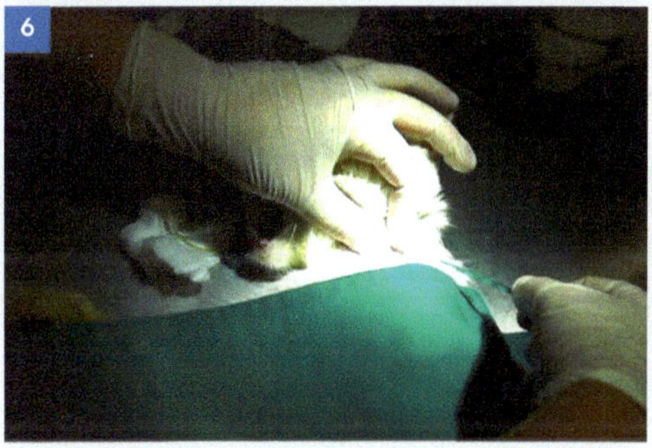

6

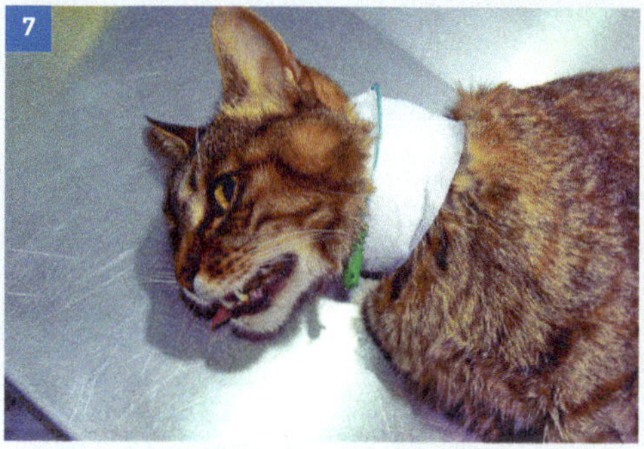

7

6. Once the entire tube has been inserted in the oesophagus, tug gently on the free end to eliminate the loop that is usually situated in the laryngopharynx (6).

7. Push or pull the free end of the tube until it is at the desired height in the oesophagus. It should not reach the stomach. Now the tube just needs fixing in position with a Roman sandal suture. Apply an antiseptic ointment or cream and bandage. A good bandage does away with the need for an Elizabethan collar (7).

Cats normally stay at the clinic for the first few days after inserting a feeding tube, as the staff should ensure that the patient tolerates the tube and type of food without any problems. The cat should receive 25 % of its nutritional needs by tube on day 1, increasing to 50 % on day 2, 75 % on day 3, and 100 % from day 4 onwards.

A specific feeding schedule should be designed for each cat. If the owner cannot follow the recommendations for any reason, they should inform the vet immediately. Box 4 lists some guidelines that should be explained to owners of cats fitted with a feeding tube.

Canine hepatic fibrosis and cirrhosis

The liver may respond to severe damage and necrosis by regenerating, mineralising, or fibrosing itself. It all depends on the severity of the lesion and level of structural damage to the supporting connective tissue. Any pathological process that causes a loss of hepatocytes and decline in the integrity of the supporting tissues can culminate in **hepatic fibrosis**. When the hepatic fibrosis is severe and includes the formation of regenerative nodules surrounded by

Box 4. GUIDELINES FOR OWNERS OF CATS WITH AN OESOPHAGEAL OR NASOESOPHAGEAL FEEDING TUBE.

1 Before feeding the animal using the tube, first make sure it is permeable by introducing a few millilitres of water.

2 If the water passes down the tube without difficulty or causing the cat discomfort or inducing a cough, the owner can start feeding. It helps if the cat is sat down or standing, as they will find it easier to swallow.

3 Periodically, after a certain volume, patients tend to make a small swallowing gesture; this is normal and even desirable, as it implies the cat is passing the food down into their stomach.

4 Feeding should take about 10 to 15 minutes – there is no rush whatsoever. The quicker the food is given, the greater the chance of regurgitation and vomiting.

5 If any medications need administering with the feed, they should be given after the first dose of food.

6 If all goes well, with no nausea or strange meowing, owners should finish giving the full ration prescribed by the vet.

7 After the feed and before closing the tube, it should be cleaned by flushing with 5 ml of water.

8 Finally, close the tube securely and place it out of the cat's reach so it cannot bite or pull on it.

fibrotic tissue it is defined as **cirrhosis**. Cirrhosis corresponds to the final stage of liver disease. Accordingly, many dogs with cirrhosis have clinical and laboratory signs of severe liver dysfunction. Over time, the cirrhosis progresses, and patients develop portal hypertension; therefore, many dogs with cirrhosis also have ascites and acquired portosystemic shunts.[1,2] Nearly all liver diseases evolve relatively slowly, and fibrosis develops as the necrosis and inflammation continue to progress.

Diagnosis

Abdominal X-rays should highlight microhepatia, while ultrasound images present a significant increase in echogenicity. Experienced ultrasound technicians can sometimes detect the presence of acquired portosystemic shunts. As is almost always the case, a definitive diagnosis can only be made following a liver biopsy and histopathology.[27]

Treatment

The vet can choose from a lot of medications in their attempt to slow the advance of liver fibrosis and cirrhosis. However, no drugs have demonstrated any efficacy in completely halting this progression.

TIP

It is best to avoid reaching such a situation by treating any liver diseases aggressively upon diagnosis and establishing long-term monitoring of patients who have had them in the past.

Treatment should focus on three aspects:

1. Treating the underlying cause of the liver disease, if any (e.g. by chelating copper).
2. Treating collagen deposition (e.g. with antifibrotic agents, see Table 4).
3. Treating the consequences of the fibrosis and cirrhosis (e.g. through diet and management of any portal hypertension, hepatic encephalopathy, and hypokalaemia).

Hepatocutaneous syndrome

While this condition is also known as superficial necrolytic dermatitis or metabolic dermatosis, the most commonly used term is hepatocutaneous syndrome. It is an uncommon clinical entity in dogs and rarely encountered in cats.[29]

Hepatocutaneous syndrome has been associated with various **hepatopathies**[30] and more recently with **glucagon-secreting tumours**.[31] The liver disease most frequently diagnosed in these cases is **idiopathic hepatocellular collapse**. Nevertheless, it is not the only cause of hepatocutaneous syndrome as the ingestion of mycotoxins that cause liver damage, drug-induced liver disease (barbiturates and primidone), and cirrhosis have all been linked to the onset of the condition.

With respect to the pathological secretion of glucagon, hepatocutaneous syndrome has been related to pancreatic adenocarcinomas,[32] gastric carcinomas, hyperglucagonaemia,[33] and glucagon-secreting hepatic metastases. Dogs with hyperglucagonaemia usually develop diabetes, and while the diabetes is believed to be the cause of hepatocutaneous syndrome, there is no concrete evidence to support this and in fact very few dogs have patent diabetes at the time of diagnosis.

The syndrome tends to affect mature or elderly dogs, with a mean age at diagnosis of 10 years. Apparently, males are more predisposed to this type of clinical entity.

Table 4. Drugs used to treat hepatic fibrosis/cirrhosis in dogs.

Drug	Dosage	Properties	Precautions
Colchicine	0.025–0.03 mg/kg PO every 24 h	Reduces collagen formation	Do not start using at the same time as azathioprine or chlorambucil. Similar side effects.[28]
D-penicillamine	10–15 mg/kg PO every 12 h	Antifibrotic action by inhibiting collagen cross-linking, which makes it more degradable	Start at low doses given 30 minutes before eating, that is, on an empty stomach.
Prednisolone	0.5–1 mg/kg PO every 24 h	Anti-inflammatory and antifibrotic	Do not administer to animals with ascites or hepatic encephalopathy.
Azathioprine	2.2 mg/kg PO every 24 h	Anti-inflammatory and antifibrotic	Use lower doses if combined with corticosteroids. After 2 weeks' treatment, reduce the frequency to every 48 h.
Zinc (elemental)	15 mg/kg PO every 24 h	Antifibrotic, hepatoprotector, and copper-chelating agent	Best given on an empty stomach an hour before eating. Some vets recommend administering it with a little tuna oil if there are signs of nausea. Target serum zinc level: 2–5 µg/ml.

All other treatments to resolve the primary cause and improve liver and biliary function should be kept in place.

Diagnosis

Skin lesions may appear weeks or months before the animal is brought for consultation. This is usually because they can be intermittent, and owners consider them insignificant.

The lesions first tend to develop on the paws and include interdigital erythematous lesions, scabs, erosions, hyperkeratosis, and fissures in the paw pads (Fig. 5). Some patients lose their claws, and the skin lesions can become pruritic and painful. These may be followed by lesions around the mouth, chin, eyes, heels, and elbows (at the pressure points), vulva, and scrotum (Fig. 5). These lesions generally consist of symmetrical erythema, alopecia, scabs, erosions, and/or ulcers. Some patients may have vesicular lesions. These blisters predominantly contain necrotic epidermal tissue and are not usually full of purulent material. The skin lesions are highly susceptible to secondary infections by *Staphylococcus* spp., *Malassezia* spp., *Candida* spp., and dermatophytes. Adequate control and treatment of the underlying cause is enough for these infections to resolve spontaneously without any specific treatment.

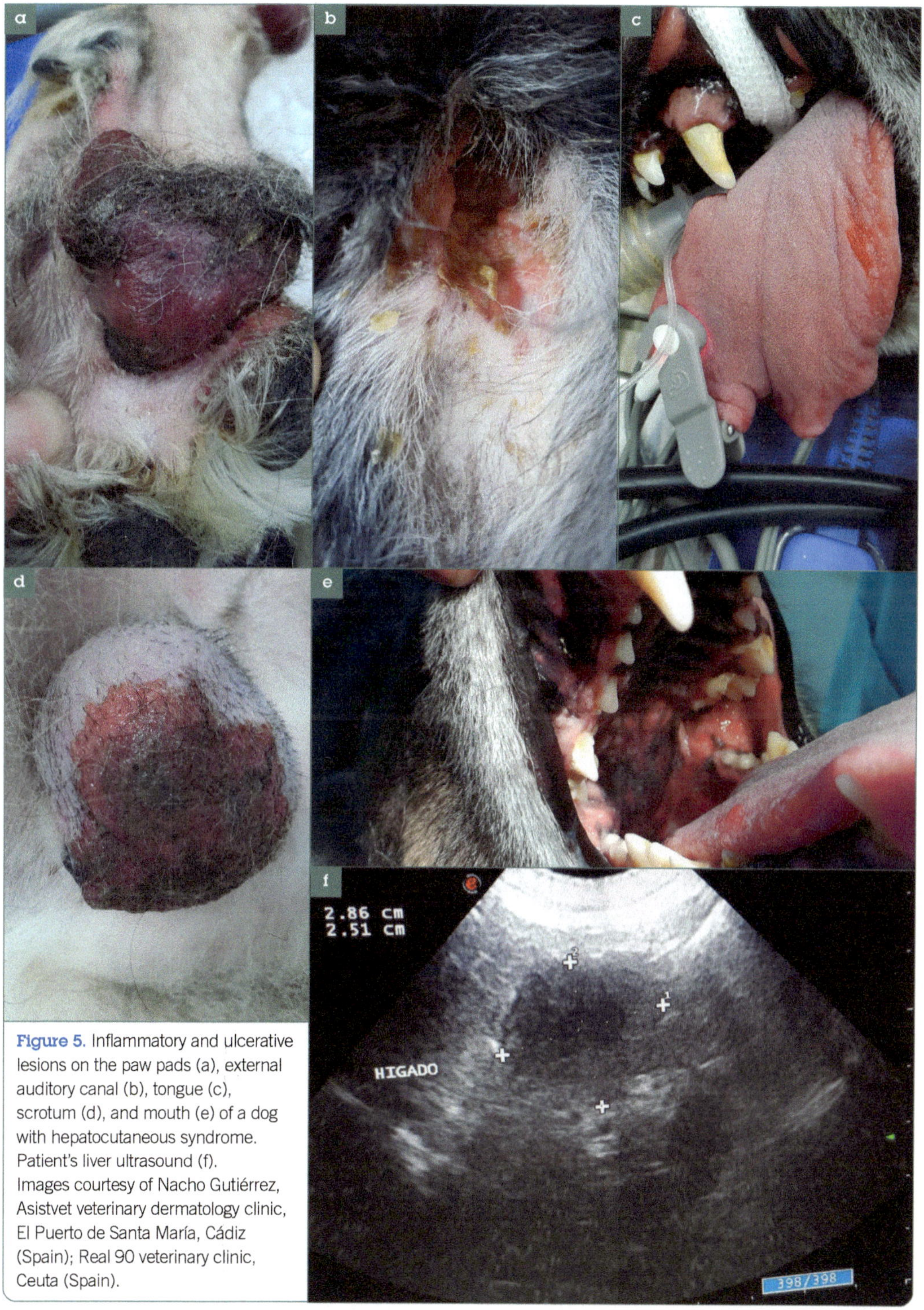

Figure 5. Inflammatory and ulcerative lesions on the paw pads (a), external auditory canal (b), tongue (c), scrotum (d), and mouth (e) of a dog with hepatocutaneous syndrome. Patient's liver ultrasound (f).
Images courtesy of Nacho Gutiérrez, Asistvet veterinary dermatology clinic, El Puerto de Santa María, Cádiz (Spain); Real 90 veterinary clinic, Ceuta (Spain).

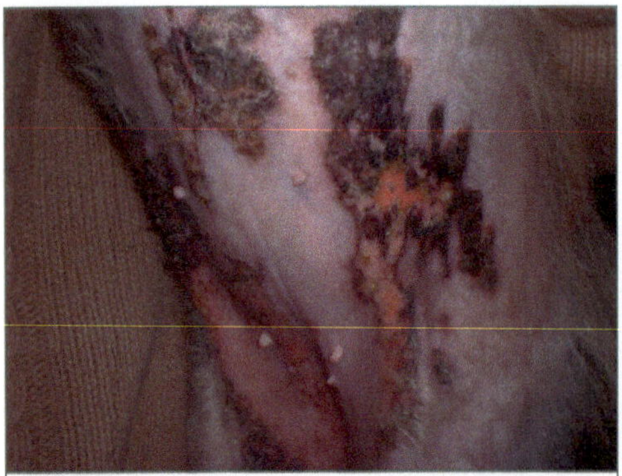

Figure 6. Skin lesions on the abdomen of a dog with hepatocutaneous syndrome.
Image courtesy of Gustavo Machicote, Fauna veterinary clinic, Pontevedra (Spain).

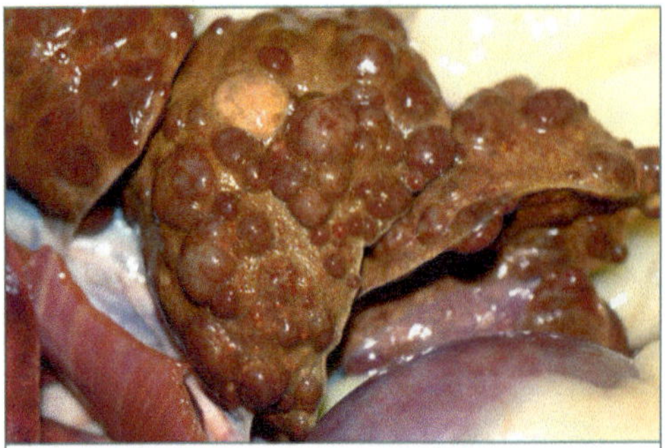

Figure 7. Photo taken during the necropsy, of the liver of a dog with hepatocutaneous syndrome.
Image courtesy of Gustavo Machicote, Dermapet, Santiago de Compostela (Spain).

These dermatological lesions possess a characteristic histopathology known as diffuse parakeratosis. This means there is marked vacuolar degeneration of the most superficial layers of the stratum spinosum (due to intra- and extracellular oedema throughout these layers of the epidermis). The oedematous extracellular spaces fill with neutrophils, necrotic epithelial cells, and detritus, creating an "eosinophilic layer". There is significant epidermal hyperplasia and slight perivascular neutrophilic infiltration of the superficial dermis.

Obviously, besides the aforementioned clinical signs of dermatitis, a lot of dogs also show signs of an underlying condition. As such, if the hepatocutaneous syndrome is the result of a hepatic problem, the patient will suffer weight loss, PU/PD, jaundice, and/or anorexia. They also tend to have mild to moderate, nonregenerative or slightly regenerative anaemia. Blood chemistry indicates an increase in serum liver enzyme activity in 95 % of cases (elevated ALT and ALP). Hypoproteinaemia and hyperglycaemia are often observed in fasting blood samples, although only a small percentage of dogs are diabetic at the time of diagnosis. In fact, if a dog with hepatocutaneous syndrome develops diabetes, it is usually because the syndrome is in an advanced stage. Around 30–40 % of dogs with hepatocutaneous syndrome have hyperglucagonaemia, and hypoaminoacidaemia is observed in 85–90 %. Altered bile acids are observed in most cases.

Liver ultrasound is generally characteristic of the condition and with solitary or multiple lesions.

HOW TO PERFORM A GOOD SKIN OR MUCOCUTANEOUS BIOPSY

The lesions should not be prepared aseptically and be careful not to destroy them if the area needs shaving. The best biopsy samples are taken from the margins of the skin lesions. The lesions should always be examined previously by cytology to record which bacteria and yeasts are present. It is also the ideal opportunity to collect good samples for a dermatophyte culture.

In patients with several lesions, the typical ultrasound image is known as the "Swiss cheese" pattern. Some clinicians believe this hepatic image is pathognomonic of the superficial necrolytic dermatitis. However, the liver in dogs with idiopathic hepatocellular collapse normally appears nodular in ultrasound imaging. Liver histopathology evidences moderate to severe hepatocellular collapse and vacuolar degeneration accompanied by nodular regeneration. The severe vacuolisation suggests a hormonal or metabolic aetiology, but the initial cause remains to be determined. In some dogs, the liver shows signs of cirrhosis.

If the hepatocutaneous syndrome is associated with a **glucagonoma** rather than liver disease, the patient's clinical signs will depend on this hormonal disorder. The clinical picture includes depression, anorexia, diarrhoea, vomiting, weight loss, and normochromic normocytic anaemia. An increase in liver enzyme activity is only observed in 40–50 % of cases and around 30 % have concurrent diabetes. In the latter case, patients commonly have hyperglucagonaemia, hypoalbuminaemia, and hypoaminoacidaemia. Bile acids levels are usually normal. Only very few cases course with pancreatic masses that can be detected with ultrasound.

TAKE NOTE!

Patients with glucagonoma have plasma glucagon levels that are between 5 and 10 times higher than the upper limit of the normal range.

Advanced imaging studies, such as magnetic resonance imaging, computerised axial tomography, or arteriography, may be required for the definitive diagnosis of cases where there is a suspicion of glucagonoma. Even so, exploratory surgery may become indispensable.

TIP

Whether the hepatocutaneous syndrome is secondary to liver disease and related to glucagon hypersecretion, always measure zinc, amino acid, and fatty acid levels before starting treatment.

Treatment

An 11-step layered treatment has been suggested for treating hepatocutaneous syndrome related to liver disease:

1. A diet rich in high-quality proteins (and also designed to facilitate recovery).
2. If the patient does not eat, insert a feeding tube or even start parenteral feeding if necessary.
3. Begin treatment for the diabetes, if present. At best, these patients respond erratically to insulin.
4. Provide symptomatic treatment of any secondary skin infections. A 3 % chlorhexidine shampoo will effectively resolve any bacterial infection, but it often falls short of treating yeasts. If the secondary infection is due to *Malassezia*, the treatment of choice is a shampoo with miconazole. Some shampoos are now available with a combination of miconazole and chlorhexidine. If there are exudative lesions, try treating them with an antiseptic and/or astringent solution (one part chlorhexidine with three parts Burow's solution).

5. Amino acid supplementation:
   - Enrichment with egg yolks (3 to 6 daily). The benefits are thought to stem from their amino acid profile. Protein concentrates for bodybuilding have also been tried with some success.
   - Intravenous amino acid therapy seems to be of some help in dogs with hepatocutaneous syndrome. Before starting the therapy, check the patient's bile acid levels, as the treatment could induce hepatic encephalopathy in dogs with abnormal levels. Recommendations in the literature are for 10 g of amino acids per 100 ml of solution. A typical dose is 25 ml/kg over 8–12 hours via a jugular central venous catheter. If the patient shows improvement, do not repeat. When there is no evident improvement after the amino acid infusion, it can be repeated every 7–10 days. Dogs can be given up to a maximum of four doses as described. If the patient still does not respond after the fourth dose, they probably never will. The amino acid IV therapy can be repeated whenever the skin lesions flare up. Some patients may need an infusion every few months, while others may require them monthly. As the disease progresses, the frequency of the infusions usually has to be increased. If hepatic encephalopathy develops following amino acid IV therapy, it normally disappears within 12 hours after the last infusion.
6. Omega-3 essential fatty acid supplementation. A commercial omega-3 solution is normally used at double the recommended amount.
7. Zinc supplementation, preferably in the form of zinc methionine at a dosage of 2 mg/kg per day.
8. Niacinamide supplementation at a dosage of 250–500 mg/dog split over two or three doses per day.
9. If there is localised inflammation, such as pododermatitis, that cannot be controlled with the treatments described above, the use of topical corticosteroids is another option. The first-choice corticosteroids are those which imply less systemic absorption (e.g. hydrocortisone aceponate, fluocortin).
10. Systemic corticosteroids (prednisolone at an initial dosage of 1 mg/kg every 24 hours) can prove beneficial in some dogs, but their use is not currently recommended.
11. Ketoconazole has been used to successfully treat secondary *Malassezia* infections and may also have a certain degree of anti-inflammatory and antipruritic effect. Normal dosages are 5 to 10 mg/kg every 12 hours. If the ketoconazole therapy is thought to be aggravating the liver disease, other possibilities are itraconazole or fluconazole, which are better tolerated by the liver.

The treatment of hepatocutaneous syndrome related to glucagonoma includes management of the diabetes (if present), surgical removal of the primary pancreatic tumour, octreotide administration (a long-acting somatostatin analogue that temporarily inhibits glucagon secretion), and, as with cases related to liver disease, fatty acid and amino acid supplementation.

TIP

Whenever possible, medications that lack a clear benefit for patients with any type of liver disease should be avoided. This is even more important in conditions such as hepatocutaneous syndrome. Therefore, always strive to use a topical treatment, and if this is not possible, ensure the drugs selected have the least possible hepatotoxicity.

Prognosis

Dogs with hepatocellular collapse generally have a poor prognosis. Even in the best of cases, patients are not expected to live beyond 2.5 years. The prognosis is poor for patients with a glucagonoma, and most dogs already have metastasis when the initial diagnosis is made.

Liver tumours

Primary liver tumours are rare occurrences in cats and dogs, representing just 0.6–1.5 % of all neoplasms found in dogs and 1.0–2.9 % of the tumours observed in cats. This proportion increases to 6.9 % in cats if we discount haematopoietic tumours.[34–37] Primary liver tumours are classified according to their histology[37] and morphological presentation[38] (Box 5 and Table 5).

TAKE NOTE!

The incidence of metastatic liver disease in dogs is 2.5 times greater than that of primary liver tumours. By contrast in cats, primary liver neoplasms are more common than secondary ones.[37]

Malignant liver tumours are more common in dogs.[35–38] In fact, the most frequent malignant primary tumour in dogs is hepatocellular carcinoma.[39] Whereas in cats, benign liver tumours are more common.[35–37,40–42]

Box 5. CLASSIFICATION OF LIVER TUMOURS IN SMALL ANIMALS.

Based on their histology:

- Hepatocellular
- Bile duct
- Neuroendocrine or carcinoid
- Mesenchymal

Based on their morphology:

- Nodular
- Single
- Diffuse

Table 5. Frequency of primary liver tumours in dogs according to their histology and morphology.[35,38,43–48]

	Nodular	Single	Diffuse
Hepatocellular	16–25 %	53–84 %	0–19 %
Biliary	0–21 %	37–46 %	17–54 %
Neuroendocrine	33 %	0 %	67 %
Mesenchymal	64 %	36 %	0 %

Clinical presentation of liver tumours

Both cats and dogs with liver tumours show vague, nonspecific signs of liver dysfunction and most patients do not develop any other signs until the disease is in a very advanced stage. The condition will progress symptomatically in 50 % of cats and 75 % of dogs with liver tumours,[34–53] especially if it is malignant.

The clinical picture comprises anorexia, lethargy, weight loss, PU/PD, vomiting, and abdominal distension. Jaundice, diarrhoea, and excessive bleeding, which are actually more indicative of liver disease, are observed much less frequently. Neurological signs in these patients, such as depression, dementia, or convulsions, may be attributed to hepatic encephalopathy, hypoglycaemia, or metastasis to the nervous system.[38,46,54] Unfortunately, these clinical signs cannot be used to differentiate between a primary and metastatic neoplasm or another type of liver disease.[36]

A physical examination may reveal hepatomegaly in up to 75 % of cats and dogs with hepatic masses, this may be accompanied by abdominal distension due to ascites or haemoperitoneum. The internal bleeding may be due to tumour rupture, which is typical of hepatocellular adenomas, hepatocellular carcinomas, and hepatic haemangiosarcomas.

Laboratory diagnosis

Table 6 shows the blood parameters that usually present alterations in patients with a liver tumour.

Leukocytosis, nonregenerative anaemia, and thrombocytosis are common laboratory findings in dogs with hepatic tumours. The leukocytosis is thought to be caused by the inflammation and necrosis of hepatic masses,[43,44] while the anaemia is likely due to chronic inflammation, erythrocyte sequestration, and iron deficiency.[55] Thrombocytosis probably develops as a paraneoplastic feature of the patient's liver tumour because it induces thrombopoietin synthesis, although the excess of platelets may also be due to the anaemia and inflammatory cytokines.[56–58] Liver enzyme activity tends to be elevated, but the magnitude of the increase is not always an accurate reflection of the degree of liver involvement.[37] In dogs with primary tumours, the greatest changes are seen in ALP and ALT, meanwhile the most notable increases in dogs with metastatic liver tumours affect AST and bilirubin.[27,59]

TAKE NOTE!

Whenever the ratio of AST to ALT is <1, it is an indication that the presence of a hepatocellular or bile duct carcinoma should be suspected, and if the ratio is >1, the vet should suspect a neuroendocrine or mesenchymal tumour.[38]

Table 6. Blood parameters usually altered in patients with liver tumours.[37,38,40–48]

Blood parameter	Cats	Dogs
Leukocytosis	Unchanged	54–73 %
Anaemia	Unchanged	27–51 %
↓ Albumin	Unchanged	52–83 %
↑ ALP	10–64 %	61–100 %
↑ ALT	10–78 %	44–75 %
↑ AST	15–78 %	56–100 %
↑ GGT	78 %	39 %
↑ Bilirubin	33–78 %	18–33 %

Besides the alterations in liver enzyme activities, other lab anomalies include hypoalbuminaemia, hypoglycaemia, hyperglobulinaemia, and elevated bile acid concentrations.[34,35,38,43–46]

In the case of cats, and in contrast to dogs, azotaemia is a common finding in animals with hepatobiliary tumours. Indeed, it may be the only abnormality in blood chemistry. Either way, liver enzymes, particularly ALT and AST, and bilirubin tend to be significantly high in most cats with malignant liver tumours.[40–42]

Diagnostic imaging

In general, X-rays provide scant information about these kinds of tumours, but it can help detect ascites or lung metastases. Having said that, ventrodorsal X-rays in both cats and dogs with large hepatobiliary tumours will generally reveal a cranial abdominal mass displacing the stomach caudally and laterally.[44,45,47] On rare occasions, mineralisation of the biliary tract may be noted in dogs suffering from a biliary tract carcinoma.[37]

Abdominal ultrasound is currently the diagnostic imaging technique of choice when assessing the morphology of the liver and biliary tract in cats and dogs alike.[51,60–64] It can also be used to collect fine-needle puncture and Tru-Cut needle biopsy samples.

Ultrasound-guided needle sampling is a minimally traumatic method of obtaining very useful histological information for the diagnosis.[61–64]

The patient's coagulation profile should be checked before performing either of the techniques, as mild to moderate bleeding can be expected in at least 5 % of all procedures.[61–64] If the coagulation profile is abnormal, give the patient two or three doses of vitamin K_1 (5 mg SC per dose) between 24 and 48 hours before the biopsy and another 3–4 days after the procedure. Fine-needle and Tru-Cut needle biopsies have a diagnostic accuracy of 60 % and 90 %, respectively. Other biopsy techniques have been refined in recent years; one example being the **keyhole technique**. Under ultrasound guidance, this method can be used to accurately collect a small sample from the correct area through a small opening in the abdominal wall (incisional biopsy). After sample collection, a cellulose sponge or gelatine can be inserted to close the site and prevent bleeding.

Lastly, advanced imaging techniques, such as magnetic resonance imaging and computerised axial tomography, provide better quality images and a more accurate diagnosis of small masses as well as a clearer picture of their relationship to adjacent structures.[65]

WHAT INFORMATION CAN BE OBTAINED FROM A LIVER ULTRASOUND WHEN A TUMOUR IS DETECTED?

Ultrasound images of a liver tumour should indicate whether it is cystic or solid and if it is focal, nodular, or diffuse. When dealing with focal tumours, it is important to determine the size and location of the mass and its relationship to surrounding anatomical structures, such as the gallbladder or caudal vena cava.[51,60–64] Additionally, Doppler techniques can be used to study the tumour's vascularisation.[37] Finally, remember to check the intra-abdominal lymph nodes for any signs of metastasis.

Treatment of primary liver tumours

Surgery is the modality of choice when the tumour is basically a localised mass limited to a single hepatic lobe. Hepatocellular adenomas and carcinomas can have a good prognosis. For instance, in a study sample of 40 dogs with hepatocellular carcinomas, the mean postoperative life expectancy was 1,460 days.[45] It is worth noting that the tumour in these dogs was located on the left side of the liver. In fact, dogs with a neoplasm on the right side have a worse prognosis, probably because the caudal vena cava is damaged during surgery.

Some of the complications typically seen after a liver lobectomy include haemorrhaging, vascular compromise of adjacent lobes, reduced liver function, and transient hypoglycaemia.[37,66]

Multiple nodular or diffuse malignant tumours generally have a very poor prognosis, and the patient's life expectancy after the lobectomy is relatively short. Chemotherapy has not proven particularly useful, and it is often hard to administer radiotherapy at sufficiently high doses, since a dog's liver cannot tolerate radiation levels above 30 Gy.[37,65]

Hepatic encephalopathy

Hepatic encephalopathy (HE) refers to changes in the nervous system that occur in patients with severe liver dysfunction. The patient's brain receives large amounts of substances that should be eliminated by the liver, and these can provoke various alterations (Box 6).[67,68] These neurological signs may appear at any given moment, but they mostly manifest following a protein-rich meal or if the patient is suffering from intestinal bleeding.

Diagnosis

The cause of the liver dysfunction and patient's treatment response must be identified during the diagnosis of HE. Provided that the HE is not the result of a congenital shunt, it is normally a new situation that owners find particularly worrying, as it tends to be the umpteenth clinical condition in pets that are already in a poor state of overall health. The best indicators of liver function are serum bile acid concentrations. Animals with HE have markedly elevated bile acids levels, including after fasting. Fasting ammonia concentrations will also be high. Liver enzyme activities depend heavily on the primary disease and the chronicity of the overall clinical picture. Hypoalbuminaemia, hypoglycaemia, and low uraemia levels are often observed in patients with HE.

Box 6. CLINICAL SIGNS OF HE ACCORDING TO SEVERITY.

Mild
- Depression
- Lethargy
- Increased docility
- Increased aggression

Moderate
- Wandering aimlessly
- Circling
- Apparent blindness
- Head pressing

Severe
- Stupor
- Seizures
- Coma

Treatment

The treatment of HE can be broken down into three steps:

1. Treat the primary disease, if it can be identified. Be sure to use appropriate dosages when administering hepatotoxic drugs or which are metabolised by the liver (see Chapter 3).
2. Reduce the production of ammonia waste.
   - Design a diet with a sufficient amount of high biological value proteins and low nitrogenous waste.
   - Control any gastrointestinal bleeding. Antacids are highly recommended (e.g. proton pump inhibitors). Sucralfate is a very practical option as it can help heal the gastroduodenal mucosa, neutralise gastric acid, and inhibit pepsin.
3. Control the anaerobic flora in the colon. This can be accomplished by either of two often complementary therapeutic approaches:
   - Lactulose: 0.1–0.5 ml/kg PO every 8–12 hours. Establish the dose according to the effect. The aim is to produce two or three soft stools per day with a so-called pudding consistency. When the dose is too high, patients suffer from flatulence, stomach cramps, severe diarrhoea, dehydration, and acidosis.
   - Antibiotics: antibiotics can be used to keep colonic bacteria levels low, which translates into less waste produced by their metabolism. The most used are ampicillin (5 mg/kg PO every 8–12 hours) or amoxicillin (2.5 mg/kg PO every 12 hours) and metronidazole (7.5 mg/kg PO every 8–12 hours).

   It has recently been suggested that probiotics may displace the ammoniagenic bacteria that have grown in the colon; nevertheless, further studies are required before their use can be fully recommended.

What should a good diet for HE consist of?

As a general rule, dogs should follow a diet with a protein content restricted to 2.0–2.5 mg/kg that is based around branched-chain amino acids and with less aromatic amino acids. Low-protein diets are recommended for cats, such as those indicated for kidney and liver diseases, and 25 to 30 % of the protein content should be a dry extract. Vegetable, egg (ovalbumin), and milk (lactalbumin) proteins with high biological value are popularly used as a source of amino acids in these cases. The calorie load usually derives from carbohydrates and fats to avoid using the protein as a source of energy. The daily ration should be split into small amounts given frequently throughout the day. Try to use low-residue nutrients to minimise the anaerobic metabolism of the ammoniagenic bacteria in the colon.

Hepatic diets are mainly indicated for diseases that induce liver dysfunction. In liver diseases that course with inflammation but no organ dysfunction, the veterinary surgeon should assess the pros and cons of a protein-restricted diet. Personally, we prefer not to restrict protein intake, instead supplementing the patient's diet with vitamin E, SAMe, and/or silymarin, among others.

MANAGING EPISODES OF HEPATIC ENCEPHALOPATHY

If the patient is experiencing a seizure: administer benzodiazepines, barbiturates, or propofol. Propofol is ideal thanks to its extrahepatic metabolism.
The other two options can produce very prolonged effects due to their exclusively hepatic metabolism.

If the patient is not having a seizure: administer an isotonic saline solution supplemented with potassium chloride and glucose at 2–2.5 %. Perform enemas with a lukewarm isotonic saline solution. Lactulose (5–10 ml, at 1 part lactulose to 3 parts saline solution, 3 or 4 times a day) or povidone iodine (use a 10 % solution and rinse after 10 minutes with lukewarm saline) can also be added to the enemas.

THE OWNER'S PERSPECTIVE

There are very marked **differences between cats and dogs** with respect to **liver diseases**, spanning from the **prevalence** of the various conditions to their eventual **prognosis**. Make an extra effort to give the owner a **detailed explanation** of what is happening to their pet, lay out the diagnostic plan, potential treatment options, and, ultimately, a realistic prognosis.

Owners can find it **hard to believe** that their pet has been ill for weeks or months **without them noticing anything**. It is important to focus on the clinical signs that most readily reveal when an animal has a liver problem. Use them to explain to the owner that the disease started some time ago and that **quick, radical action** is required to obtain the maximum benefit from the treatment options.

Diet is a **key component** of the treatment of liver diseases. A **feeding tube** is a simple tool that can be used to significantly improve the quality of life, and often the duration, of a patient with liver disease. But owners should still be given a **detailed explanation** of what feeding tubes involve and stress that in most cases they will be used for a limited period.

KEY POINTS VETERINARY PRACTITIONERS SHOULD BEAR IN MIND

When most patients with liver disease are brought to a clinic, they have already been ill for days or weeks but their owners did not notice sooner. So as the vet, you must be clear in your mind and avoid wasting time on therapeutic tests. You should implement a **well-organised, complete diagnostic plan** before promptly initiating the **most comprehensive treatment possible**. Do not be afraid to propose tests, biopsy, or the insertion of a feeding tube, as **time is particularly of the essence** in patients with liver disease.

The **prognosis** for liver disease **in dogs is usually worse than that for cats**. As such, do not let yourself become too optimistic when treating dogs or lose hope when treating cats.

Caring for liver disease can involve some complex pharmacological treatments. **Diligently select the drugs that most easily mark the difference** and dismiss those which are really just "complementary", at least when starting therapy.

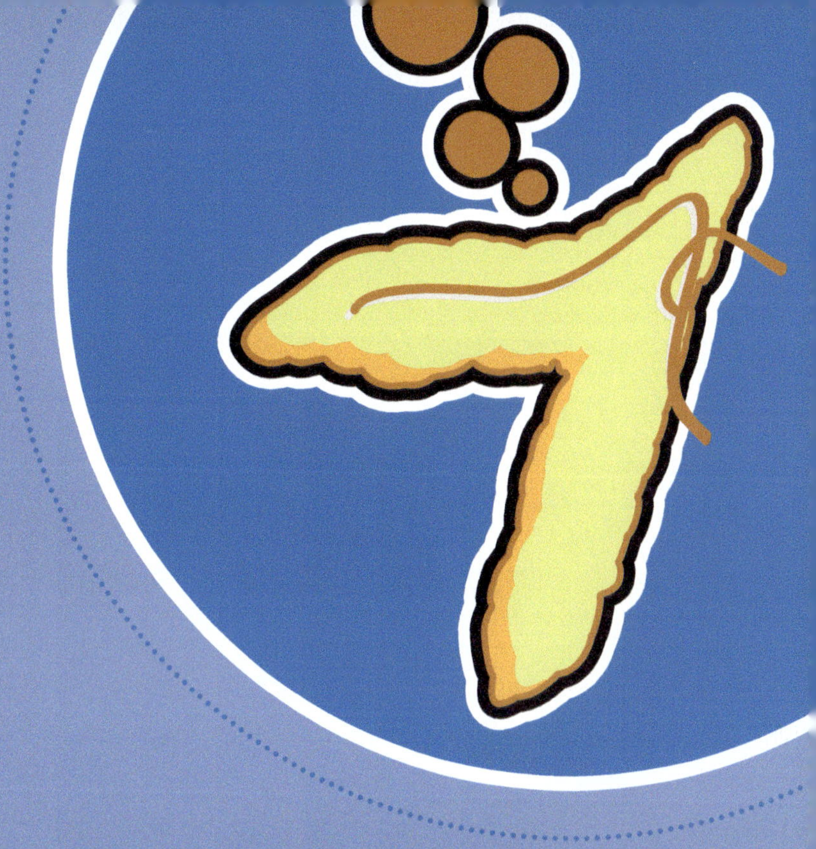

10 Endocrine problems in senior patients

10

Endocrine problems in senior patients

The study of hormonal diseases is one of the cornerstones of small animal medicine when dealing with older patients. While these conditions can affect young or even paediatric animals (e.g. patients with congenital hypothyroidism), they are much more frequent in senior animals. While there are many types of hormonal disturbances, for the purposes of this chapter we will discuss three specific diseases: diabetes mellitus, which affects both cats and dogs; hyperadrenocorticism, which mainly affects dogs; and hyperthyroidism, which mainly affects senior cats. Unfortunately, covering other endocrine diseases of increasing importance (e.g. canine hypothyroidism, hyperaldosteronism, feline acromegaly) is beyond the scope of this chapter. For further information on these diseases, we urge the reader to consult texts devoted entirely to endocrinopathies of cats and dogs.

Diabetes mellitus

Diabetes mellitus (DM) is an endocrine disease characterised by an inability to maintain blood glucose levels within the species' normal range. This can be due to an inadequate secretion (congenital or acquired) of insulin by the pancreas (type I DM), inadequate action of insulin at the insulin receptor (type II DM), or antagonism caused by other substances (type III DM).

Epidemiology

Just over 30 years ago, diabetes was diagnosed in 19 out of 10,000 dogs. By 1999, prevalence had tripled, with DM affecting 58 per 10,000 dogs. A similar increase was observed for feline diabetes, which was a rare disease in cats up until the 1970s, but currently affects 1 per 50–100 cats, depending on the country.[1,2] Today, DM is considered one of the most common endocrinopathies of dogs and the second most common in cats.

Pathophysiology

Box 1 lists the known predisposing factors for DM in dogs and cats.

Canine diabetes mellitus

DM (type I) in humans is characterised by destruction of the β cells of the islets of Langerhans, or pancreatic islets, due to chronic pancreatitis or immune-mediated disease, resulting in hyperglycaemia and glycosuria.[3] In dogs, loss of the β cells of the pancreas usually occurs rapidly due to immune-mediated damage, vacuolar degeneration, or pancreatitis. Interestingly, natriuresis and dehydration induced by water loss are not typical characteristics of DM in diabetic dogs, in contrast to human and feline patients.[4]

In intact female dogs, transient or permanent DM can occur during the dioestrus phase due to progestogen-induced insulin resistance.[5]

Box 1. PREDISPOSING FACTORS FOR DM.

In dogs:

- Samoyed, Cairn Terrier, Golden Retriever, German Shepherd Dog, Miniature Schnauzer, Keeshond, Poodle, and Cocker Spaniel breeds.[7]
- Neutered animals (possibly because these are overrepresented), both female and male.
- Obesity.
- Hypothyroidism or immune-mediated diseases.
- Cocker Spaniel breed with pancreatitis.

In cats:

- Burmese breed with predisposition,[6] and Maine Coon, Siamese, and Russian Blue breeds.
- Castrated males.
- Obesity (Fig. 1).
- Concurrent diseases such as hyperadrenocorticism or acromegaly.
- Chronic hyperglycaemic therapy (e.g. corticosteroids or progestogens).

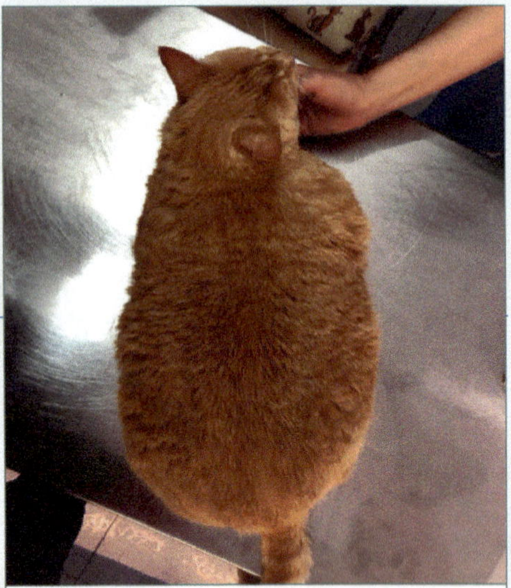

Figure 1. Domestic shorthair cat with obesity and a body condition score of 9/9. Obesity predisposes both cats and dogs to diabetes.

Feline diabetes mellitus

The processes underlying the development of hyperglycaemia in feline DM are listed below.[8]

- Presence of the phenomenon known as **insulin resistance**: absence of the desired effect on insulin receptors. Unlike diabetic dogs, in which rapid and direct destruction of pancreatic β cells occurs, DM in cats is characterised by insulin resistance.
- **Reduced or absent insulin production.** This occurs due to exhaustion of β cells and glucose toxicity, which leads to the accumulation of amylin in the islets of Langerhans and apoptosis of β cells.
- Presence of **chronic lymphoplasmacytic pancreatitis**.

There is a fourth process that appears to be critical to the establishment of DM in some cats. It involves the liver's role as a stabiliser of glucose levels, both during and after the period in which insulin exerts its hypoglycaemic effect. Further research will be required to determine the importance of this fourth process.

Diagnosis

History and physical

Before beginning additional tests, the veterinary surgeon must be fully aware of the basic clinical signs that all (or almost all) DM patients will present. These are polyuria, polydipsia, polyphagia, weight loss, and poor haircoat. Other less frequent or obvious clinical signs are hepatomegaly, plantigrade stance in cats, and cataracts in dogs. We should also bear in mind that this endocrinopathy will be accompanied by other pathologies that can be as important as DM itself: this occurs frequently in dogs and very often in cats.

Laboratory diagnosis

The laboratory tests most commonly used for the diagnosis of DM are blood tests. While urinary tests (Fig. 2) remain useful and can complement the results of blood tests, they have been largely replaced by the latter.

All patients with suspected DM should undergo a complete blood count; a complete biochemical workup including electrolytes; urinalysis with urine culture and determination of the urine protein:creatinine (UPC) ratio; determination of triglyceride levels (more important in dogs) and total T_4; and blood pressure measurement.

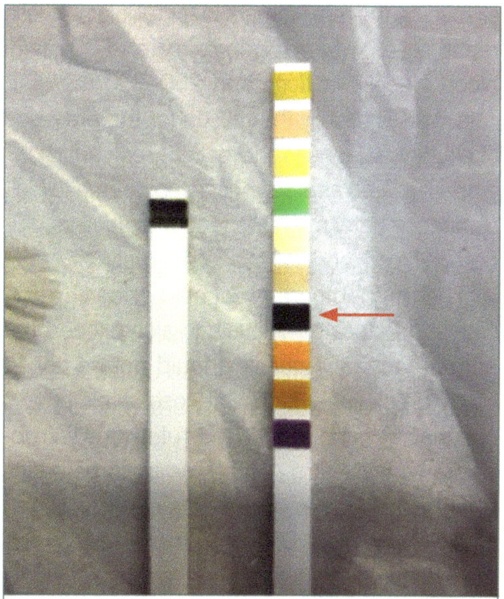

Figure 2. Urine strips with a positive result for glycosuria. For diagnosis of DM, urinary tests should be supported by blood tests such as measurement of blood glucose and fructosamine levels.

Table 1. Types of insulin for maintenance treatment of dogs or cats with DM.

Type of insulin	Description	Nadir and duration of effect	Initial dose	Comments
Intermediate action	Insulin of porcine origin (65 % in crystalline form and 35 % in amorphous form), 40 IU/ml	Cats: • Nadir: 2–8 h • Duration: 8–14 h Dogs: • Nadir: 1–10 h • Duration: 10–24 h	Cats: 0.25–0.5 IU/kg every 12 h (without exceeding 3 IU/cat) Dogs: 0.25–0.5 IU/kg every 12 h	More used in dogs than in cats
PZI (long acting)	Recombinant insulin of human origin, 40 IU/ml	Cats: • Nadir: 5–7 h • Duration: 8–24 h Dogs: • Duration: 8–12 h	Cats: 1–2 IU/cat every 12 h Dogs: 0.25–0.5 IU/kg every 12 h	More commonly used to treat cats than dogs, for which it was authorised later
Insulin glargine (long acting)	Recombinant insulin of human origin, 100 or 300 IU/ml	Cats: • Nadir: 12–14 h • Duration: 12–24 h Dogs: • Nadir: 6–10 h • Duration: 12–20 h	Cats: 0.25–0.5 IU/kg every 12 h Dogs: 0.3 IU/kg every 12 h	More used in cats than in dogs

Adapted from Behrend E et al. 2018 AAHA diabetes management guidelines for dogs and cats. *J Am Anim Hosp Assoc*, 2018, 54(1):1–21.

Diabetic patient monitoring

Good control of diabetic patients is defined as the "absence of clinical signs of hyperglycaemia in the absence of signs of hypoglycaemia". Therefore, the clinician's goal should be to keep the patient's blood glucose below the renal threshold for tubular reabsorption for as long as possible. The clinician should not be overly concerned if blood glucose exceeds this threshold at any time during the day, or does so intermittently. What is concerning is a failure to avoid the most important clinical signs such as PU/PD, polyphagia, or weight loss.

To achieve good control of the diabetic patient, it is necessary to apply as complete as possible a monitoring system, bearing in mind the limitations of the owner and the tolerance of the patient. Next, we will describe some of the most commonly used monitoring methods in veterinary medicine: glucose curves, urine strips, and fructosamine determination. It should be noted that there is no perfect monitoring system in either dogs[16] or cats.[17]

Box 2. DIETARY RECOMMENDATIONS FOR CATS AND DOGS WITH DM.

In diabetic cats:

- High-protein diets (≥40 % metabolisable energy, ME) have been shown to be effective in controlling blood glucose, minimising the risk of hepatic lipidosis, reducing muscle loss, and optimising palatability.
- Feline diabetic diets should be low in carbohydrates (approximately 12 % ME) to reduce postprandial hyperglycaemia.
- Diets for diabetic cats are supplemented with arginine, which appears to stimulate insulin secretion.
- Feline diabetic diets are not usually high in fibre, as its effect against postprandial hyperglycaemia appears not to be as marked in cats as in dogs, and higher fibre content can affect the palatability of the diet.
- Diabetic cats fed wet food tend to have better control of hyperglycaemia: this type of food appears to have a greater satiating effect, and can have a lower proportion of carbohydrates than dry food.

In diabetic dogs:

- Diabetic dogs with a healthy body weight can be fed a normal physiological diet as long as the number of feeds is regulated to reduce postprandial hyperglycaemia.
- Diets rich in fibre have a strong satiating effect that improves postprandial glycaemic control and reduces the amount of calories ingested by the patient, which is particularly interesting if the patient is overweight or obese.

Glucose curves

What are they for?

Glucose curves can help resolve some of the most common doubts of small animal clinicians:

- Although the patient is clinically well, is there underlying hypoglycaemia that can be detected with laboratory tests but is not yet evident? This provides us with a certain capacity to predict the next steps.
- How correct is the change in insulin dose that I have proposed? This gives us peace of mind and trust in our own decisions.
- When does the maximum effect or glucose nadir occur (i.e. the point at which blood glucose is lowest), and how pronounced is the decrease in blood glucose? This tells us whether the insulin dose is adequate, too low, or too high.
- How long will the patient's blood glucose level remain above the recommended upper limit for its species? This helps us to foresee whether the clinical signs will subside and tells us whether the insulin dose and dosage regimen are correct, and whether the type of insulin administered is appropriate.

TAKE NOTE!

On a glucose curve, the ideal nadir is between 80 and 150 mg/dl blood glucose, both in dogs and cats. On the other hand, maximum blood glucose values are approximately 200 mg/dl in dogs and 250–300 mg/dl in cats.

When should glucose curves be performed?

- When we begin insulin treatment (or change insulin type).
- 7–14 days after changing insulin treatment.
- At least every 3 months, even in apparently well-controlled diabetic patients.
- Every time clinical signs reappear.
- Every time we know or suspect that our patient is experiencing hypoglycaemia.

How are glucose curves performed? (Fig. 3)

1. Perform an initial blood glucose test before administering insulin. The result is known as the preinsulin blood glucose value.
2. Inject insulin at the usual dose and time. If applicable, also provide the patient with the normal amount of food.
3. In patients treated with PZI or intermediate-acting insulin, draw a blood sample every 2 hours. In cats treated with insulin glargine, this can be done every 3–4 hours.[5]
4. Continue with this protocol until the first 12 hours have elapsed. In patients that receive insulin once daily, it may be necessary to continue throughout the day until the next dose.
5. If at any time the patient's blood glucose drops below 150 mg/kg, blood samples should be taken every 60 minutes thereafter, regardless of the type of insulin or the time of administration.

TIP

Although there are numerous portable glucometers for measuring blood glucose in cats and dogs, those that are specifically calibrated for these species may be more reliable. However, the most important thing when using these glucometers is to always use the same device on the same patient.[85,86,88]

How are glucose curves interpreted?

The first objective in treating a diabetic patient is to achieve a correct glucose nadir. If a glucose curve indicates a nadir <80 mg/dl, the insulin dose should be reduced, regardless of how good the glucose curve or the preinsulin blood glucose value are.

The second objective, provided a correct glucose nadir has been established, is to estimate the duration of effect of insulin. This in turn will indicate whether the patient should be treated every 12 hours (like the vast majority of diabetic cats and dogs) or every 24 hours.

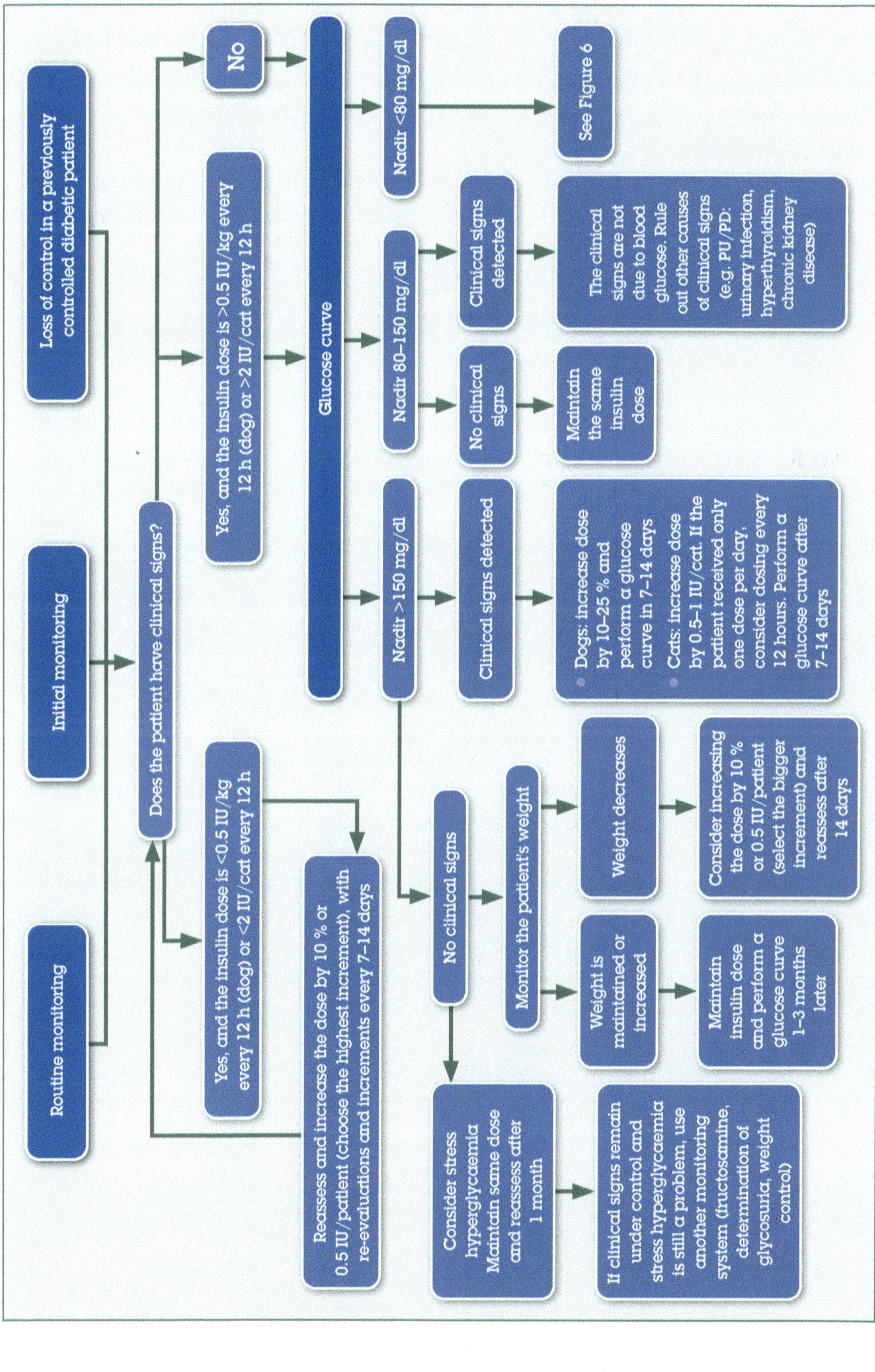

Figure 3. Algorithm for monitoring glucose levels in diabetic cats and dogs.

HOW IS INSULIN THERAPY IN DIABETIC PATIENTS ADJUSTED ACCORDING TO THE NADIR OBTAINED IN THE GLUCOSE CURVE?

Nadir <80 mg/dl:

- If the patient has clinical signs of **hypoglycaemia** (drowsiness, lethargy, and weakness in mild cases, shock and coma in severe cases), treat these signs and withdraw insulin therapy.
- If, after interrupting insulin therapy, blood glucose levels again exceed 250 mg/dl, restart insulin therapy.
- In dogs, reduce the starting dose by 10–25 % if there are no clinical signs of hypoglycaemia or by 50 % if there are.
- In cats, reduce the dose to 0.5 IU/cat if there are no clinical signs of hypoglycaemia or to 1 IU/cat if there are.
- Perform a second glucose curve the next day to check for hypoglycaemia. If hypoglycaemia is observed, reduce the dose and repeat the next day. If not, re-evaluate in 7–14 days.
- If blood glucose does not return to <250 mg/dl, consider remission (especially in cats). Schedule follow-up visits to control recurrence.

Nadir 80–150 mg/dl:

- If the patient does not have clinical signs of hypoglycaemia, make no changes.
- If the patient has clinical signs, make changes, but keep in mind that:
  - Glucose curves change from day to day.
  - The effect of insulin may not last long enough: if insulin is administered once a day, a switch can be made to administration every 12 hours; if insulin is already administered every 12 hours, consider changing the type of insulin.
  - If you switch to a regimen of administration every 12 hours, ensure that the effects of the two insulin doses do not overlap, as the effect of the second dose combined with the first can cause hypoglycaemia (this may require lowering the dose given in the afternoon/evening).
  - Consider the presence of another disease that may be causing the clinical signs.

Nadir >150 mg/dl:

- If the patient has clinical signs of **hyperglycaemia** (PU/PD are the most important, but also polyphagia and weight loss), increase the dose by 10–25 % in dogs or 0.5–1 IU in cats (increase the dose based on the size of the patient and the degree of hyperglycaemia). If the insulin was administered once per day, switch to twice per day.
- If the patient has no clinical signs:
  - Consider stress hyperglycaemia or a placebo effect on the owner's part.
  - If the patient's weight has been maintained, do not modify the dose and reassess in 1–3 months. If the weight has dropped, increase the dose and reassess in 14 days.
- Consider the presence of insulin resistance if:
  - In dogs, an insulin dose >1 IU/kg per dose does not produce a response or a dose >1.5 IU/kg fails to lower blood glucose levels below 300 mg/dl.
  - In cats, the insulin dose is >5 IU/cat per dose.

WHAT IS THE SOMOGYI EFFECT?

The Somogyi effect, or hypoglycaemia-induced hyperglycaemia, refers to the "rebound" of blood glucose to hyperglycaemic levels after hypoglycaemia caused by administration of an excessive amount of insulin. This is due to the physiological action of counterregulatory hormones (e.g. epinephrine, cortisol, glucagon) released in response to the hypoglycaemia that normally occurs after excessive administration of exogenous insulin.

The Somogyi effect is more common in dogs than in cats, in which this effect may not occur.[87] If the Somogyi effect is detected, the insulin dose should be reduced. Normally, if the nadir rises above 80 mg/dl, the Somogyi effect disappears.

Where are glucose curves performed?

Glucose curves can be performed in the clinic or hospital or at home. Whenever possible glucose curves should be performed at home, as they are more reliable, especially if blood samples are taken correctly. Doing this at home avoids stress-induced hyperglycaemia in cats. Moreover, the patient will be able to continue with its normal daily routines, eating and drinking at the usual times and consuming the same amounts as normal. We will not discover anything new if we say that our patients are not happy in our centres, no matter how friendly we have designed them. Our patients prefer to be at home, in the same way that we, when hospitalised, miss our own beds and just want to be with our family.

Urine strips for determination of glycosuria

Urine strips are one of the simplest methods by which owners can monitor diabetic patients (Fig. 4). However, it is important to be aware of their limitations.

The first and clearest limitation is that glycosuria will only be evident when the renal threshold for tubular reabsorption is exceeded. This means that the urine strips can give us an idea of blood glucose levels when they exceed 200 mg/dl in dogs and 250–300 mg/dl in cats. If the patient is below this limit, the urine will not contain glucose, but patients with a blood glucose concentration close to the lower limit may be dangerously close to developing hypoglycaemia.

The second limitation is that, in contrast to blood sample analysis, the result does not reflect glucose levels at a specific point in time. Urine glucose values constitute an average of actual levels in the preceding minutes or hours. Therefore, making therapeutic decisions based on this value is clearly less accurate than measuring blood or interstitial glucose levels.

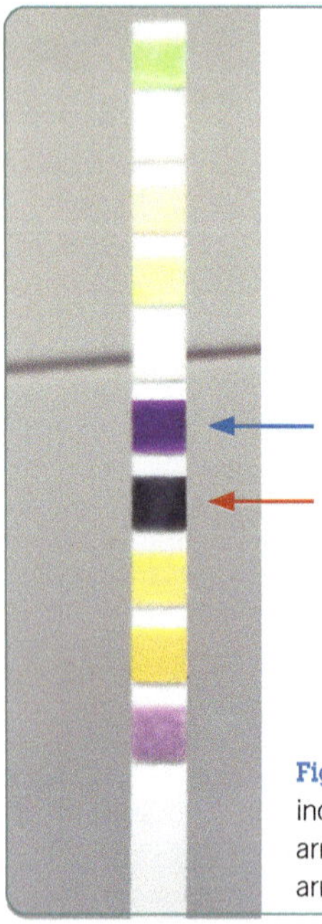

Figure 4. Urine strip indicating ketonuria (blue arrow) and glycosuria (red arrow).

Finally, it should be noted that, in general, a well-controlled diabetic patient will have intermittent low-grade glycosuria and periods of negative glycosuria.

Fructosamine

Fructosamine refers to glycosylated proteins that are formed nonenzymatically when proteins such as albumin bind irreversibly to glucose. For clinicians, it is very important to understand that the fructosamine concentration depends on blood glucose levels during the life of albumin. In other words, in situations of hypoalbuminaemia or high albumin turnover, fructosamine concentration may be abnormally low despite high blood glucose levels. For example, in uncompensated hyperthyroid patients who are also diabetic, fructosamine levels can be normal or even low.

Fructosamine can provide information on blood glucose levels in the preceding week or 2 weeks in cats and dogs, respectively.

The best way to use fructosamine values is to analyse their progression over multiple readings. This is much more useful than considering individual readings.

Other data to monitor

A good way to make the owner feel involved in managing their pet's DM is to assign them tasks. These do not have to be very complex or extremely strict, but are of undoubted utility for the clinician. An online spreadsheet shared between the veterinary surgeon and the owner will significantly facilitate therapeutic decision-making. On this spreadsheet, the owner should indicate the following:

- The patient's weight (weekly) (Fig. 5).
- The weight of the different foods that the patient eats.
- The volume of water consumed or urine produced (this can be done by weighing the litter box in the case of cats).
- The patient's behaviour (appetite, need for water, mood).
- The dose of insulin administered, the time of administration, and whether any problems occurred with injection or storage of the insulin.
- The result of urine test strips for glycosuria (if used).

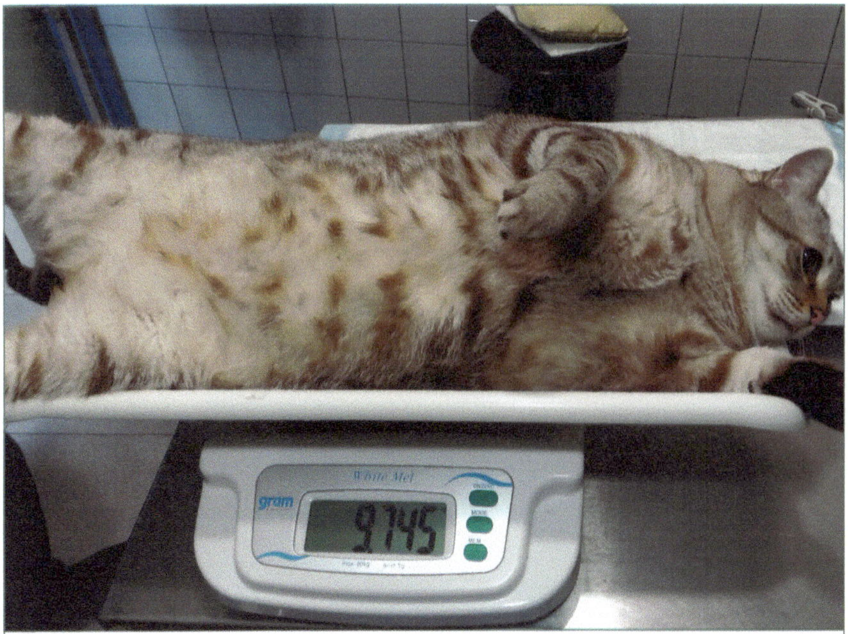

Figure 5. Diabetic cat before undergoing a procedure under anaesthesia to resolve oral problems. Weight monitoring is essential in this type of patient.

HOW DO WE MONITOR OUR DIABETIC PATIENTS AND WHAT DECISIONS SHOULD WE MAKE?

Monitoring on the first day of treatment:

- Start insulin therapy.
- Measure the level of fructosamine in the blood.
- If possible, perform a glucose curve to avoid hypoglycaemia. If the nadir is <150 mg/dl:
  - In dogs, reduce the dose by 10–50 %.
  - In cats, reduce the dose to 0.5 IU/cat.
  - In both species, perform a new glucose curve the next day until a nadir >150 mg/dl is achieved.

  If the nadir is >150 mg/dl, send the patient home and re-evaluate in 7–14 days (do not change the dose until after re-evaluating).

Monitoring until DM is controlled:

- If you have never seen the owner inject their pet with insulin, ask them to do so in front of you.
- Perform a new glucose curve every 7–14 days until glycaemic control and adequate insulin dose are achieved. Evaluate fructosamine.
- Review the other data that the owner has recorded on the shared sheet.
- Weigh the patient and perform a complete physical examination.

Long-term actions:

- Review the shared sheet with other recorded monitoring data.
- Weigh the patient and perform a complete physical examination.
- Perform a new glucose curve and test for fructosamine.
- Every 3–6 months perform a complete blood and urinary analysis.
- If the insulin dose needs to be changed, perform a glucose curve after 7–14 days.
- Taking individual glucose measurements is not usually recommended when increasing the insulin dose, but is advisable when it is necessary to lower it.

What if the diabetic patient is not well controlled? Action protocol for patients with poorly controlled DM

The patients we will discuss in this section fall into one of four categories:

- Patients with hypoglycaemia (Figs. 6 and 7).
- Patients with hyperglycaemia.
- Patients with insulin resistance (defined as >1.5 IU/kg per dose in dogs, and >5 IU per dose in cats).
- Patients that need frequent readjustments of insulin dose.

The following protocol should be applied to any patient with clinical signs (PU/PD, polyphagia, and unintended weight loss):

- Investigate causes related to the owner's handling of the insulin. Ask the owner to prepare and administer the dose in front of you. Check the syringe type and ensure that the insulin has not expired, has been kept cold, and has not changed colour, turned cloudy, or flocculated.
- Check the diet and amounts of food administered, including feed and human food or table scraps.
- Ask about other medications that the patient may be taking, or to which they may have access, that cause insulin resistance. Glucocorticoids (administered by any route), progestogens, and cyclosporine are the most common products.
  - If the medication is to be administered for a short time or can be withdrawn for 2 weeks, do not alter the insulin dose and reassess 2 weeks after finishing or withdrawing the medication.
  - If the medication cannot be withdrawn, increase the insulin dose. On these occasions, it is advisable to consult with a specialist endocrinologist.
- Rule out hypoglycaemia by performing a new glucose curve at home. If hypoglycaemia is detected, the Somogyi effect should be suspected, and the insulin dose should therefore be reduced.
- Rule out concurrent diseases:
  - Look for oral diseases, and perform an ovariohysterectomy in intact females (ensure the absence of ketoacidosis before anaesthetising).
  - If recent blood or urinary test results are unavailable, repeat the tests. Here, the tests described earlier in this chapter ("Laboratory diagnosis" section) will suffice.
  - If control of the patient is still not achieved, consider performing second-level diagnostic tests, such as abdominal ultrasound, chest X-rays, and quantification of pancreatic-specific lipase (remember that this is species-specific), serum trypsin-like immunoreactivity (TLI), folate, cobalamin, and symmetric dimethylarginine (SDMA). The aforementioned laboratory tests combined with these second-level tests will help confirm or rule out previously unidentified diseases such as chronic kidney disease, pancreatitis, urinary infections, and tumours.
  - Consider performing specific tests to rule out hyperadrenocorticism, acromegaly, and hyper- or hypothyroidism. Generally, hyperadrenocorticism or acromegaly should not be investigated before spending 4–6 weeks trying to control DM: doing so earlier can yield false positives in the case of hyperadrenocorticism and false negatives in the case of acromegaly.

Hyperadrenocorticism is a complex disease that deserves specific mention. Interested readers can skip ahead in this chapter to delve further into the diagnosis and treatment of canine and feline hyperadrenocorticism. It should be noted that in both dogs and cats this syndrome can occur due to endogenous or iatrogenic causes. In addition to insulin resistance, this disease can lead to PU/PD due to other causes, as well as dermatological disorders including thinning of the skin, alopecia and, in the case of cats, skin fragility. Diagnosis in dogs is established using ACTH stimulation, which is more specific (fewer false positives) but less sensitive (more false negatives) than the low-dose dexamethasone suppression test.[18] In cats, the low-dose dexamethasone suppression test is preferred, although it should be noted that the dose used in cats is 10 times higher than that used in dogs.[19]

Just a few years ago, **acromegaly** was considered a rare endocrine disease. However, recent studies have shown that in more than 30 % of cats diabetes may be due to underlying acromegaly.[20,21] Feline acromegaly is due to a pituitary tumour that produces abnormally high amounts of growth hormone (GH). This hormone causes insulin resistance, which initially leads to a diabetic state in which the patient loses weight, which is usually regained or even exceeded during the course of the disease. The high doses of exogenous insulin required to control these patients are often a sign that makes the veterinary surgeon suspect that another condition underlies the patient's DM. Definitive diagnosis is usually achieved by determining somatomedin C or insulin-like growth factor 1 (IGF-1). For this test to be reliable, the patient must have received insulin for at least 6 weeks; otherwise, a false negative may be obtained.

Both **hyperthyroidism** (more common in cats) and **hypothyroidism** (more common in dogs) can lead to insulin resistance. In both cases, the diagnosis can be complicated due to euthyroid sick syndrome. This syndrome implies that when a patient has another primary disease (apart from the thyroid problem) levels of total T_4 are usually lower than would otherwise be expected. Thus, in the case of a dog with uncontrolled DM, total T_4 levels can be lower than normal due to the DM, giving the impression that we are dealing with a hypothyroid patient, which is not actually the case. On the other hand, in cats with uncontrolled DM, measurement of total T_4 to diagnose hyperthyroidism may reveal normal values when the patient is actually hyperthyroid. In these cases, in addition to initially trying to control DM for a few weeks (limiting the euthyroid sick syndrome), we can measure total T_4 together with cTSH (see "Feline hyperthyroidism" section below) or free T_4 (by equilibrium dialysis).[22,23]

Hyperadrenocorticism or Cushing's syndrome

Hyperadrenocorticism (HAC), or Cushing's syndrome, is a clinical condition caused by excess levels of corticosteroids or other steroid hormones in the blood. This can be due to a variety of causes, such as a benign pituitary tumour, an adrenal tumour, or iatrogenic causes (usually due to chronic administration of corticosteroids or progestogens) (Fig. 8). HAC caused by a pituitary tumour, usually an adenoma, is known as Cushing's disease. This adenoma secretes corticotropin (ACTH) in excess, resulting in bilateral hyperplasia of the adrenal glands, which in turn secrete an excessive amount of cortisol. Some cases, usually those involving adrenal tumours, may involve secretion of cortisol precursors such as progesterone, 17-OH-progesterone, androstenedione, testosterone, and oestrogens, all of which exert steroidal effects. It is important to take this into account, as clinicians are often obsessed with cortisol levels, which may be normal, despite oversecretion of some cortisol precursors.[24]

Epidemiology and pathophysiology

Canine HAC

HAC is a common endocrine disease in dogs: every year 1–2 per 1,000 dogs are diagnosed with this condition.[25-27] The majority of cases (85 %) of HAC in dogs correspond to the pituitary form. HAC due to benign or malignant tumours of the adrenal glands (adrenal HAC) accounts for the remaining 15 % of cases.[28]

Pituitary HAC tends to occur more frequently in middle-aged and older dogs. Although cases have been described in patients aged 6 months to 20 years, the majority of cases occur in animals aged 6 years and older.[28] The Poodle, Dachshund, Boxer, and various Terrier breeds appear to be predisposed to pituitary HAC.[28] Although no sexual predisposition has been described for pituitary HAC, female dogs may be at greater risk of adrenal HAC.[28] Finally, pituitary HAC appears to occur more frequently in smaller dogs: 75 % of diagnosed patients weigh less than 20 kg.[28]

Cases of HAC caused by ectopic ACTH secretion by a nonpituitary tumour or by food-dependent hypercortisolaemia are rare.[29,30]

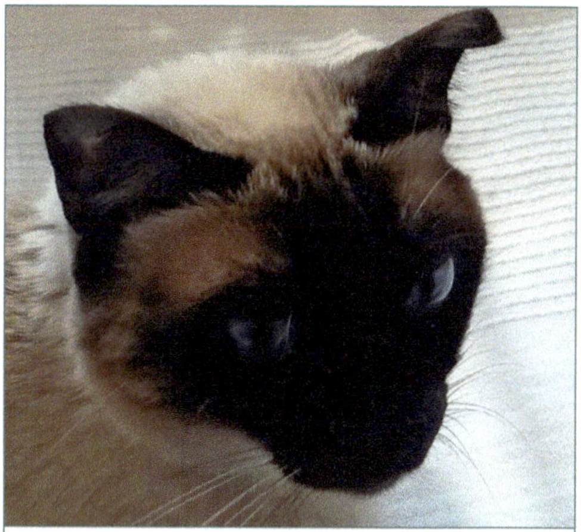

Figure 8. Mixed-breed cat (Siamese cross) with the ears folded forward, a typical sign of HAC in this species. The cat had received several injections of methylprednisolone acetate to control inflammatory bowel disease, resulting in iatrogenic HAC.

Feline HAC

Feline HAC is much less common than the canine form, and usually affects cats that are slightly older than dogs with HAC: the mean age at diagnosis reported in one study was 10 years.[31] In terms of the origin of endogenous HAC, 80 % of cases are due to pituitary tumours and 20 % due to adrenal tumours.[31] Most cases (pituitary and adrenal) are due to adenomas, while carcinomas are very rare in both locations.[31]

Diagnosis

History and physical examination

The clinical signs most commonly reported by owners of dogs or cats with HAC are PU/PD and polyphagia.[28,31,32] Other clinical signs such as panting or weight gain are typical in dogs,[28] while abdominal distension and skin atrophy are more common in cats (Box 3).[31]

Box 3. MOST COMMON CLINICAL SIGNS IN PATIENTS WITH HAC.[28,31]

In dogs:

- PU/PD (90 %)
- Polyphagia
- Panting
- Abdominal distension
- Alopecia
- Hepatomegaly
- Muscle weakness
- Systemic hypertension

In cats:

- PU/PD (81 %)
- Abdominal distension
- Polyphagia
- Skin atrophy
- Loss of muscle mass
- Weight loss
- Lethargy
- Alopecia

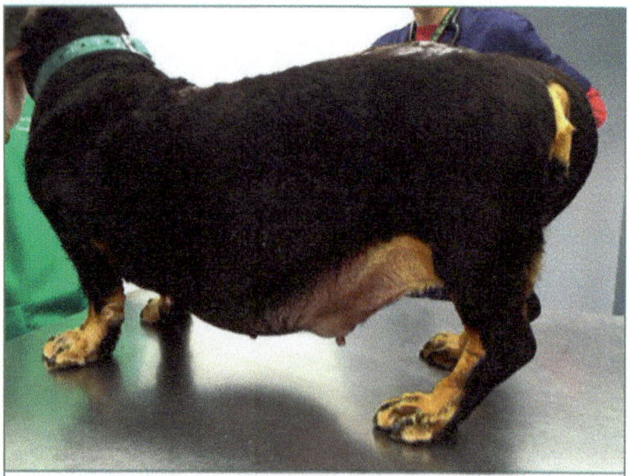

Figure 9. Mixed-breed dog (Dachshund cross) with the typical pendulous abdomen characteristic of patients with hyperadrenocorticism. This patient also had dermal lesions on the back (barely visible in this image). Image courtesy of Eliseo A. Zuriaga, Anicura Valencia Sur Veterinary Hospital, Silla (Valencia, Spain); Global Veterinary Hospital, Puerto de Sagunto (Valencia, Spain).

A distended abdomen is one of the characteristic findings in the physical examination of dogs with HAC (Fig. 9), and probably occurs due to loss of abdominal muscle tone, hepatomegaly, accumulation of fat in the abdomen (due to a redistribution of stored fat in the body), and distension of the urinary bladder. Skin abnormalities include endocrine alopecia (bilateral, symmetric) (Fig. 10), thinning of the skin, pyoderma, comedones and, less commonly, hyperpigmentation and calcinosis cutis (Fig. 11). In some patients with pituitary macroadenomas, altered mental status or even stupor may be observed.[28,33]

Due to a lower prevalence of HAC in cats (in which slightly less than 200 cases are described in the literature between 1973 and 2015), the clinical picture can vary slightly between individuals. Nonetheless, PU/PD, abdominal distension, polyphagia, and skin atrophy can be expected in cats with HAC. Weight loss, commonly associated with a loss of muscle mass, is a characteristic clinical sign in cats, but not dogs, with HAC.[31]

Laboratory diagnosis

In dogs and cats with suspected HAC, it is important to request and perform, to the extent possible, basic blood tests including a complete blood count, a biochemical workup including electrolytes, determination of fructosamine, and, in cats (which are usually already over 10 years of age), total T_4 levels. Urinalysis should also be performed, including a urine test strip, determination of urine specific gravity, a urine sediment test, urinary culture, and measurement of the UPC.

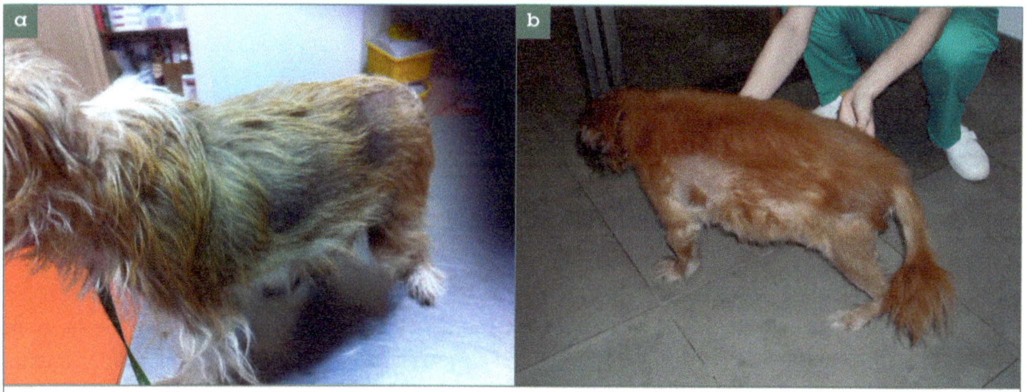

Figure 10. Typical endocrine alopecia pattern in two dogs with HAC. Images courtesy of Eliseo A. Zuriaga, Anicura Valencia Sur Veterinary Hospital, Silla (Valencia, Spain); Global Veterinary Hospital, Puerto de Sagunto (Valencia, Spain).

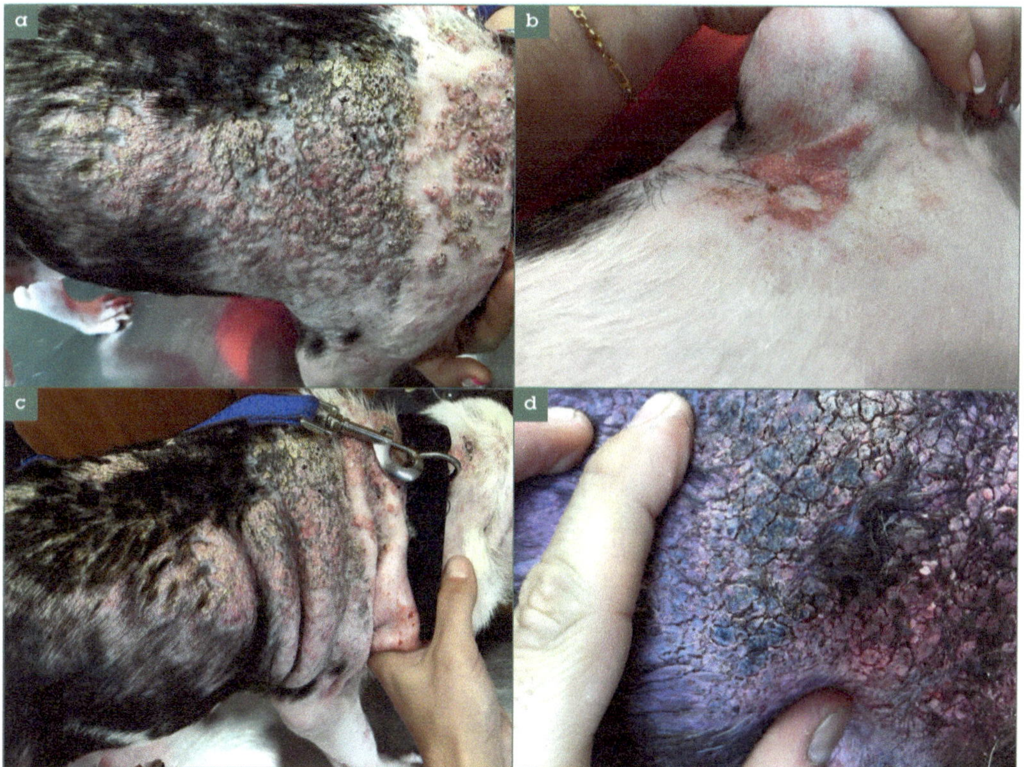

Figure 11. Calcinosis cutis in a dog with HAC, a consequence of not diagnosing and treating the initial skin lesions in time. Images courtesy of Eliseo A. Zuriaga, Anicura Valencia Sur Veterinary Hospital, Silla (Valencia, Spain); Global Veterinary Hospital, Puerto de Sagunto (Valencia, Spain).

In dogs with HAC, findings include a stress leukogram (with mature neutrophilia, lymphopenia, eosinopenia, and monocytosis), thrombocytosis, and, less frequently, mild erythrocytosis. The biochemistry profile of these patients reveals an increase in alkaline phosphatase in more than 85 % of cases, in some cases accompanied by a moderate increase in ALT, fasting hyperglycaemia (due to insulin resistance), hyperlipidaemia, and low levels of urea and phosphorus in the blood (probably due to PU/PD). Finally, urinalysis usually reveals a urine specific gravity <1,020, although this parameter can vary considerably between individual cases. Urinary tract infections at the time of diagnosis are common, affecting 40–50 % of dogs with HAC.[34] It should be noted that these canine patients do not usually present with pyuria, stranguria, or haematuria due to the anti-inflammatory effect of steroid hormones.[28,32,35]

In cats with HAC a stress leukogram is also observed, although monocytosis is not a consistent finding in this species. Of all biochemical findings, only hyperglycaemia is common (80 %) in cats with HAC. Only 30 % show a slight increase in ALT, and, given that cats lack the corticosteroid-induced isoenzyme alkaline phosphatase, only 24 % show slight increases in this parameter. Another difference with respect to dogs is that in 30 % of feline HAC cases blood urea (BUN) is increased, probably due to dehydration or underlying kidney disease. In most cats with suspected HAC, urinary analysis reveals a urine specific gravity >1,020, although this can be because many cats with HAC are glycosuric and have concomitant DM.[31]

Definitive diagnosis

In both dogs and cats definitive diagnosis is based on the presence of clinical signs and laboratory findings compatible with HAC (after ruling out exogenous administration of products with a steroidal effect) and the results of adrenal function tests. These tests are usually divided into screening tests and differentiation tests. The objective of the former is to confirm or rule out the presence of elevated blood cortisol levels, while the objective of the latter is to determine whether hypercortisolaemia is due to a pituitary, adrenal, or iatrogenic problem. If HAC is suspected but screening tests do not yield compatible results, it is advisable to screen again 1–3 months later using a different type of screening test, especially if clinical signs persist over time.

Next, we will describe the different screening tests and how to interpret the results obtained. Tables 2 and 3 provide a summary of how to perform each of these tests.

Screening tests

- **Low-dose dexamethasone suppression (LDDS):**
  - Explanation: demonstrates decreased pituitary sensitivity to negative feedback from glucocorticoids.
  - Indications: most authors and consulted sources consider the LDDS the test of choice for diagnosis of HAC, unless iatrogenic HAC is suspected, in which case ACTH stimulation is preferred.
  - Interpretation of the test: diagnosis of HAC is confirmed if no inhibition of cortisol secretion occurs 8 hours after dexamethasone administration.
  - Sensitivity and specificity: 85–100 % and 44–73 %, respectively (varies by study).

TAKE NOTE!

The clinician should take into account that the dose of dexamethasone used in LDDS is 10 times higher in cats than in dogs. Currently, this test is considered the most appropriate to initially diagnose HAC in cats.[31]

- **ACTH stimulation:**
  - Explanation: measures the adrenocortical reserve, i.e. the amount of cortisol contained in the adrenal glands. Due to its higher purity and better quality control, use of synthetic ACTH is recommended.
  - Indications: this is the best test for diagnosis of iatrogenic HAC and spontaneous Addison's disease (hypoadrenocorticism).
  - Interpretation of the test: diagnosis of HAC is confirmed if cortisol levels are elevated after ACTH administration (based on the reference range established by the laboratory).
  - Sensitivity and specificity: varies depending on the study consulted. The sensitivity of this test for the diagnosis of all forms of spontaneous canine HAC ranges from 57 to 95 %. In dogs with pituitary HAC, the sensitivity is around 80 %, while specificity ranges from 59 to 93 %.

TAKE NOTE!

Although ACTH stimulation is less effective in diagnosing spontaneous HAC, this test is still widely used because it requires less time to perform and its initially low sensitivity can be improved following interpretation of the patient's history and physical examination and with a thorough ultrasound examination of the adrenal glands.

TAKE NOTE!

Due to its low sensitivity and moderate specificity, ACTH stimulation is not a good initial screening test for spontaneous HAC in cats.[19]

- **Urine cortisol:creatinine ratio (UCCR):**
  - Explanation: provides an overall readout of cortisol production, adjusted for fluctuations in blood concentrations. Baseline UCCR can be measured alone or with other endocrine tests.
  - Indications: can be used to detect hypercortisolaemia, although the clinician should not overestimate the diagnostic power of a single positive result. The LDDS test can be combined with UCCR tests to potentially demonstrate both increased cortisol production and decreased sensitivity to glucocorticoid feedback.

- Sensitivity and specificity: this test is very easy to perform and has high sensitivity. When a single urine sample is collected randomly, sensitivity and specificity for the diagnosis of HAC are 75–100 % and 20–25 %, respectively.[36,37] One study reported that this test has great intra-individual variability; however, in patients that had physical examination findings and laboratory results compatible with HAC, and had two baseline UCCR measurements above the cut-off value, sensitivity and specificity increased to 99 % and 77 %, respectively.[38]

TIP

UCCR has good sensitivity but low specificity in cats, and therefore can be used as a simple test to screen patients with suspected HAC.[89]

Table 2. Tests for the screening of patients with suspected HAC.

Test	Active substance used	Procedure
LDDS	Dexamethasone (sodium phosphate): • Dogs: 0.01 mg/kg IV • Cats: 0.1 mg/kg IV	Blood samples are collected: • Before administration • 4 hours after administration • 8 hours after administration
ACTH stimulation	Tetracosactide: 5 µg/kg IV or IM, in both dogs and cats. For cats, there is also a dose of 125 µg/cat. In cats, the cortisol peak occurs at 60 minutes (IV route) or 45 minutes (IM route).	Blood samples are collected: • Before administration • 60 minutes after administration
UCCR	-	2–3 urine samples are collected at home (spontaneous urination) several days after the visit to avoid the effect of stress. Samples must be taken in the morning and on consecutive days.

Author's note: during the LDDS and ACTH stimulation tests it is best to keep the patient fasting, although the effect of food ingestion on test outcomes is unknown. Prior fasting is not necessary, unless lipaemia interferes with reading of the test results.

Differentiation tests (pituitary versus adrenal HAC)

The clinician must understand that while it is useful to know whether or not a patient has HAC, it is essential to reach the end of the diagnostic path and determine whether the patient has pituitary or adrenal HAC, since the treatment options and, above all, the prognosis will be different. To determine which form of HAC we are dealing with, the differentiation tests described below are used.

- **Determination of endogenous ACTH:**
  - Explanation: canine ACTH (cACTH) is a pituitary hormone secreted in pulses in healthy dogs and those with pituitary HAC.
  - Indications: cACTH concentrations do not differ between healthy dogs and those with pituitary HAC, and therefore measurement of this parameter is not useful for the diagnosis of HAC. Nonetheless, cACTH measurement is the most accurate independent biochemical test to differentiate pituitary from adrenal HAC. A normal or high concentration of cACTH is compatible with pituitary HAC, while a low or undetectable value is compatible with adrenal HAC.
  - Sensitivity and specificity: this test has a low sensitivity, although this depends on the determination method used. A two-site solid-phase immunochemiluminescent method is currently recommended, and shows excellent discrimination between pituitary and adrenal HAC.[39] This test can give lower than expected values in patients with pituitary HAC due to the pulsatile secretion of ACTH in dogs, and degradation of this hormone by proteases present in plasma can be a problem if the sample is not handled correctly. Due to problems with the methods used and the lack of validation in cats, this test is not considered adequate for this species.
- **High-dose dexamethasone suppression (HDDS):**
  - Explanation and indications: if dexamethasone is administered to a healthy dog, it will cause rapid and moderately prolonged suppression of cortisol secretion. Cortisol production is not suppressed in a patient with adrenal HAC and is suppressed inadequately at low doses (0.01 mg/kg) in patients with pituitary HAC. In 75 % of dogs with pituitary HAC the secretion of both cortisol and ACTH is suppressed at high doses (0.1 mg/kg). In the other 25 % (not suppressed at high doses), the most likely cause is a macroadenoma.[40,41] In dogs that show no cortisol suppression in response to low-dose dexamethasone, determination of cACTH rather than HDDS is recommended to differentiate pituitary from adrenal HAC: although suppression in response to dexamethasone supports a diagnosis of pituitary HAC, a dog with resistance to high-dose dexamethasone may have either adrenal or pituitary HAC. This test is rarely used in cats, in which it can distinguish the origin of HAC in only 50 % of cases.

TAKE NOTE!

For HDDS in cats, dexamethasone is administered at a dose of 1 mg/kg. The test is performed the same way. However, only in 40–50 % of cats with pituitary HAC is cortisol secretion suppressed by at least 50 %.[90]

Table 3. Differentiation tests in patients with HAC.

Test	Active substance used	Procedure
HDDS*	Dexamethasone (sodium phosphate): • Dogs: 0.1 mg/kg IV • Cats: 1 mg/kg IV	Blood samples are collected: • Before administration • 4 hours after administration • 8 hours after administration
Determination of endogenous ACTH (only recommended in dogs)	-	1. A blood sample is obtained and placed in a tube with EDTA. 2. The tube is centrifuged for 15 minutes (ideally in a refrigerated centrifuge). 3. The EDTA plasma sample is transferred to dry plastic tubes and frozen. 4. The samples are kept frozen until the reading is taken.

* HDDS is performed when HAC has been demonstrated using LDDS.

TIP

In cats, the dexamethasone suppression and ACTH stimulation tests are best used to diagnose HAC. In cats with HAC, there is inadequate dexamethasone suppression and an exaggerated response after ACTH stimulation (1–2 hours after administration). To diagnose iatrogenic HAC it is generally sufficient to stimulate with ACTH.

Diagnostic imaging

A large number of imaging tests can be used to establish diagnosis in patients with suspected HAC. This is because this endocrinopathy produces a plethora of clinical signs, and therefore almost any imaging modality will yield useful data that can be borne in mind when establishing diagnosis, treatment, and even prognosis.

Radiography

Although perhaps considered old-fashioned, radiography, especially thoracic radiography, provides relevant information with minimum investment of time and money. When HAC is suspected in a patient and radiography is performed, the clinician should check for the following:

- Mineralisation of the trachea and main bronchi.
- Lung lesions compatible with metastasis (possible in patients with adrenal HAC).
- Hepatomegaly (detected in 80–90 % of dogs with HAC).
- Adrenal calcification (detected in 50 % of dogs with HAC). This finding is unimportant in geriatric cats.
- Presence and location of calcium oxalate uroliths throughout the entire urinary system.
- Pulmonary embolism. Chest radiography can aid diagnosis of this disease, although it is rare in dogs and even more so in cats.

Abdominal ultrasound

Many authors use this diagnostic imaging technique to differentiate between pituitary and adrenal HAC. This is because in adrenal HAC one of the adrenal glands usually presents a mass that causes an increase in the size of the gland and loss of its normal shape. The contralateral adrenal gland is usually of normal size, or smaller due to atrophy. However, in pituitary HAC symmetric bilateral adrenal hyperplasia is usually detected, with normal or slightly enlarged glands.

One of the advantages of diagnosing adrenal masses by ultrasound is being able to discern whether they cause vascular invasion, based on which a future adrenalectomy can be scheduled if necessary. Furthermore, this technique can detect metastases in abdominal organs.

Advanced imaging techniques

Magnetic resonance imaging (MRI) and computed tomography (CT) are two of the modalities used to visualise the pituitary gland in patients with suspected HAC. They are used to reveal the presence of pituitary tumours. MRI is usually recommended, as it is more sensitive than CT for the detection of these tumours. CT does not typically detect pituitary tumours smaller than 1 cm.

Both techniques can be used to assess the presence of adrenal tumours and detect metastasis in other organs, as well as vascular invasion.

The fact that both techniques require anaesthesia means that they are not first-choice techniques for the diagnosis of HAC, and are only used when other tests fail to demonstrate the presence of the disease. However, there are two occasions when these tests are necessary: in the case of neurological clinical signs compatible with a pituitary macroadenoma; and when programming hypophysectomy or pituitary radiotherapy.

Treatment

There are various treatment options depending on the origin of the HAC. Nonetheless, certain guidelines must be followed in the vast majority of cases, as follows:

- Treatment of HAC should only be considered once diagnosis has been established with complete certainty. For this reason, therapeutic tests for this diagnosis are discouraged.
- Not all patients with HAC should be treated immediately. Some patients without obvious clinical signs or with mild clinical signs, such as increased alkaline phosphatase, hepatomegaly, or even mild alopecia, do not require treatment. In other words, the pros of the treatment do not outweigh the cons. Rather, patients that should be treated are those with very marked PU/PD, severe dermatologic manifestations, or recurrent infections. Patients with hypertension or proteinuria should be treated for HAC, and may also require specific treatment to reduce blood pressure or the degree of proteinuria.

Medical treatment

Medical treatment is the most commonly used approach in dogs and cats with pituitary HAC. Furthermore, it can be used in patients with adrenal HAC if adrenalectomy is not possible due to vascular invasion by the tumour, metastasis, or excessive cost. The active ingredients most commonly used are trilostane and mitotane. Both have similar efficacy for the treatment of pituitary and adrenal HAC. Let's delve a little further into the characteristics of these two drugs:

- **Trilostane** is a competitive inhibitor of 3β-hydroxysteroid dehydrogenase. This enzyme converts pregnenolone and 17α-OH-pregnenolone into progesterone and 17α-OH-progesterone, respectively. The drug disruptors) stimulate the growth of this subpopulation of thyrocytes. Although not all these factors have been identified to date, those that appear to contribute to the development of FHT include: dietary causes (alterations in dietary iodine content, fish); the presence of endocrine disruptors such as bisphenol A (BPA) and other polychlorinated biphenyls (PCBs); lifestyle; and flame retardants used in furniture.[52–55] Table 4 shows some of the causes of FHT.

Diagnosis

History and physical examination

Most cats with FHT are over 10 years old,[53,56] although this endocrinopathy has also been described in younger cats.[57]

Although none of the clinical signs of FHT are pathognomonic, the most notable is marked weight loss despite polyphagia and hyperactivity. Some patients also show clinical signs related to impaired digestion and cardiac dysfunction caused by myocardial hypertrophy (Fig. 12), and even congestive heart failure in severe cases. These signs manifest in the form of apathetic FHT, in which appetite and activity are decreased.[50,58]

Hyperthyroid cats are often more irritable than normal and less tolerant of stressful situations, and easily pant or show signs of tachypnoea. A more aggressive or youthful character is observed in some cases. Meowing or increased vocalisations, especially at night, are also commonly reported at the time of diagnosis by owners of cats with FHT. Muscle weakness may be evident (and severe in some cases), and can be exacerbated in cats with hypokalaemia.

Some cats can develop a hyperthyroid crisis (also known as a thyroid storm in human medicine). This is an acute manifestation of thyrotoxicosis, with high mortality, characterised by altered mental status (ranging from agitation to coma), cardiovascular signs, and multiple organ dysfunction syndrome, without the characteristic hyperthermia described in humans.[59,60]

The frequency of PU/PD in cats diagnosed with FHT has changed over time. This suggests that cats with FHT do not present PU/PD until advanced disease stages or when there is concomitant chronic kidney disease. By increasing the glomerular filtration rate, FHT causes a decrease in the levels of kidney markers in the blood, and therefore FHT can sometimes mask chronic kidney disease: the true cause of PU/PD can only be established after treatment.[61–63]

Careful palpation of the thyroid gland is of great importance in the diagnosis of FHT. Two techniques are used, both of which detect the presence of a thyroid nodule with comparable efficacy: the classic technique (Fig. 13) and the Norsworthy technique.[65]

Finally, cardiac abnormalities associated with FHT include tachycardia, murmur, arrhythmias, and the presence of a gallop rhythm. Some hyperthyroid cats develop congestive heart failure or even aortic thromboembolism.[66]

Table 5 shows the most frequent clinical signs in cats with FHT.

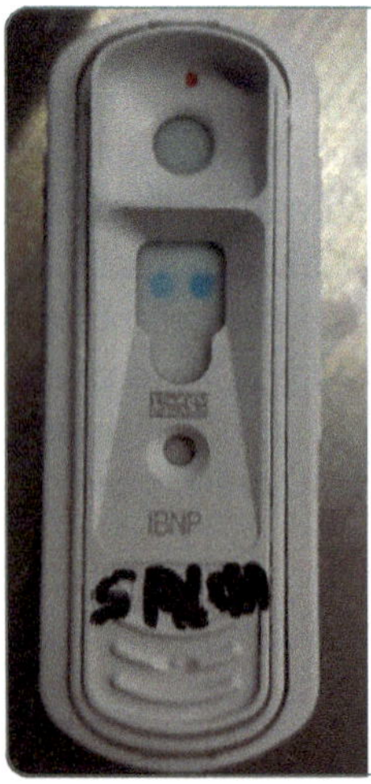

Figure 12. Rapid test for determination of feline brain natriuretic peptide (proBNP). The blue circle on the right (sample) is more evident than that on the left (control), implying a positive result, which indicates myocardial distress, in this case in a 22-year-old cat with concomitant arterial hypertension.

Table 4. Causes of FHT.

Cause	Mechanism of action	Effect	Location
Iodine deficiency	Deficiency in iodine, which is necessary for the synthesis of thyroid hormones	Decreased synthesis of T_4 and T_3 Increase in TSH levels	Thyroid gland
Soy isoflavones **Herbicides** **Methimazole (thiamazole)**	Inhibition of thyroid peroxidase in the follicles	Decreased synthesis of T_4 and T_3 Increase in TSH levels	Thyroid gland
PCBs **Flame retardants** **Phthalates**	Competitive binding to thyroid hormone transporter protein	Decreased availability of thyroid hormones in the brain	Circulatory system
Polybrominated diphenyl ethers (PBDEs)	Alteration of membrane transport	Increased biliary elimination of thyroid hormones	Liver
Erythrosine (dye) **PCB** **Selenium deficiency**	Inhibition of deiodinase activity	Decreased peripheral synthesis of T_3	Kidney and liver
Phthalates **Polybrominated diphenyl ethers (PBDEs)** **PCB**	T_3 receptor antagonism	Altered binding of T_3 to its receptor	Brain Pituitary gland Peripheral tissues
Pesticides **PCB**	Inhibition of the TSH receptor	Decreased synthesis of T_4 and T_3	Pituitary gland

Adapted from Feldman EC, Fracassi F, Peterson ME, eds. *Feline Endocrinology*, Milan, Edra, 2019.

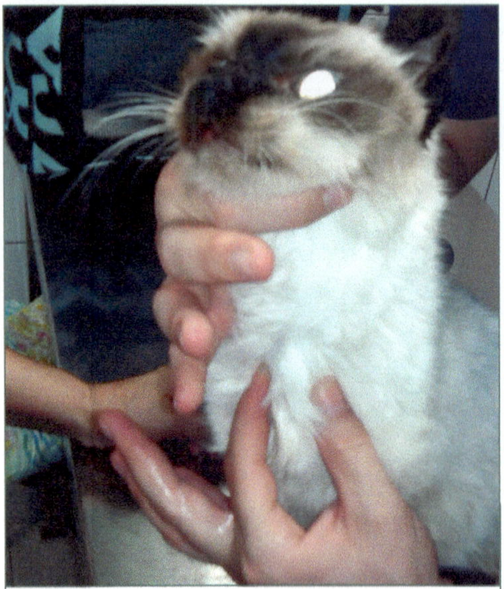

Figure 13. The photograph shows the correct posture for detecting thyroid nodules using the classic technique, placing the thumb and forefinger on either side of the trachea. In the Norsworthy technique the index finger of each hand is placed on either side of the trachea.

Table 5. Clinical signs of FHT.[64]

Clinical sign	Frequency (%)
Palpable thyroid nodule	98
Loss of muscle mass	77
Thinness	35
Tachycardia (>240 bpm)	31
Heart murmur	29

Laboratory diagnosis

The laboratory diagnosis of a cat with suspected FHT is based on the combination of blood test results (complete blood count and serum biochemistry with determination of ions, fructosamine, and total T_4) and urinalysis findings. Table 6 summarises the most frequent findings in blood and urine analyses in FHT.

Diagnosis of FHT is straightforward when high total T_4 levels are detected in serum or plasma. Increased total T_4 levels are observed in 90–95 % of cases. In the remaining 10 % levels of this hormone remain within the normal range, although often in the upper half of this range. Measurement of T_3 is of no diagnostic benefit in cats with FHT. In fact, measurement of this parameter can result in false negatives, as up to a third of the cats with FHT have normal T_3 values.

Measurement of free T_4 levels was considered an ideal solution for the diagnosis of FHT in cats with total serum T_4 levels within the normal range. However, it has since been observed that 10–30 % of healthy cats may have high levels of free T_4. In fact, measurement of free T_4 for the diagnosis of FHT is more sensitive but less specific than measurement of total T_4. Thus, the current recommendation is to measure free T_4 in cats with clinical signs compatible with FHT and total T_4 values in the upper half of the normal range. It is not advisable to measure free T_4 without simultaneously measuring total T_4.[68] Until recently it was considered essential to use equilibrium dialysis to determine levels of free T_4. However, it has been recently discovered that other immunoassays constitute reliable alternatives.

TSH determination is one tool to consider in the diagnosis of FHT. Currently, we measure the canine (cTSH) rather than the feline (fTSH) form, due to greater availability in laboratories, lower cost, and a (relatively) good correlation with fTSH, although it is known that this approach detects only 35 % of fTSH. The TSH concentration is practically undetectable in cats with FHT, whereas this occurs in only 10 % of healthy cats.[23]

Table 7 summarises the interpretation of thyroid hormone levels in euthyroid and hyperthyroid cats.

Table 6. Summary of the most frequent blood count, serum biochemistry, and urinalysis findings in cats with FHT.[67]

Alteration	Frequency	Comments
Polycythaemia and macrocytosis	<50 %	Usually mild to moderate and without clinical consequences.
Leukocytosis, neutrophilia, lymphopenia, and eosinopenia	Frequent	Reflection of the stress response.
Lymphocytosis and eosinophilia	Rare	Due to cortisol deficiency induced by hyperthyroidism.
Increased liver enzyme levels	>90 %	Most significant finding in biochemical workup. Enzyme activity values increase or decrease as T_4 levels do.
Hyperphosphataemia	Up to 40 %	Unknown origin.
Ionised hypocalcaemia	Up to 50 %	Unknown origin.
Azotaemia	2–10 %	Mild to moderate. Preexisting chronic kidney disease. Negatively affects the prognosis.
Hyperglycaemia	Sometimes	Usually due to stress. Decreases sensitivity to insulin.
Hypokalaemia	Rare	Should be taken into account, especially in the presence of muscle weakness.
Increased SDMA	10 %	Marker of possible occult chronic kidney disease. Subsequent azotaemia upon reestablishment of euthyroidism.
Hypocobalaminaemia	40 %	Does not usually require supplementation.
Increase in β-hydroxybutyrate levels	20 %	Reflects the catabolic state of hyperthyroidism.
Decreased urine specific gravity	Variable	If <1,035, may indicate increased risk of posttreatment azotaemia.
Proteinuria	Frequent	Moderate.
Urinary tract infection	12 %	Can occur in the absence of clinical signs.

Table 7. Interpretation of thyroid hormone levels in cats.[67]

Status	Total T_3	Total T_4	Free T_4	TSH
Euthyroid				
Healthy	RV	RV	RV	RV or ↓
Nonthyroid disease	↓ or RV	↓ or RV	RV, ↓ or ↑	RV or ↓
Hyperthyroid				
Subclinical	RV	RV	RV	↓
Mild	RV	RV or ↑	RV or ↑	↓ or RV
Moderate with nonthyroid disease	RV	RV or ↑	↑	↓ or RV
Moderate-severe	↑	↑	↑	↓ or RV

RV, reference value.

Diagnostic imaging

Thyroid scintigraphy is the most valuable imaging tool for the diagnosis of FHT. It allows evaluation of the size, location, and functionality of thyroid tissue, and is considered the gold standard for diagnosis of FHT (Fig. 15). Scintigraphy consists of the injection of pertechnetate (^{99m}Tc), a radioactive isotope, and comparison of its uptake by the thyroid gland versus the salivary glands (T:S ratio). Some experts, such as M. E. Peterson in the United States and P. Xifra in Spain, use the pertechnetate technique to calculate the dose of radioactive iodine (^{131}I) required by each patient and thereby individualise the treatment dose.[69]

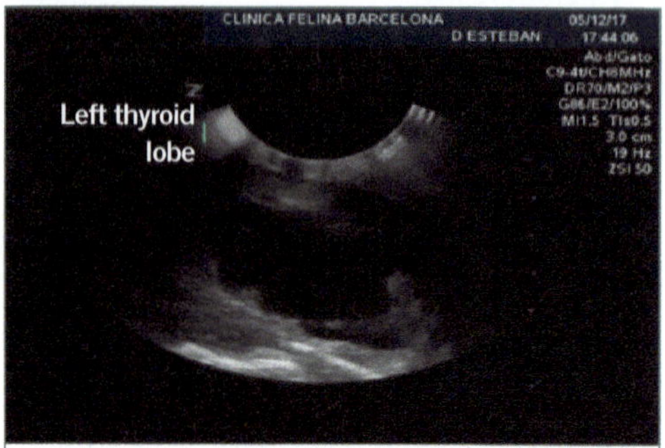

Figure 14. Ultrasound of a thyroid nodule. Although not used much, it can be interesting to perform an ultrasound of a thyroid nodule for the sake of orientation in cases involving a large cervical mass. Image courtesy of Diego Esteban, Clínica Felina Barcelona (Spain).

Treatment

FHT can be treated in several ways, although there are four main approaches: medical, dietetic, surgical, and radioactive iodine (^{131}I) treatment. Each approach has both advantages and disadvantages (Table 8). The first two are reversible but only palliative, while the last two can be curative but are irreversible. When dealing with FHT caused by a malignant transformation of the thyroid gland (thyroid carcinoma), curative treatments should be the only ones considered.

When recommending one treatment or another, two main factors should be taken into account: **concurrent illnesses** and the **owner's preferences**.

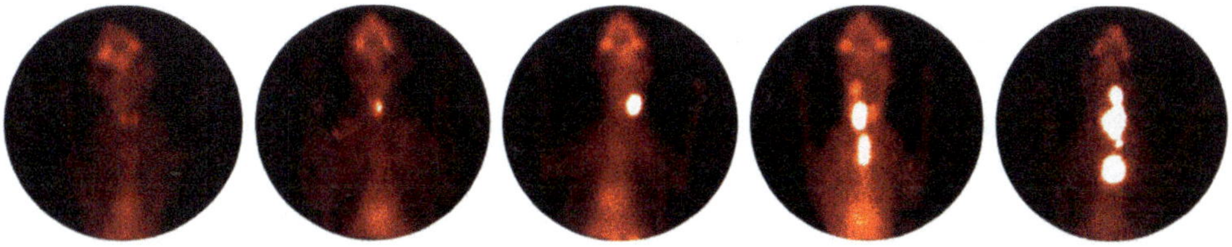

Figure 15. Images obtained by scintigraphy in different cats. Images show a normal thyroid gland and thyroid masses ranging from small to giant. Images courtesy of Iodocat, Pilar Xifra.

Among the concurrent diseases:

- **Chronic kidney disease** is the most common concurrent condition that will affect the treatment of FHT. The clinician should consider FHT as a nephrotoxic state. Traditionally, it is recommended to start medical treatment with methimazole or carbimazole for 30 days and reassess both kidney function and total T_4 levels, which allows assessment of the risk of applying a definitive treatment. Currently, in cats with stable IRIS stage 2 or 3 chronic kidney disease there are no contraindications to definitive treatment.
- **Liver disease** in cats with FHT can be a real challenge for the clinician, who will find it very difficult to determine at the time of diagnosis whether increases in transaminases are due to FHT or concurrent liver disease. In these cases, it is recommended to begin nondefinitive treatment with carbimazole or methimazole: this will allow us to clarify this doubt and determine the appropriate next step. In addition, the clinician must remember that drugs to control FHT can cause hepatotoxicity in cats.
- **Cardiomyopathies** are another group of diseases that make surgical treatment or iodotherapy less advisable, as they increase the associated risk. Nowadays it is considered uncommon to observe **arterial hypertension** associated with FHT before starting treatment. However, it can be caused by both chronic kidney disease and cardiomyopathy if either are present or develop due to FHT. Therefore, blood pressure should be monitored in all patients with FHT.[70]

Regarding the owner's preferences, we must take into account the reluctance of many owners to hospitalise their cat for a long period of time, the cost of definitive treatments, and difficulties administering medication. Some centres use lower doses of ^{131}I (2–3 mCi) to reduce hospitalisation time to less than 1 week. The costs of iodotherapy are similar to those of long-term control with medical treatment (€2,000–€3,000). There are products available with excellent palatability and ease of administration.

Medical treatment

Medical treatment can be considered in the short term, in order to stabilise the patient before a thyroidectomy or before treatment with radioactive iodine, or in the long term. The advantage of chronic treatment is that surgical anaesthesia can be avoided, and no specialised facilities or permits are required.

Unfortunately, this type of treatment does not stop the growth of thyroid adenomas because it lacks cytotoxic activity, and over time up to 20 % of these adenomas can transform into carcinomas.[72] For this reason, it is not considered the best possible treatment.

There are two active principles of the thioamide family that help restore euthyroidism in cats:

- **Methimazole.** Also known as thiamazole. Currently, there are different formulations authorised for the treatment of FHT, sold in tablet form and as oral solutions. After administration, the drug accumulates inside the thyroid gland and inhibits thyroid peroxidase and

Table 8. Pros and cons of the different therapeutic measures for FHT.[71]

Factor	Medical treatment	Low-iodine diet	Thyroidectomy	Radioactive iodine (^{131}I)
Initial cost	Low	Low	High	High
Total cost	Moderate	Moderate	Low	Low
Requirements	None	Cat without outdoor access Exclusive diet	Surgeon's experience	Specialised facilities for handling radioactive substances
Ease for the owner	Medium in case of tablets, easy in case of liquid/transdermal	Easy	Easy, except for the hospital stay	Easy, except for hospitalisation and radiation protection measures
Anaesthesia	No	No	Always	Yes, if prior scintigraphy is performed
Time to euthyroidism	2–4 weeks	6–8 weeks	24–48 h	Days or weeks
Hospitalisation	No	No	1–3 days	3 days to 4 weeks, depending on relevant legislation
Hypocalcaemia	No	No	Frequent	No
Limitations	Daily medication Adverse effects Iatrogenic hypothyroidism	Poor palatability Persistent hyperthyroidism in some cats	Recurrence in case of unilateral thyroidectomy Iatrogenic hypothyroidism	Iatrogenic hypothyroidism Persistent hyperthyroidism

consequent formation of thyroid hormones. Notably, it does not inhibit iodine uptake or the secretion of preformed thyroid hormones. There is also the option of administering methimazole transdermally with an ointment consisting of pluronic acid and lecithin. This route provides demonstrated absorption, and may be helpful in some cats when treatment cannot be administered otherwise. However, methimazole ointment is not as effective as oral methimazole, and blood tests are required to confirm its effect.[73]

- **Carbimazole.** Carbimazole is sold for the treatment of FHT in the form of tablets and slow-release tablets. This drug, once administered orally, is metabolised to methimazole (5 mg of carbimazole is equivalent to 3 mg of methimazole).[74] The slow-release tablet formulation allows administration every 24 hours. The main advantage of carbimazole is palatability, as it lacks the bitter taste of methimazole.

The recommended starting dose of methimazole is 2.5 mg/cat every 12 hours, and some cats can be controlled with 0.625–1.25 mg daily.[75] For carbimazole, the recommended dose is 5 mg every 12 hours,[76] or, in the case of the slow-release formulation, 15 mg every 24 hours. The first checkup is scheduled for 2–4 weeks to check if euthyroidism has been restored.

Until total T_4 levels are restored to the middle of the reference range, checks should be performed every 2–3 weeks and the dose increased or decreased as necessary in increments or decrements of 1.25–5 mg. The time that elapses between administration of the medication and sample collection has no bearing on monitoring.[56]

As time passes, the thyroid nodule (or nodules) increases in size, requiring a corresponding increase in the dose of methimazole or carbimazole.[72]

Table 9 lists the adverse effects of thioamide administration in cats and their frequency of appearance. Some of the adverse effects, including gastrointestinal signs, are temporary and disappear without needing to withdraw the medication. Others, such as facial excoriations, appear during the first weeks, while liver disease and blood dyscrasia appear in the medium or long term.[78]

Table 9. Adverse effects of thioamides in cats.[77]

Adverse effect	Oral methimazole	Transdermal methimazole	Oral carbimazole
Gastrointestinal signs, lethargy	23 %	3.7 %	33 %
Mild haematological abnormalities (leukopenia, eosinophilia, lymphocytosis)	16.4 %	-	34.9 %
Excoriations of the face, itching	4 %	8 %	11.6 %
Generalised peripheral lymphadenopathy	Few cases	-	-
Liver disease	2.6 %	4 %	-
Haemorrhagic diathesis (epistaxis, oral bleeding, increased PIVKA)	2.5 %	-	-
Severe thrombocytopenia (<75,000/µl)	2.8 %	8 %	-
Agranulocytosis and neutropenia (severe leukopenia, granulocytes <500/µl)	2.7 %	6.1 %	-
Myasthenia gravis	Few cases	Single case	-
Anaemia	Few cases	-	-

PIVKA, proteins induced by absence or antagonism of vitamin K.

Surgical treatment

The first and perhaps most important issue before performing a thyroidectomy is to stabilise the patient so that the surgery, and above all anaesthesia, does not pose an insurmountable challenge. After a period of stabilisation and euthyroidism, anaesthesia of the cat should be possible without any greater risk relative to other cats of the same age. In patients with hyperthyroid cardiomyopathy it may take several months, and several echocardiograms, to resolve the cardiac lesions caused by thyrotoxicosis. Before surgery, it is recommended to treat with thioamides and beta-blockers (atenolol) if necessary, to reduce the surgical risk.

To plan the intervention, it is necessary to know whether the disease is uni- or bilateral (70 % of cases are bilateral). If the owner's budget and the patient's cardiovascular status allow it, prior scintigraphy can be performed to detect hyperfunctional lobes and the presence of ectopic foci, which, if present, could affect the outcome.

Two surgical techniques are used: extracapsular (Fig. 16) and intracapsular thyroidectomy. In both cases, the goal is to remove all abnormal thyroid tissue while preserving the parathyroid glands. Postoperative complications include hypoparathyroidism and associated hypocalcaemia, laryngeal paralysis, and Horner's syndrome.[79]

The hypocalcaemia that accompanies hypoparathyroidism usually appears between 1 and 3 days after bilateral thyroidectomy, and is mild in most cases (total calcium, 6.5–7.5 mg/dl). As such, supplementation is not necessary in the

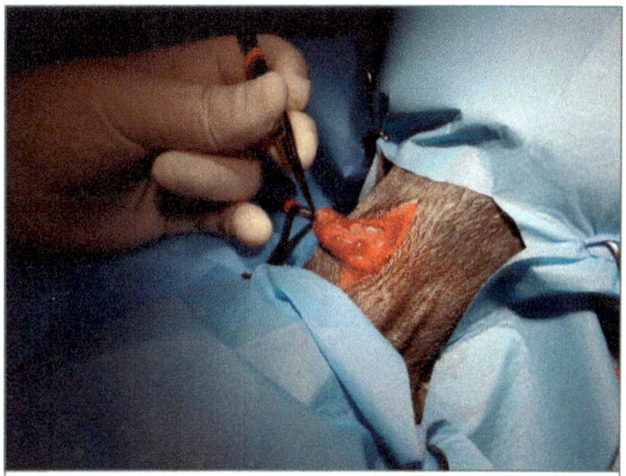

Figure 16. Intraoperative image of an extracapsular thyroidectomy in a cat with unilateral involvement of the thyroid gland.

absence of tremors, tetany, or seizures. If any of these signs are observed, calcium gluconate and vitamin D should be administered.

Hypothyroidism resulting from thyroidectomy, if it occurs, is usually temporary (2–3 months), and requires treatment only if the patient shows lethargy and worsening of azotaemia. This point is of vital importance: as previously stated, hyperthyroidism is considered a nephrotoxic state, but sustained hypothyroidism should also be considered a cause of kidney damage. In the event of sustained hypothyroidism, thyroid hormones should be administered (levothyroxine 20–40 µg/kg PO every 24 hours). This treatment can almost always be interrupted several months after surgery, since the thyroid tissue attached to the parathyroid glands is usually sufficient to maintain euthyroidism.

Total T_4 levels should be measured every 6–12 months to monitor for possible recurrence of FHT after surgery.

Radioactive iodine treatment

Radioactive iodine for the treatment of FHT is simple, safe, and effective, and is the best curative treatment for most patients. It will not be necessary to medicate the cat for the rest of its life (unless it develops hypothyroidism or other diseases that necessitate such treatment) and radioactive iodine avoids the risk associated with surgery and, in some cases, anaesthesia (if scintigraphy is not performed). In 95 % of cats, FHT can be resolved with a single injection of ^{131}I. The main drawbacks are a long hospitalisation period and the need for radioprotective measures and specialised facilities with specific permits. The cost is high, although not much greater than that of the multiple checkups required during medical treatment.

Iodotherapy is based on the selective uptake of radioactive isotopes of ^{131}I by the thyroid gland, which does not distinguish between these forms and dietary iodine. This results in the destruction of neoplastic cells through the action of the β particles emitted for an average of 8 days. These particles travel up to a maximum of 2 mm, thereby respecting the surrounding tissue.

The administered dose of ^{131}I can be fixed or adjusted according to total T_4 levels and the results of scintigraphy (thyroid gland volume or radioactive isotope uptake).[69] The choice of one method over another depends on the veterinary centre. However, a key disadvantage of a fixed dose is overdose and consequent iatrogenic hypothyroidism. On the other hand, variable doses are calculated based on formulas that are yet to be standardised.

Radioactive iodine is also the treatment of choice for patients with functional **thyroid carcinomas**. Higher doses are administered (e.g. 30 mCi) and longer hospitalisation periods are required.[80]

In some cases, iatrogenic hypothyroidism may develop. If after the first few months (when low total T_4 levels are common) this condition does not resolve spontaneously or the clinical signs are severe, treatment with levothyroxine (20–40 µg/kg PO every 24 hours) should be instituted. During this time, until euthyroidism is achieved, it is advisable to monitor levels of total T_4 and TSH, as well as renal parameters.

Dietary treatment

A diet deficient in iodine deprives the patient of the essential element for activation of thyroid hormones. According to initial studies of the Hill's diet y/d, 70 % of cats with FHT will be euthyroid at 4 weeks, 90 % at 8 weeks, and practically 100 % at 12 weeks. While these results are in line with real-life observations in patients with moderate FHT, cats with severe FHT rarely achieve euthyroidism.[81,82]

Dietary treatment is primarily indicated in cats that cannot be medicated or have adverse reactions to drugs, are not candidates for curative treatment (surgical or iodotherapy), and must be fed exclusively (and accept) a diet deficient in iodine.

Problems or disadvantages associated with dietary treatment include the following:

- Many cats do not accept the diet.
- The diet should be the only source of food. No other food or treats can be offered.
- Outdoor access must be limited (to prevent hunting).
- It controls, but does not cure, the disease.
- The thyroid tumour will continue to grow.
- The long-term effects of iodine deficiency are not known.
- Clinical signs may not resolve (e.g. weight loss).

When switching from medical to dietary treatment, methimazole therapy must be completely withdrawn before introducing the iodine-deficient diet so as not to cause marked hypothyroidism. When transitioning from a dietary treatment to a medical treatment, the patient can switch to an adequate diet while starting the new medication.[83]

Table 10 shows the results of the main studies investigating the effects of an iodine-deficient diet for the treatment of FHT.

Table 10. Scientific evidence supporting the use of an iodine-deficient diet in cats with FHT.

Study	No. of cats	T_4 normalised at 30–60 days	T_4 normalised at 60–90 days	Changes in clinical signs or physical examination
van der Kooij et al. (2014)[84]	225	56/88 (62.5 %)	51/68 (75 %)	Improvement No monitoring of weight No significant decrease in heart rate
Fritsch et al. (2014)[85]	18	5/12 (41.7 %)	6/12 (50 %)	No change in weight No monitoring of heart rate
Hui et al. (2015)[86]	49	20/48 (41.7 %)	39/47 (83 %)	No change in weight No monitoring of heart rate
Scott-Moncrieff et al. (2015)[87]	8	6/8 (75 %)	7/8 (87.5 %)	No change in weight No monitoring of heart rate
Vaske et al. (2016)[88]	17	6/15 (40 %)	6/15 (40 %)	No change in weight No improvement in muscle condition No monitoring of heart rate
Loftus et al. (2019)[89]	8	6/8 (75 %)	4/7 (57.4 %)	No change in weight No monitoring of heart rate
Grossi et al. (2019)[90]	14	3/8 (37.5 %)	3/6 (50 %)	Weight improvement (no significant difference relative to two other groups treated with methimazole)
Total of 7 studies	341	102/187 (54.5 %)	116/163 (71.2 %)	A diet deficient in iodine does not restore euthyroidism in all cats

THE OWNER'S PERSPECTIVE

Endocrine diseases can rarely be cured, and even if there is a cure, the patient must be **monitored** for recurrences. This will entail a considerable increase in the owner's **veterinary costs**.

We must provide the owner with a clear **explanation** of the **disease** and describe how are we going to **orient the treatment** with their help, and schedule **regular monitoring**. If we do not have the **trust and complicity of the owner**, these cases are more doomed to failure than many other internal medicine cases.

These diseases can often be **controlled or alleviated** but they are seldom cured. To control or alleviate them it is necessary to **administer drugs**: some must be injected and many others can be given orally. The **normal, adverse, and secondary effects** must be explained so that the owner can recognise them and act quickly. If the owner concludes that the prescribed therapy causes more **problems** than it solves, the **temptation to abandon** it can become too much to bear for many clients, who stop treating their sick pets.

KEY POINTS VETERINARY PRACTITIONERS SHOULD BEAR IN MIND

Endocrinopathies are one of the most complex diseases that the veterinary clinician will treat. This is because its effects have consequences in a **multitude of organs and systems** that are initially unrelated to the affected gland.

Arriving at a **correct diagnosis** and beginning **appropriate treatment** is as important as **monitoring** possible comorbidities that accompany these diseases.

In general, an early diagnosis and prescription of adequate treatment can result in a favourable or very favourable prognosis. However, as we have emphasised, there are many comorbidities that can sometimes remain hidden at the time of diagnosis. This is why the veterinary clinician should be **very cautious about assigning a favourable prognosis** to a patient with an endocrinopathy. A good strategy is to maintain a **reserved prognosis** until treatment has started, no comorbidities or secondary or adverse effects occur, the patient accepts the treatment and necessary monitoring at home, and the owner is willing to cooperate.

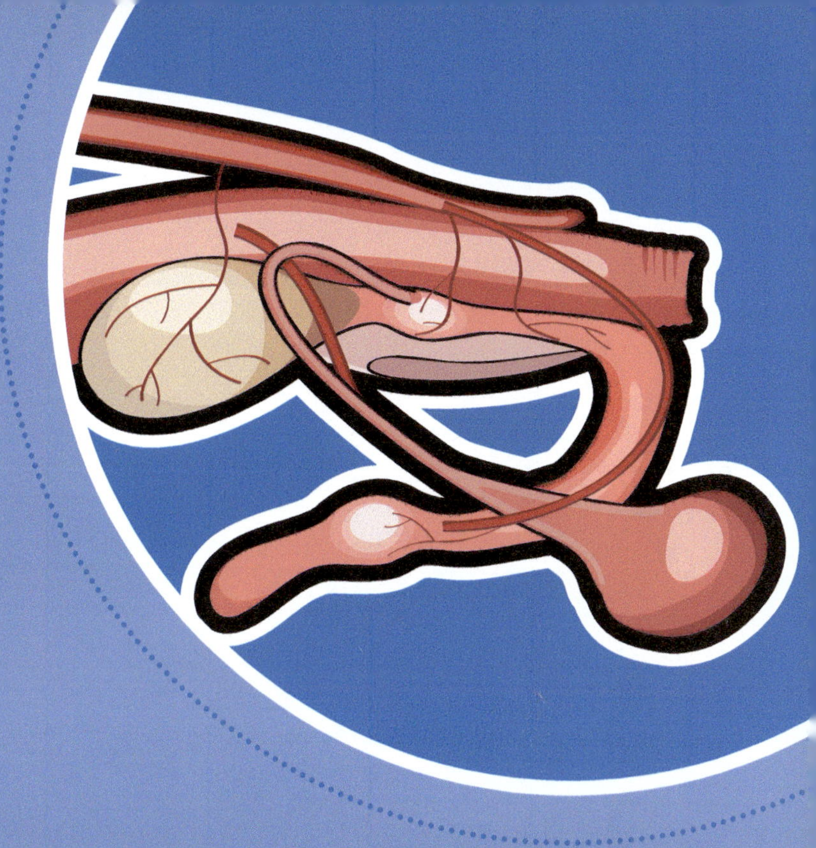

11 Reproductive diseases in senior patients

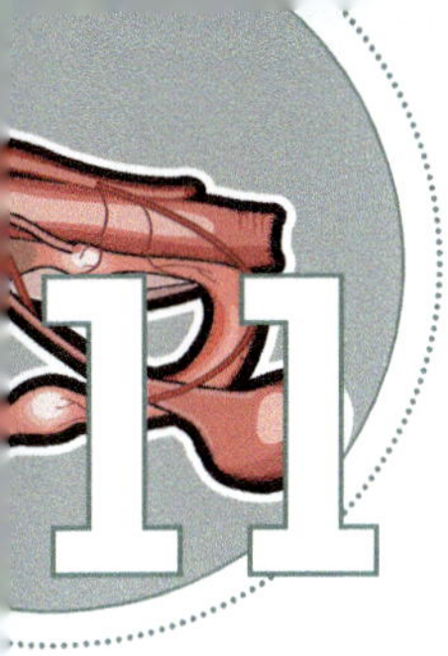

Reproductive diseases in senior patients

A large variety of diseases can affect the reproductive system of senior cats and dogs. However, limiting our discussion to the most prevalent reduces this number to three: pyometra and mammary tumours in females of both species and benign prostatic hyperplasia in male dogs.

As always, the objective of this chapter is to understand the pathophysiology to help orient the diagnosis and complete or improve the treatment of these diseases.

This chapter is subdivided into the three major diseases, as described below.

Benign prostatic hyperplasia

Benign prostatic hyperplasia (BPH) refers to an exaggerated growth of the prostate gland due to continuous hormonal stimulation, which is typical in intact adult male dogs. The prevalence of this disease increases almost linearly with age, with rates of 95 % reported in dogs >9 years of age[1] and up to 80 % in dogs aged 5 years and older.[2] Although more common in older dogs, it is not uncommon to detect this form of glandular hyperplasia in animals as young as 2.5 years.

The disease can be divided into two phases:[3]

- Dogs aged <5 years: BPH is basically epithelial, also known as the **glandular form**.
- Dogs aged >5 years: usually affected by the **complex form**, which consists of atrophic epithelial areas in addition to hyperplasia.

BPH affects this gland diffusely, causing it to expand dorsally.[4]

Pathophysiology of BPH

This alteration is characterised by an increase in the number and size of prostate cells induced by testicular hormones. Specifically, testosterone is reduced to dihydrotestosterone (DHT) by the action of 5α-reductase. This reduced testosterone or DHT is recognised as the hormone responsible for BPH (i.e. for the growth of both the stroma and the prostatic parenchyma).[5] However, this relationship is not straightforward. In fact, even though serum levels of testosterone and DHT decrease as the dog ages, the prostate continues to grow. This is due in part to the action of the hormone oestradiol, levels of which remain constant in the dog's blood throughout the aging process.[6,7] Oestradiol induces synthesis of DHT receptors in prostate cell nuclei, which leads to sensitisation of these cells, attenuating the effects of the serum concentrations of this hormone.[8,9]

TAKE NOTE!

As the dog ages, levels of DHT and its receptors increase in prostate tissue.

Other hormones play an important role in the development of this disease in humans and rats. For example, humans with acromegaly have a tendency to develop BPH due to serum concentrations of growth hormone.[10] Prolactin, another pituitary hormone, plays an important role in the proliferation and differentiation of the prostate epithelium in these species.[11–13]

Clinical signs

Although obvious clinical signs are absent in many BPH cases, others present with frequently inconspicuous signs. Some cases involve intermittent urethral discharge that can range from pale yellow to red or haemorrhagic. This secretion often goes unnoticed by the owner, especially in animals that live outdoors or those that are particularly scrupulous about hygiene. It is important to differentiate haematuria from haemorrhagic urethral discharge. Although both can present in patients with BPH, they have distinct differential diagnoses.

Defecation is only affected when prostatomegaly causes compression of the colon. Tenesmus and constipation may develop as a result.[14] Ventrodorsally flattened stools will appear when the prostate compresses the rectum, which only happens occasionally due to the anatomical location of the prostate. It is statistically more likely for the hyperplastic prostate to "fall" towards the abdomen than to "grow" towards the caudal zone.

In contrast to what happens in humans, dogs with BPH do not usually experience urinary retention, despite the growth of the prostate towards the lumen of the urethra.[15] The most common complication in these patients is bacterial prostatitis.[16] Perianal hernia, although possible, is much less common.

Diagnosis

Great strides have been made in the diagnosis of this disease. The widespread availability of ultrasound and specific serological testing greatly facilitates this task.

Traditionally, diagnosis of prostate disease involves rectal palpation. This technique should be used whenever possible, as it provides a large amount of information at a very low cost (Box 1). Unfortunately, the position of this gland can vary depending on the degree of distension of the urinary bladder and the patient's age and disease. Therefore, training in this technique should be a priority in order to obtain the maximum information from rectal palpation.

Alterations in blood test results (blood count and traditional biochemical workup) are uncommon. However, a commercial ELISA test to measure CPSE (canine prostate-specific arginine esterase) can be used. CPSE is a hormone of the kallikrein family and can be found in both ejaculate and blood. It is secreted by prostatic epithelial cells when under androgenic stimulation.

Box 1. FINDINGS ON RECTAL PALPATION OF THE PROSTATE GLAND IN A PATIENT WITH BPH.

- Increase in size towards the dorsal area
- Slightly mobile
- Smooth surface
- Uniform
- Symmetric
- Painless

CPSE can be used as a marker for canine BPH.[17] Serum concentrations of this hormone do not appear to be altered in other prostate diseases. The sensitivity and specificity of this test are around 97 % and almost 93 %, respectively.[18]

Urinalysis can be normal or may reveal haematuria without pyuria or bacteriuria.

TIP

The best samples for cytology and culture are ejaculate samples and those collected by prostate massage or aspiration biopsy.

The technique used to collect samples by prostate massage is described in Box 2 and Figure 1.

Imaging has become a common and often vital tool for evaluating prostate structure and size. Dogs with BPH typically have prostates 2 to 6 times larger than those of unaffected dogs.[19-23]

It is not easy to evaluate the prostate using simple X-rays: it is usually easier to identify it using contrast radiography (urethrocystography) in animals with a distended bladder.[24] Nonetheless, mild to moderate prostatomegaly can be identified in cases of dorsal displacement of the colon and cranial displacement of the bladder (Fig. 2).

TAKE NOTE!

A patient is considered to have prostatomegaly if, in the laterolateral projection of the caudal abdomen, the prostate occupies more than 70 % of the distance between the sacral promontory and the pubis.[25]

Box 2. TECHNIQUE FOR PROSTATIC MASSAGE.

1 Catheterise and fully empty the dog's urinary bladder.
2 Gently massage the prostate rectally or transabdominally (for 1–2 minutes).
3 Gently withdraw the catheter and as it passes through the prostate, aspirate to collect the material.

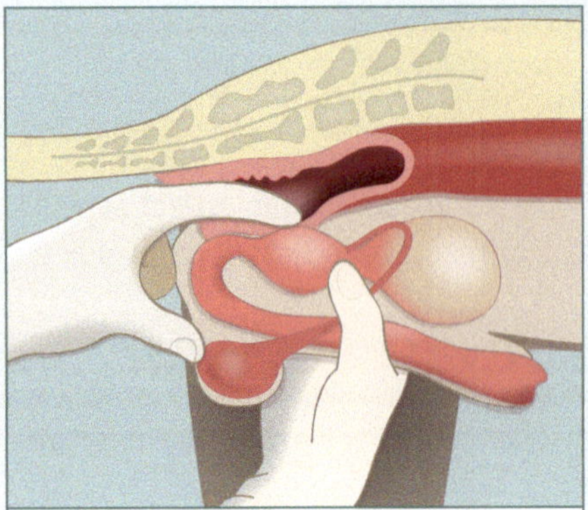

Figure 1. Technique for performing prostate massage in dogs.

Currently, ultrasound is the tool most commonly used to evaluate this gland. Ultrasound examination of the hyperplastic prostate shows a well-defined, enlarged gland with an isoechoic to hyperechoic image. Small hypoechoic areas may be observed if cystic hyperplasia is present.[16]

Definitive diagnosis can only be established after fine-needle aspiration (FNA) or biopsy. FNA is usually the most widely used definitive method. Puncture, whether transrectal or transabdominal, should not be performed in patients with abscesses.

The most common differential diagnoses include, in addition to BPH, squamous metaplasia and chronic prostatitis. Cytology of BPH typically shows mild chronic interstitial inflammation.[16]

Treatment

Traditionally, treatment has been reserved for animals with clinical signs caused by BPH. This was due to a lack of safe or temporary treatments for this disease. However, because treatment of BPH has since evolved substantially, withholding treatment in these situations may no longer be necessary. All treatments aim to reduce prostate size to alleviate clinical

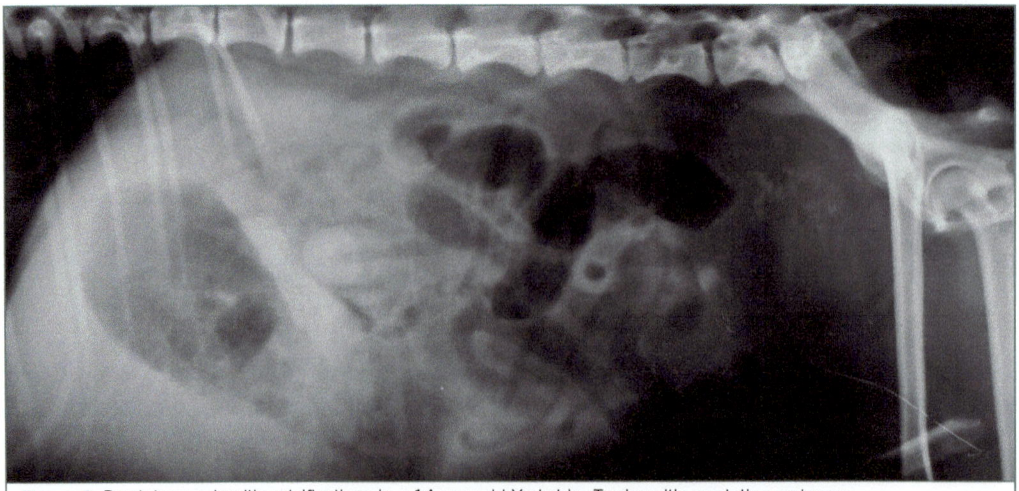

Figure 2. Prostatomegaly with calcifications in a 14-year-old Yorkshire Terrier with prostatic carcinoma.

signs. The main differences between treatment types are duration and possible adverse effects. Table 1 shows a list of the different treatments described in the literature.

Table 1. Hormonal treatments in senior patients.

Family of origin	Active substance	Dosage	Treatment duration	Secondary or adverse effects
Oestrogens	Diethylstilbestrol	0.2–1 mg PO every 2–3 days	3–4 weeks	• Bone marrow suppression • Squamous metaplasia
Progestogens	Medroxyprogesterone	3 mg/kg SC	Once a month	• Possible growth of mammary masses • Onset of diabetes mellitus
	Cyproterone	1.25–2.5 mg/kg PO once daily	15 days	
	Delmadinone	1–2 mg/kg SC once daily	Once a month	
	Chlormadinone	2 mg/kg PO once daily	3–4 weeks	
GnRH analogue	Deslorelin	4.7 mg or 9.4 mg SC	An implant with a 6–12-month duration of effect, depending on the dose	Possible change in behaviour in the first days due to an increase in testosterone in the blood
Testosterone and/or DHT antagonist	Osaterone	0.25–0.5 mg/kg PO once daily	7 days	• Polyphagia • Polydipsia • Anxiety or increased calmness
	Flutamide	5 mg/kg PO once daily	Safe for 7 weeks	-
5 α-reductase inhibitor	Finasteride	0.1 mg/kg PO once daily	3–4 weeks to observe the effect. Stopping treatment is not recommended.	-

Before the advent of new pharmacological treatments, castration was the most commonly used treatment. It is still one of the most common therapeutic approaches in dogs as it is the only definitive measure. After surgery, the size of the prostate is reduced by 50 % after 3 weeks and 70 % after 9 weeks.[26]

Recently authorised pharmacological treatments offer a temporary alternative, avoiding the risk associated with anaesthesia and causing significantly fewer side effects than their predecessors. The three main products are: osaterone, delmadinone, and deslorelin.

Osaterone

This is a powerful antiandrogen that works by blocking androgenic products in sensitive prostate tissue. Both osaterone and its main metabolite (PB-1) have antiandrogenic effects. This hormonal blockade is responsible for the reduction in prostate size (Fig. 3). Osaterone and PB-1 exert a dual effect: on the one hand they block the entry of testosterone into prostate cells, reducing the substrate for 5α-reductase and therefore the production of DHT, and on the other hand they block DHT receptors, preventing the synthesis of cellular material.

The usual dose of osaterone is between 0.25 and 0.5 mg/kg daily for 7 days, every 6 months. This is due to its pharmacokinetics and the peculiar anatomy of the target gland. With the doses described, prostate size is reduced by 27 % 1 week after starting treatment and by 40 % after 2 weeks. Clinical signs usually remit within 2 weeks of treatment.

Delmadinone

This is a progestogen with powerful antiandrogenic and antiestrogenic effects. It is injected subcutaneously in both dogs and cats. The usual doses are 1–2 mg/kg SC every 30 days.[27] This progestogen appears to be safe for use to treat BPH. However, due to the hormonal nature of the active ingredient, it is worth checking the patient's mammary tissue for masses, as well as measuring blood glucose or fructosamine levels to prevent the onset of diabetes mellitus, especially in patients receiving prolonged treatments.[28,29] Although the effect is similar to that achieved after administration of osaterone, the latter appears to reduce prostate size significantly faster.[30] Delmadinone has also been used to treat hypersexuality, anal adenoma, and certain cases of canine aggression linked to sex hormones.

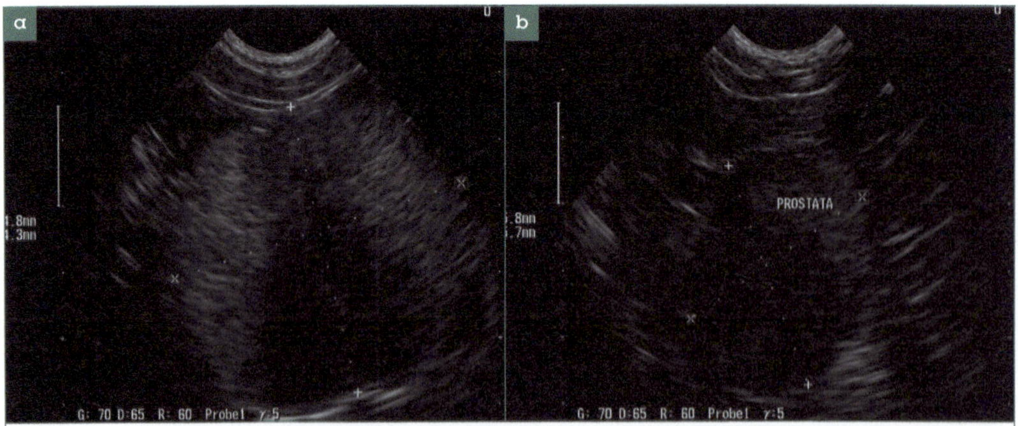

Figure 3. Ultrasound of benign prostatic hyperplasia (a). Image obtained 1 month after starting osaterone treatment (b). Images courtesy of Ana Prats and Antoni Prats, Rocaberti veterinary clinic, Barcelona (Spain).

Deslorelin

This product is administered in the form of biannual or annual implants. It primarily acts by causing desensitisation of gonadotropin-releasing hormone (GnRH) receptors and by blocking the production of sex hormones. In other words, it produces or mimics the effects of surgical castration in a prolonged but reversible manner. The great advantage of this product is the novel excipients it contains.

GnRH agonists have been around for a long time, but most have very short half-lives. For example, buserelin has a half-life of 72–80 minutes, regardless of the route of administration.[31]

TAKE NOTE!

Thanks to their biocompatible and lipophilic matrix, these implants allow deslorelin to be released progressively over 6–12 months.

The main effects of deslorelin in males are due to a drastic reduction in serum testosterone levels. In adult males the level of this hormone is approximately 2–4 ng/ml.[32] After administration of this GnRH agonist, testosterone falls to concentrations <0.1 ng/ml.[33] This decrease is not immediate: it takes about 12 days to occur, and suppression of testosterone secretion is actually preceded by an increase in its production. Once testosterone secretion is reduced, the decrease in prostate size is accompanied by a marked reduction in ejaculate volume, sperm production and quality, libido, and testicular diameter.[34]

Pyometra

Pyometra is a bacterial infection of the womb or uterus. This is one of the most common and serious infectious diseases of adult female dogs and cats. It is more common in intact and nulliparous females aged over 6 years. In fact, there seems to be greater likelihood of pyometra in females with increasing age.

TAKE NOTE!

It is important to remember that hysterectomised females can develop stump pyometra.

A look at our records indicates that pyometra is much more prevalent in female dogs than female cats, although in Spain many more cats than dogs undergo ovariohysterectomy at the decision of their owners. This prevents accurate assessment of the incidence of pyometra in both species. In any case, the reproductive physiology of dogs does not work in their favour. Below we will briefly review the pathophysiology of pyometra.

Pathophysiology

Traditionally, it was assumed that purulent infection of the womb was almost totally dependent on the presence of cystic endometrial hyperplasia (CEH). CEH is a progressive pathological change, promoted by sex hormones, in the uterine endometrium. Repeatedly, during heat, elevated levels of oestrogens in the blood combined with the hormonal effect of dioestrus (progesterone) favour the development of CEH. In female dogs dioestrus lasts about 2 months. During this time progesterone levels in the blood are similar to those found during pregnancy. The repeated presence of progesterone in the absence of pregnancy leads to the development of CEH. The secretion of the endometrium provides an ideal culture medium for bacterial infections, and the bacteria reach the uterus after the cervix has remained open during proestrus and oestrus. In this context, once CEH is established, pyometra can be considered an almost logical consequence.[35]

However, more recent evidence suggests that this is not always so, since cases of pyometra without CEH are not uncommon. Therefore, it may be more accurate to consider CEH and pyometra as separate diseases, rather than components of a complex. Some studies have shown that sustained high levels of progesterone produce typical signs of CEH but not pyometra.[36] Other studies have reported that levels of sex hormone receptors in the canine endometrium are increased in females with CEH but not in those with pyometra.[37–39] Currently, there are insufficient data to confirm whether pyometra is caused by production of sex hormones or by the uterine response they induce.

One requirement for pyometra to occur is colonisation of the uterus by bacteria. The most common of these bacteria is *Escherichia coli*, with a prevalence ranging from 59 % to 95 % depending on the study consulted. Other bacteria isolated from infected uteruses include *Streptococcus*, *Klebsiella*, *Pseudomonas*,

WHAT HAPPENS IN CATS?

Because female cats are induced ovulators, progesterone levels are not usually high unless that cat has been mounted or a progestogen has been administered iatrogenically. If mounting without fertilisation has occurred or a progestogen has been administered, the chances of pyometra are increased (Fig. 4). Other infections or diseases that alter the antibacterial response in cats can also promote pyometra in intact females.

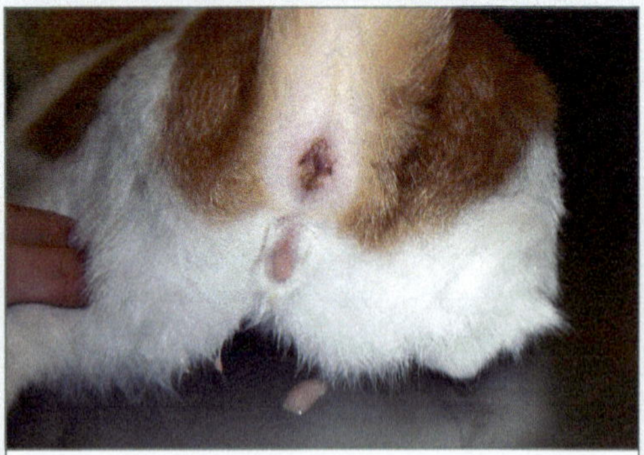

Figure 4. Detail of the perianal area of a 2-year-old female cat with purulent vaginal discharge due to pyometra. This cat had received oral progestogens.

Staphylococcus, and anaerobic bacteria.[40–43] In fact, one study[42] found that *E. coli* had an affinity for progesterone-stimulated endometrial receptors. This would explain the great prevalence of these bacteria in canine uterine infections. *E. coli* can reach the uterus via faecal, vaginal, or bladder colonisation.[44–46]

Clinical signs

The plethora of clinical signs normally found in females with pyometra can be reduced to those described in Tables 2 and 3.[35,40,45,47,48]

This clinical picture and its severity can vary depending on the degree of opening of the cervix. Pyometras are usually described as either open or closed, depending on whether the cervix is open or closed. This parameter is sometimes considered a question of chance, when this is not in fact the case: the cervix can be open or closed to varying degrees within the same infectious episode. This means that vaginal discharge is intermittent and that the female's condition improves or worsens depending on the drainage capacity of the cervix.[35]

Treatment

Ovariohysterectomy continues to be the most common and definitive treatment (Figs. 5 and 6). Unfortunately, not all senior cats or dogs with pyometra will arrive at our centre in adequate conditions to undergo anaesthesia and emergency surgery. Thus, for each patient, we must determine the ideal moment to enter the operating room, or whether action is required sooner rather than later, before the patient's condition deteriorates further. To this end, it is essential to know how to recognise the clinical signs of systemic inflammatory response syndrome (SIRS). This is the formal name for septic syndrome, sepsis, or septic shock.[51] For diagnosis of SIRS, a patient must fulfil at least two of the four inclusion criteria. These criteria are listed in Table 4.

To properly treat these patients, SIRS must be treated before addressing the pyometra. It is important to remember the rule of 20, depicted in Box 3.

Once the patient is stabilised, there are two possible options. The primary, and definitive,

Table 2. Most common clinical signs in dogs with pyometra.[49,50]

Clinical sign	%
Vaginal discharge	85
Lethargy/depression	62
Inappetence/anorexia	42
Polyuria and polydipsia	28
Vomiting	15
Nocturia	5
Diarrhoea	5
Abdominal enlargement	5

Table 3. Most common clinical signs in cats with pyometra.[49,50]

Clinical sign	%
Copious vaginal discharge	100
Palpable uterus	100
Fever	24
Anorexia	24
Lethargy	24
Weight loss	14
Unkempt appearance	9
Polyuria and polydipsia	9

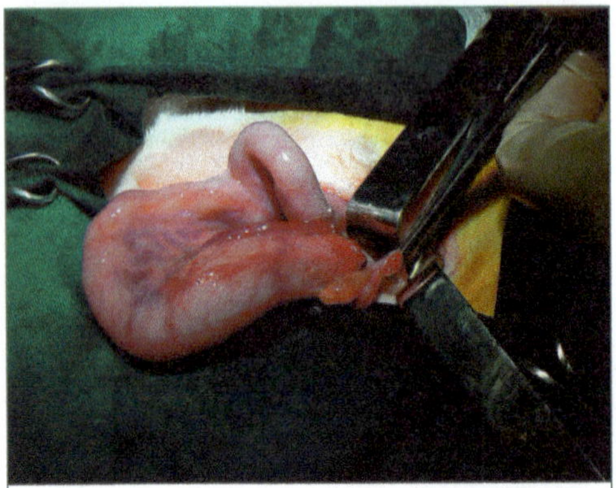

Figure 5. Image taken during ovariohysterectomy of the cat in Figure 4.

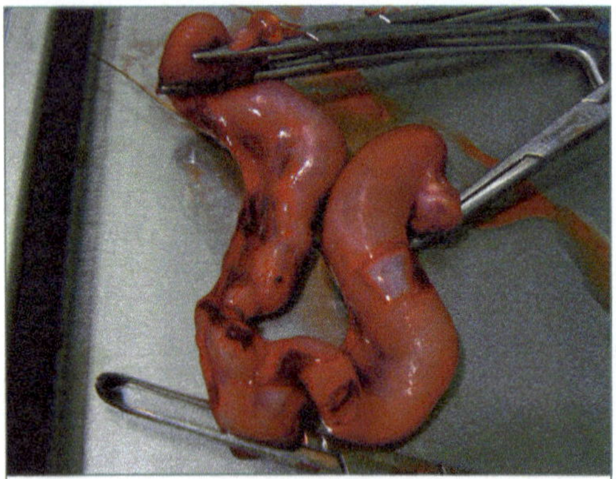

Figure 6. Appearance of the uterus and ovaries after excision.

option is ovariohysterectomy. However, new drugs have opened new therapeutic avenues based on medical rather than surgical treatment. This treatment consists of the use of prostaglandin $F_{2\alpha}$ or its analogues (cloprostenol, dinoprost), aglepristone (a blocker of uterine progesterone receptors), and appropriate antibiotic therapy. Table 5 shows the recommended doses for each species. The objective of these drugs is to reduce progesterone levels through luteolysis, diminish its effect by blocking its receptors, and open the cervix to release the purulent content. Combination therapy has proved more effective than monotherapy.

Currently, the combination of aglepristone and prostaglandins or even ergotamines is commonly used.[54]

Table 4. Inclusion criteria for sepsis in cats and dogs.[52,53]

Criterion	Cats	Dogs
Temperature (°C)	<37.7 or >39.4	<37.7 or >38.8
Respiratory rate (bpm)	>40	>20
Heart rate (bpm)	<140 or >225	>120
Leukocytosis or leukopenia (10^3/µl)	>19,500 or <5,000	>16,000 or <6,000

TIP

The use of $PGF_{2\alpha}$-type prostaglandins has been associated with numerous side effects, and it is advisable to be aware of these effects in order to prepare accordingly and explain them to the owner before beginning treatment.

Misoprostol is an analogue of PGE_1. An advantage of this product is that it is administered orally and its side effects are usually restricted to the gastrointestinal region. Compared with other prostaglandins, misoprostol appears to cause less frequent adverse effects.

Box 3. TWENTY PARAMETERS THAT SHOULD BE MONITORED DURING SIRS.

1 Balanced fluid therapy
2 Perfusion/blood pressure
3 Cardiac function
4 Albumin
5 Oncotic pressure
6 Oxygenation/ventilation
7 Glucose
8 Electrolytes/acid-base balance
9 Mental state
10 Coagulation
11 Haematocrit
12 Kidney function/urine production
13 White blood cell count/antibiotic therapy
14 Gastrointestinal motility and integrity
15 Drugs and their metabolism
16 Nutrition
17 Pain control
18 Catheter care/mobilisation
19 Dressing and care thereof
20 Care of the affected patient

Mammary tumours

Mammary tumours are one of the most common types of tumours in both dogs and cats. They account for about 50 % of cancer cases in dogs and about 17 % in cats.[58,59] In both species, the mean age of appearance is around 10–12 years. Multiple mammary tumours are present at the time of diagnosis in 50 % of female dogs (Fig. 7) and 60 % of female cats. However, the big difference between these species is the degree of malignancy of mammary tumours. In female

Table 5. Medical treatment of pyometra in cats and dogs.

Drug	Dose in cats	Dose in dogs
$PGF_{2\alpha}$ (natural)	0.1–0.25 mg/kg SC every 12 or 24 h for 5 days.[57]	• Day 1: 0.1 mg/kg SC. • Day 2: 0.2 mg/kg SC. • Days 3–7: 0.25–0.5 mg/kg SC.
Aglepristone	10 mg/kg SC, days 1, 2, 7, and 14.[55]	10 mg/kg SC, days 1, 2, and 8.[56]
Cloprostenol ($PGF_{2\alpha}$ analogue)	1–5 µg/kg SC every 24 h up to 21 days.	1 µg/kg SC, days 3–7 or days 3 and 8.
Dinoprost ($PGF_{2\alpha}$ analogue)	0.1 mg/kg SC on day 1 and then 0.25 mg/kg SC daily for 5 more days.	25 µg/kg SC every 8 h, days 3–7; or 25 µg/kg SC every 8 h, days 3, 6, and 9.
Misoprostol (PGE_1 analogue)	-	10 µg/kg PO every 12 h, days 3–12.

dogs half of these tumours are classified as malignant, while in female cats this proportion can be as high as 80 % or even 96 %, depending on the study consulted (Figs. 8 and 9).

Predisposing factors

Nowadays, it is well accepted that the age at which a female undergoes ovariohysterectomy plays a vital role in the development of mammary tumours (Tables 6 and 7). This is probably due to consistent and repeated exposure of mammary tissue to sex hormones (oestrogens and progestogens).

In terms of breed predisposition, the Poodle, Terrier, Cocker Spaniel, and German Shepherd Dog breeds are more likely to develop mammary tumours. Siamese cats are 4 times more likely to develop mammary tumours (Fig. 10). The domestic shorthair cat may also be predisposed to this tumour type.

Diagnosis

Small animal veterinary surgeons have been waiting years for a tool that is less invasive but as reliable as biopsy for the diagnosis of these tumours. However, it appears that we must continue to wait, as the results obtained using alternative methods (usually FNA) are not usually as definitive or reliable as those obtained by biopsy.[62] This small difference is important for many owners of females with these tumours, who view this diagnostic approach as overly invasive compared with the simple cytology and mammogram used in human medicine.

Without doubt, the standard response when a veterinary surgeon discovers a lump in the

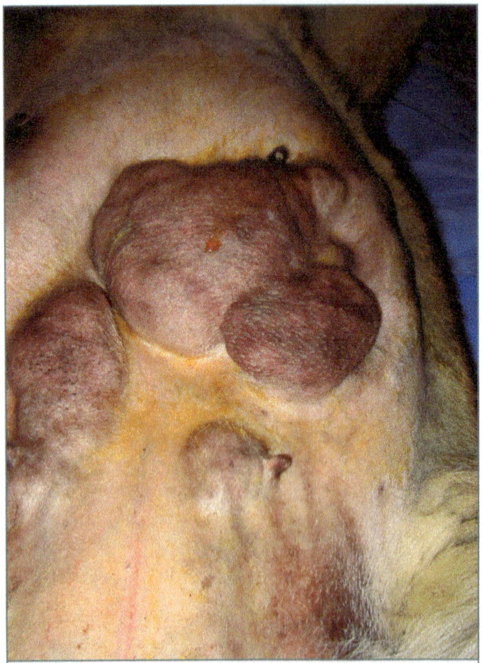

Figure 7. Multiple mammary tumours in a female dog. Image courtesy of Ana Prats and Antoni Prats, Rocaberti veterinary clinic, Barcelona (Spain).

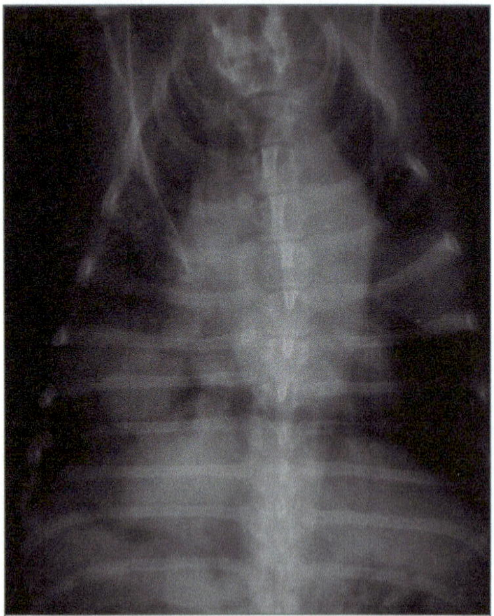

Figure 8. Chest X-ray of a 16-year-old female dog with a mammary adenocarcinoma diagnosed 4 years earlier, showing lung metastases. Image courtesy of Ana Prats and Antoni Prats, Rocaberti veterinary clinic, Barcelona (Spain).

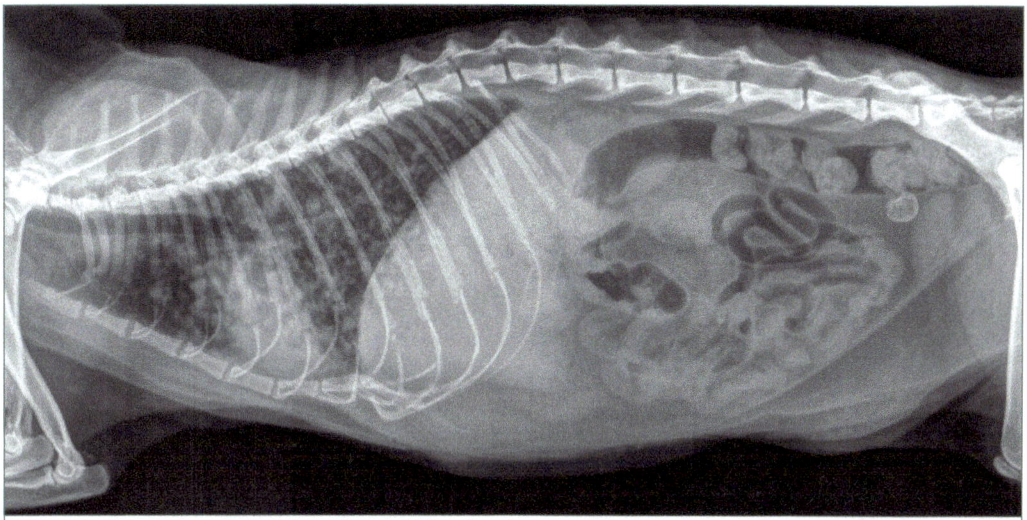

Figure 9. Pulmonary metastasis in an 8-year-old female cat as a consequence of a mammary adenocarcinoma.

mammary gland is to recommend a biopsy. And biopsy is the only method that can reveal exactly what type of tumour it is. Unfortunately, owners are not always in agreement with this approach, and therefore should be provided with a simple but clear explanation as to why biopsy of the mass is required. Macroscopic signs of malignancy can be useful to help convince the owner (Box 4); the more signs the tumour in question exhibits, the more likely it is to be malignant.

If this is explained but the owner is still not totally convinced, FNA cytology can always be performed. In any case, we must remind the client that cytology will very likely provide only a partial result, indicating whether the lesion is a tumour or not, without providing a definitive diagnosis or a reliable prognosis.

Table 6. Effect of ovariectomy on the appearance of mammary tumours in female dogs.[60,61]

Timing of ovariectomy	Risk of malignant mammary tumour in female dogs
Before the first oestrous cycle	0.05 %
Between the first and second oestrous cycle	8 %
After the second oestrus	26 %
After 2.5 years of age	No difference

Table 7. Effect of ovariectomy on the appearance of mammary tumours in female cats.[60,61]

Timing of ovariectomy	Risk of malignant mammary tumour in female cats
Before 6 months	9 %
6–12 months	14 %

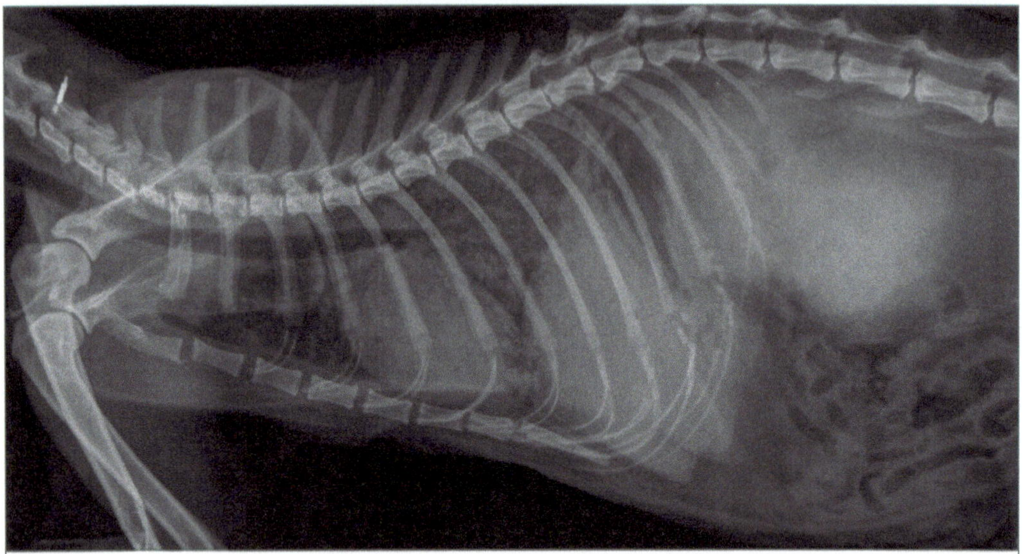

Figure 10. Renal metastasis in a 14-year-old Siamese cat as a consequence of mammary carcinoma.

Treatment

Surgical treatment

The optimal treatment for a mammary tumour is always surgery. The results obtained using other therapeutic approaches (chemotherapy and radiotherapy) do not improve the results obtained with surgery.

Box 4. GROSS SIGNS OF MALIGNANCY.

- Size >3 cm in diameter
- Presence of ulceration (Fig. 11)
- Invasion of nearby tissues, poor mobilisation
- Lymph node metastasis
- Distant metastasis

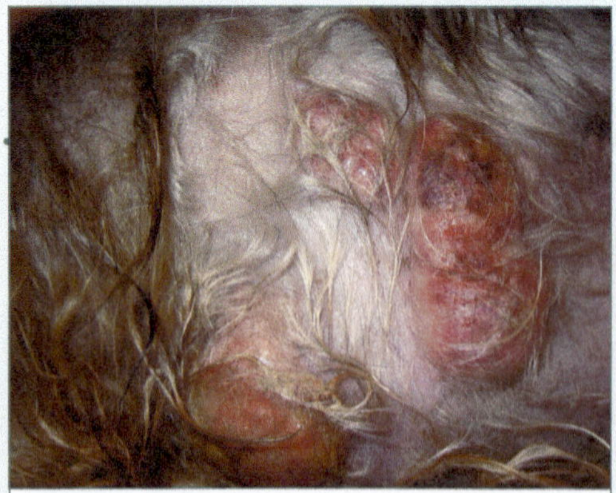

Figure 11. Slightly ulcerated canine mammary tumour. Image courtesy of Ana Prats and Antoni Prats, Rocaberti veterinary clinic, Barcelona (Spain).

HOW CAN THE MAXIMUM INFORMATION BE OBTAINED FROM A BIOPSY?

Biopsy request forms must be correctly completed, and should be accompanied by detailed information on all the nodules sent, regardless of whether they are tumours or lymph nodes.

It is helpful to make a mark or insert a suture in the sample for the purposes of orientation.

Biopsy specimens should be shipped in a suitable formaldehyde solution. If the sample is >1.5 cm, it is recommended to make several cuts into the specimen to ensure homogeneous penetration of the fixative solution.

It is advisable to send at least one cytology sample of the regional lymph nodes, or ideally an incisional or excisional lymph node biopsy sample.

Once the sample has been sent, a thorough examination of the margins of the sample, in the correct orientation (taking the mark or suture as a reference), should be requested. This will be very useful if the patient needs to undergo reintervention. Examination of infiltration into blood and/or lymphatic microvessels should also be requested.

Before excising a mammary tumour the following must be taken into account:

- Its location and lymphatic drainage
- Its size
- Any macroscopic signs of malignancy observed
- If available, histopathological diagnosis prior to surgery (e.g. old tumours, FNA cytologies)

Tumour staging can also be used (Table 8). Depending on these factors, the most appropriate surgery can be scheduled. This brings us to the next great debate in this chapter:

- What is the most appropriate way to perform a mastectomy?
- How many mammary glands should be removed?
- Should the lymph node always be removed?

We will try to answer these and other questions below.

In **female dogs**, more extensive surgery does not appear to be associated with a longer survival. For this reason, at least initially, radical mastectomy of the entire chain is not recommended. On the other hand, it would certainly make sense to carry out a **regional mastectomy** following lymphatic drainage of the affected mammary gland. It is typically assumed that mammary glands 1 to 3 drain into the axillary lymph node and that mammary glands 3 to 6

Table 8. Staging of mammary tumours (modified from Owen LN. *Classification of Tumours in Domestic Animals*, Geneva, WHO, 1980).

	Dogs (modified system)	Cats (modified system)
T: primary tumour		
T1	<3 cm maximum diameter	<2 cm maximum diameter
T2	Between 3 and 5 cm in diameter	Between 2 and 3 cm in diameter
T3	>5 cm maximum diameter	>3 cm maximum diameter
N: regional lymph node		
N0	No metastasis on cytology or histology	No metastasis on cytology or histology
N1	Metastasis present on cytology or histology	Metastasis present on cytology or histology
M: distant metastasis		
M0	No metastases detected	No metastases detected
M1	Metastases detected	Metastases detected
Staging		
Stage I	T1, N0, and M0	T1, N0, and M0
Stage II	T2, N0, and M0	T2, N0, and M0
Stage III	T3, N0, and M0	T1–2, N1, and M0; or T3, N0–1, and M0
Stage IV	Any T, N1, and M0	Any T, N1, and M0
Stage V	Any T, any N, and M1	-

drain into the inguinal lymph node. Here the problem appears when one of the affected mammary glands is 3. In these cases it is difficult to determine whether it is necessary to remove only up or only down the chain. When this happens, perhaps the optimal approach is to perform a good regional mastectomy, correctly label the sample for the pathologist, and properly explain the different possibilities to the owner.

Another option is a single lumpectomy, although this is only recommended for very small, firm, nonadherent tumours. An individual mastectomy can be performed in cases of tumours of 1 cm or little more, located in the centre of the mammary gland.

TAKE NOTE!

Ideally, all surgeries for the excision of mammary masses should include, in addition to the tumour, 2 cm of healthy tissue around the entire tumour and even the abdominal muscle tissue. The wall of the abdominal cavity is usually not touched unless there is a clear infiltration.

In **cats** this is different. The presence of microtumours at the time of surgery is very likely. Accordingly, **radical mastectomy** of the entire affected mammary chain is recommended in these cases.

Adjuvant treatments

Many adjuvant treatments have been recommended over the last 30 years. However, few have proven effective in studies. Below, we will discuss the most common adjuvant therapies to surgery used in our daily practice.

Ovariohysterectomy at the moment of mastectomy

Several studies have evaluated the effect of ovariohysterectomy after diagnosis of a mammary tumour. While some reported increases in survival time in 45 % of patients, other studies found no differences between patients that underwent ovariohysterectomy and those that did not. It seems clear that in female dogs the presence of hormone receptors in tumours is a positive prognostic factor: tumours with receptors are more benign than those without. Thus, when operating on these dogs, we have to bear in mind that the tumours prevented by ovariohysterectomy will be mostly benign tumours. Therefore, everything is left in the hands of the veterinary surgeon responsible for the case.

Finally, it should be remembered that in cases in which chemotherapy will be administered, ovariohysterectomy is recommended to prevent pyometra during treatment.

TIP

If ovariohysterectomy is performed, it should be done before mastectomy and all instruments and gloves changed to avoid surgical infection.

Chemotherapy protocols for mammary tumours

Chemotherapy is not very common in these cases due to its limited efficacy as a sole therapy. However, it is indicated and has beneficial effects in certain circumstances. It is recommended if there are macroscopic or microscopic signs of malignancy. There are many possible chemotherapy protocols for these tumours, but the most widely used consists of doxorubicin with or without cyclophosphamide (Box 5).[63–65]

Use of COX-2 inhibiting agents

Multiple recent studies have recognised that some mammary tumours (especially canine inflammatory mammary carcinomas; Fig. 12) express the enzyme COX-2. This enzyme exerts its activity through the production of PGE_2, which plays a role in inflammation and carcinogenesis in human tumours, although it was not until 2003 that it was first identified in canine mammary tumours.[66] In human medicine overexpression of the COX-2 enzyme, and the consequent increase in PGE_2 concentration, inhibits apoptosis, promotes cell proliferation, stimulates angiogenesis, and decreases immunity.[67–70] The first tumour in which COX-2 activity was detected was human colorectal cancer, after which multiple studies and trials concluded that low doses of acetylsalicylic acid can be beneficial in both the prevention and treatment of this tumour type.[71]

In veterinary medicine, studies have shown that healthy mammary tissue does not express this enzyme, although tumours tend to express it and its presence and concentration are negative prognostic factors.[66,72]

Boxes 6 and 7 summarise the tumours in which COX-2 expression has been demonstrated in dogs and cats, respectively.

Unfortunately, not all tumours express COX-2 equally; not even tumours of the same class express this enzyme in comparable concentrations. Thus, when reviewing the literature it is important to distinguish quantitative studies from qualitative studies (i.e. those that do not quantify the number of cells expressing this enzyme).

Box 5. COMMON PROTOCOLS FOR TREATING MALIGNANT MAMMARY TUMOURS IN FEMALE CATS AND DOGS.

In female dogs:

- Doxorubicin: 30 mg/m² IV every 21 days.
- Cyclophosphamide: 50 mg/m² PO, on days 3–6 of the first week of each treatment cycle.

In cats:

- Doxorubicin: 25 mg/m² IV every 21 days.
- Cyclophosphamide: 50–100 mg/m² PO, on days 3–6 of the start of each cycle.

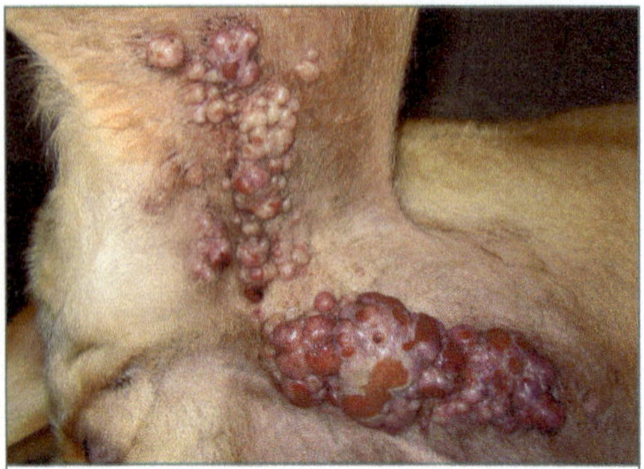

Figure 12. Canine inflammatory mammary carcinoma. Image courtesy of Ana Prats and Antoni Prats, Rocaberti veterinary clinic, Barcelona (Spain).

For example, some studies have reported COX-2 overexpression in tumours, while others have reported COX-2 negativity because the enzyme is expressed in less than 10 % of cells. This occurs for example in the case of canine osteosarcoma.[86,94]

There is a marked difference in COX-2 expression between dogs and cats. In general, with the exception of mammary carcinomas, the data available to date indicate that feline tumours express much lower levels of this enzyme, even in tumour types in which high concentrations of COX-2 are found in dogs.

It seems reasonable to assume that selective inhibition, in addition to exerting anti-inflammatory effects, should prevent or slow tumour growth. However, there is not always a good correlation between the level of enzyme expression and the effects of its inhibition. Thus, while small animal clinicians with patients with this type of tumour currently prescribe an NSAID to achieve anti-inflammatory and analgesic effects, a reliable "chemotherapeutic" effect should not be expected.

Box 6. CANINE TUMOURS WITH DEMONSTRATED COX-2 EXPRESSION.

Mammary tumours
- Tubulopapillary carcinoma
- Anaplastic carcinoma
- Inflammatory carcinoma[72–75]
- Squamous cell carcinoma
- Carcinosarcoma

Prostate tumours
- Carcinoma and adenocarcinoma[76,77]

Bladder tumours
- Transitional cell carcinoma[78]

Epithelial tumours
- Squamous cell carcinoma[79]

Nasal tumours
- Carcinoma and adenocarcinoma
- Squamous cell carcinoma, transitional cell carcinoma, and anaplastic carcinoma[80–82]

Other tumours
- Kidney carcinoma,[83] ovarian carcinoma,[84] oral melanoma,[85] osteosarcoma,[86] and meningioma[87]

Box 7. FELINE TUMOURS WITH DEMONSTRATED COX-2 EXPRESSION.

Mammary tumours
- Carcinoma[88,89]

Epithelial tumours
- Squamous cell carcinoma[90–92]

Bladder tumours
- Transitional cell carcinoma[90]

Pancreatic tumours
- Adenocarcinoma[93]

Use of antioestrogens such as tamoxifen

Use of these agents is not recommended owing to the many potential side effects.[95] Moreover, in female dogs and cats the expression of oestrogen receptors appears to be associated with reduced tumour malignancy, in contrast to findings in human medicine.[96–98]

Other

Various products are proposed to exert antitumour effects in the mammary glands in both dogs and cats. However, for the moment their efficacy is anecdotal, and no clear recommendation can be made. These products include ω-3 fatty acids and punicic acid (extracted from the pomegranate seed), as well as toceranib, a tyrosine kinase inhibitor that appears to exert antiangiogenic and immunomodulatory effects in patients with tumours, even those that do not express tyrosine kinase.[99,100]

THE OWNER'S PERSPECTIVE

Many owners may not remember the advice they were given during the first visits to our clinic when their pet was still a puppy or kitten. It is therefore useful to reinforce this advice using **information sheets for the owner**.

Owners may feel guilty when they realise that their pet has a serious disease (e.g. mammary tumours or pyometra). Exploiting this feeling can have serious consequences for our centre and for the animal, which is not to blame. Phrases like: "it doesn't matter why we are here, the important thing is **to do what is necessary to try to resolve this situation as quickly as possible"** can help in these circumstances.

If the owners are not fully convinced of the need for treatment (often surgical), we must be tactful enough to provide them with options that buy time and **demonstrate to the owners that this approach is more valid** and often less costly than other therapeutic options.

KEY POINTS VETERINARY PRACTITIONERS SHOULD BEAR IN MIND

These diseases are very common in our centres. This is due in part to the high frequency of **late gonadectomy** in Spain. However, it is important not to assume that all mammary tumours are equal, that all pyometras end well (although many do), or that prostatic hyperplasia almost never predisposes the patient to bacterial prostatitis or prostate abscesses. We should remove emotion from the conversation and **calmly explain the situation** to the owner before deciding not to intervene.

If we want to establish or have established a **prepubertal gonadectomy** programme in our centre, we must ensure that clinicians inform all owners about the **advantages and possible disadvantages**. Puppy or kitten owners should always receive complete and accurate information. This can help avoid further problems in the long run. To ensure that owners are appropriately informed, all veterinary staff should adhere to a **script**: this way there is no doubt as to the information that should be provided on the pet's first visits. Later, owners should be provided with **information sheets**, which help to reinforce the advice provided during the visit. The specific information sheets given to the owner should be recorded in the **patient's clinical file**.

Nowadays there are many **medical treatments** for these diseases that did not exist a few years ago. However, surgical treatment is still both common and necessary. The fact that a patient is senior is not an excuse for not anaesthetising and operating. Such an exception should only be made for animals with serious problems, in which anaesthesia could pose a threat to life. If we do not have sufficient confidence in our anaesthetic abilities, or do not have the necessary monitoring systems and personnel, the owner will undoubtedly appreciate being put in contact with a **referral centre** with the necessary resources. Remember: "there are no patients that don't survive anaesthesia, only patients that don't survive the anaesthetist".

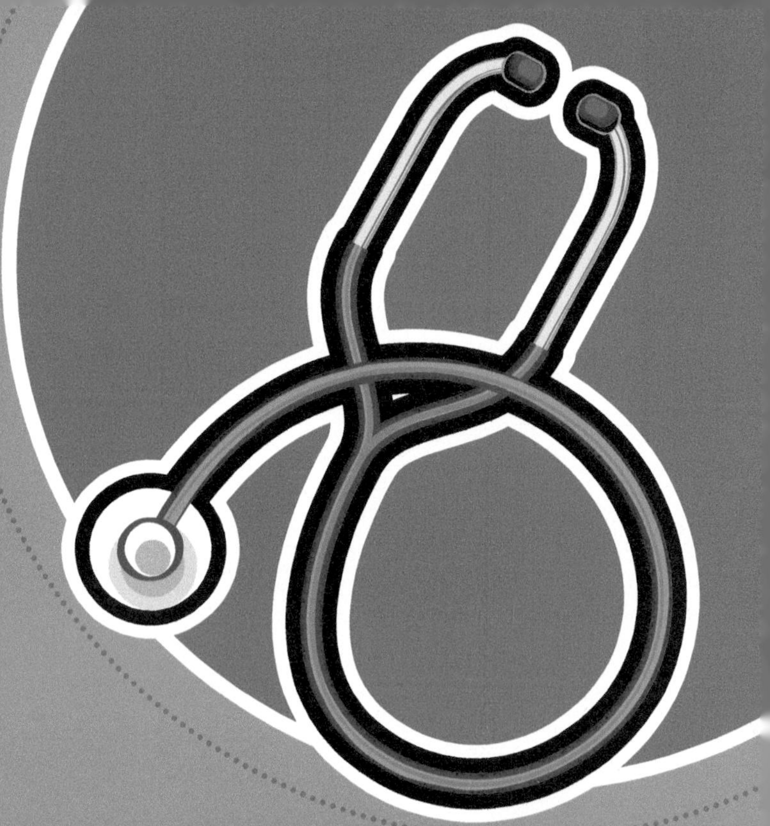

12 Senior cardiovascular disease

12

Senior cardiovascular disease

In this chapter we will provide a simple, ordered, and above all useful overview of the main diseases of the cardiovascular system in small animals. These diseases, of which there are many, can be complex in terms of aetiology and the various, often highly specialised diagnostic techniques used. Echocardiography has become the cornerstone of modern cardiac diagnosis. Unfortunately, discussion of this complex technique is beyond the scope of this book. For this reason, we will focus on the fundamental aspects of the cardiovascular examination, leaving aside echocardiography.

However, before discussing the most frequent cardiovascular diseases in senior patients, we will first review the cardiovascular examination. This review provides a good opportunity to emphasise the utility of a good cardiac examination.

Cardiovascular physical examination

In the era of diagnostic imaging techniques, physical examination of patients with possible heart or cardiovascular problems may seem somewhat obsolete. However, the basic physical examination remains important, as this forms the basis of the appropriate diagnostic plan, and avoids unnecessary tests. Below, step-by-step, we will attempt to create a useful protocol that can be easily incorporated into the veterinary surgeon's routine.

Step 1: first, observe the patient

Before even placing the patient on the table, it is helpful to observe the animal from a certain distance. This can easily be done while we present ourselves to the owner and collect the clinical data. It can be particularity informative and helpful to let the patient wander around the room, especially in the case of cats; this tends to relax them, ensuring that the examination provides us with more reliable results.

TIP

At this point, it is useful to observe the patient's respiratory pattern and to check for the presence of orthopnoeic postures, cough, and fatigue.

Step 2: evaluate the eyes, mucous membranes, and neck

By examining the eyes we can easily qualitatively evaluate the presence of arterial hypertension. Retinal vessels that are thicker than usual or tortuous indicate the need for quantitative blood pressure measurement. Acute blindness, especially in cats, is a relatively common clinical sign in animals with untreated hypertension, which can ultimately lead to retinal detachment. Patients with hypertension may also exhibit retinal haemorrhage, papilloedema, or hyphaema.

The oral (and ocular) mucosa may show changes in the normal colouration. Thus, instead of the moist, bright pink appearance of the normal mucosa, cyanotic colouration may be observed when the concentration of deoxygenated haemoglobin exceeds 5 g/dl.[1] The presence of cyanotic mucous membranes implies arterial hypoxaemia or markedly reduced perfusion of the peripheral vascular beds (although in these cases arterial hypoxaemia is absent). Cyanosis may also be observed in the digital or interdigital areas and on the tips of the ears. This cyanosis is usually related to very low cardiac output, marked arterial vasoconstriction, or vascular obstruction. The clearest example of vascular obstruction is feline aortic thromboembolism, while arterial vasoconstriction due to shock or hypothermia can cause marked cyanosis.

When examining the neck, we should pay attention to two structures: the thyroid gland and jugular veins. The thyroid gland is often enlarged in senior cats as a consequence of thyroid adenoma. These adenomas produce a hyperthyroid state that causes concentric hypertrophy and a state of high cardiac output.

The jugular veins should be inspected for distension and pulsation. This helps to provide a basic estimate of systemic venous pressure. Normal jugular veins should be easily collapsible with gentle finger compression. The jugular pulse does not usually extend beyond the first third of the neck in a standing patient. The presence of a pulse in more cranial areas or the detection of jugular distension (Box 1) usually implies right heart failure.

Finally, before completing the examination of the neck, we can apply pressure to the abdomen to check for **hepatojugular reflux**. When this reflux is present, jugular distension is observed during application of abdominal pressure. The presence of hepatojugular reflux implies one of three possibilities: systolic or diastolic right ventricular dysfunction; tricuspid valve disease; or pericardial disease.

Step 3: evaluate the thorax

At this point, each hemithorax should be carefully auscultated. However, it should be remembered that chest palpation and breathing assessment are equally important.

The hands should be passed over each hemithorax to check for abnormalities in the sternum or the ribs. It is useful to record data on the respiratory rate and respiratory pattern, and on the regularity, depth, and level of exertion during the respiratory cycle. One hand is used to search for the point of maximum heartbeat intensity, as well as the presence of

Box 1. CAUSES OF JUGULAR DISTENSION.

- Tricuspid regurgitation
- Dilated cardiomyopathy
- Pericardial effusion or cardiac tamponade
- Obstructive pericarditis
- Atrioventricular dissociation
- Obstruction of the cranial vena cava
- Hypervolaemia

vibrations (thrills). The point of maximum heartbeat intensity is an ideal place to begin cardiac auscultation. However, before beginning, it is worth performing thorough pulmonary auscultation. This is an effective and valuable tool for identifying fluid lines, rhonchi, crepitation, wheezing, and rattling.

Cardiac auscultation should be performed using a good stethoscope with which the user is familiar, in a quiet environment without much external noise, and, above all, without rushing.

If the reader is looking for a faster approach to chest auscultation, the basic elements of the auscultation procedure are detailed at the end of this comprehensive description (see Box 3 below).

Three types of sounds can be detected during cardiac auscultation: normal heart sounds and alterations thereof; murmurs; and arrhythmias.

Heart sounds

Within heart sounds, which are relatively brief, we must distinguish intensity or volume, frequency or pitch, and quality or timbre.[2] The heart sounds that we can normally hear are identified as S_1, S_2, S_3, and S_4 (Fig. 1). Below we will review each and discuss their clinical significance.

Normal heart sounds

Normal sounds are S_1 and S_2. These indicate the onset and end of systole, and bookend an intervening period in which we must classify other sounds and murmurs. Both are high-frequency sounds. S_1 is produced by closure of the mitral and tricuspid valve leaflets, while S_2 occurs when the semilunar valve leaflets of the aorta and pulmonary valves close. Owing to the participation of these two pairs of valves, the point at which the maximum S_1 intensity is detected is in the left apical region of the heart (where the mitral valve is located).

PROPER STETHOSCOPE USE

Since its invention by René Théophile Hyacinthe Laënnec in 1816, the stethoscope has undergone various modifications. With a few exceptions, stethoscopes consist of a bell and a diaphragm. The bell is used to detect low-frequency sounds, while the diaphragm amplifies high frequencies. Gentle pressure should be applied when using the bell, as otherwise the skin can act as a diaphragm and amplify high-frequency sounds.

On the other hand, maximum S_2 intensity is detected at the left base of the heart (location of the aortic and pulmonary valves). This information allows us to identify the point at which the murmurs are strongest and determine whether they occur at the base or the apex of the heart.

The intensity of S_1 will largely depend on the position of the anterior leaflet of the mitral valve at the beginning of ventricular systole, as this is the largest of the leaflets that participate in S_1. Thus, in general, S_1 will be more intense the deeper this leaflet is in the left ventricle. This can occur more easily in patients with high heart rates, short PR intervals, or high sympathetic tone. However, other causes that may contribute to the increase in S_1 intensity include anaemia, systemic hypertension, and thinness. Conversely, S_1 intensity can be reduced in patients with pleural or pericardial effusion, severe obesity, or lesions occupying the space between the heart and the rib wall (tumours or herniated contents). Similarly, the volume of S_1 is diminished in cases of myocardial failure, prolonged PR interval, premature closure of the mitral valve, patients with shock, and various arrhythmias (e.g. atrial fibrillation).[1,2]

Occasionally the tricuspid and mitral leaflets close asynchronously, allowing detection of a split S_1. This finding can be normal in large- or giant-breed dogs, can be due to a delay in ventricular conduction (e.g. bundle branch block, artificial pacemakers, or ventricular arrhythmias), or can occur in patients with mitral or tricuspid valve stenosis.[1]

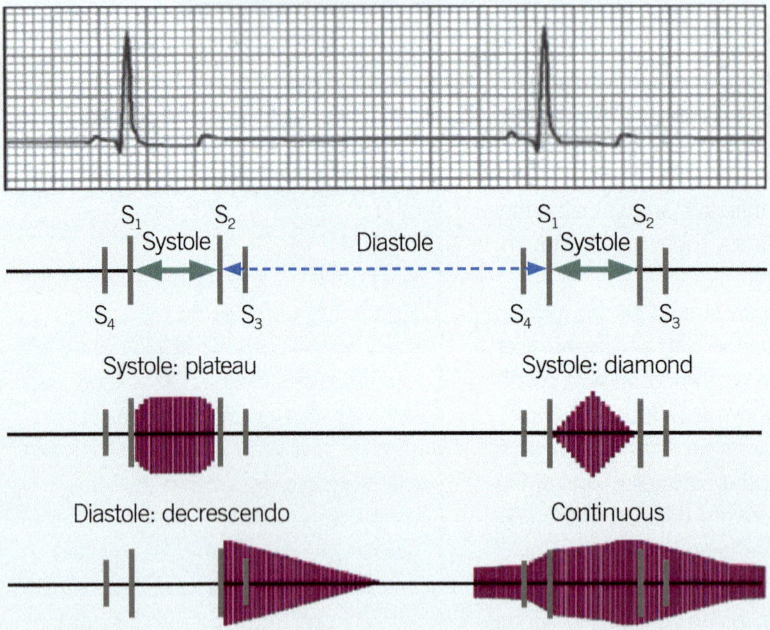

Figure 1. Relationship between heart sounds, the electrocardiographic trace, and the corresponding shape on the phonocardiogram.

The individual components of S_2 can be detected more easily. This is because during inspiration, the aortic component of S_2 precedes the pulmonary component as a consequence of the variations in the capacity of the pulmonary vascular bed and in the inspiratory increase in the volume of the right ventricle.[2] Thus, splitting of S_2 is rarely detected in normal dogs with large fluctuations in intrapleural pressure.[3] As also occurs for S_1, splitting of S_2 occurs pathologically in patients with delayed pulmonary valve closure. This is typically observed when right ventricular ejection is prolonged in cases of pulmonary hypertension, in patients with atrial or ventricular septal defects or pulmonary stenosis, or due to right bundle branch block.

TIP

Normal heart sounds (S_1 and S_2) are better detected using the diaphragm of the stethoscope, as they are high-frequency sounds. By contrast, S_3 and S_4 are low-frequency sounds and therefore better detected using the bell.

Abnormal heart sounds

While S_1 and S_2 are usually easily detected in small animals, it is also possible to identify two additional sounds: S_3 and S_4. The presence of these two sounds lends the heart a typical gallop rhythm. These rhythms usually appear due to problems associated with myocardial hypertrophy or high filling pressures.

S_3 is also known as the **ventricular gallop** or **protodiastolic gallop** and becomes audible when the ventricular rapid filling phase of diastole ends prematurely.[3] Detection of S_3 in dogs and cats has pathological implications. The diseases in which S_3 is most easily detected are those that cause ventricular dilation or eccentric hypertrophy, including dilated cardiomyopathies, atrioventricular valve insufficiency, and large left-to-right shunts.

TAKE NOTE!

Maximum S_3 intensity typically occurs in the left apical area. This sound may be the only auscultatory abnormality in patients with dilated cardiomyopathy.

The S_4 sound is also known as the **atrial gallop** or **presystolic gallop**. This sound most often occurs when increased atrial contraction is required to fill a rigid and concentrically hypertrophied ventricle. It can also occur in patients with semilunar valve stenosis.

TAKE NOTE!

S_4 may be the only auscultatory abnormality in patients with hypertrophic cardiomyopathy, systemic hypertension, or hyperthyroidism.

Murmurs

Murmurs are defined as prolonged, vibrating heart sounds produced when blood flow changes from laminar to turbulent (Fig. 2) This turbulence occurs when the blood encounters abnormal communications between the cardiac chambers or insufficient or stenotic valves. Murmurs are often detected when the blood loses its normal characteristics (e.g. in anaemia) or when the vascular diameter is very large (the larger the vessel, the greater the turbulence). These murmurs can be characterised based on their maximum intensity and their duration relative to the cardiac cycle, intensity, frequency, configuration (pattern or shape), location, and direction of radiation.[2]

Parameters useful for characterisation of murmurs

- **Point of maximal intensity (PMI) of the murmur:** based on this characteristic we can define three types of murmur: systolic murmurs start at or immediately after S_1, and extend to S_2, or just before. By contrast, diastolic murmurs, which are much less common, start at or immediately after S_2 and extend to S_1, or just before. Finally, continuous murmurs begin in systole (S_1) and extend beyond S_2, without interruption through all or part of diastole (Box 2).
- **Intensity:** the first and most important point to note is that the intensity of the murmur does not always correlate with the severity of the disease. However, classifying intensity using a scale will allow us to determine whether a murmur increases or decreases over time in a given patient, and refer it to colleagues or describe it on a report or paper (Table 1).
- **Frequency:** from a clinical point of view, murmurs can be of high or low frequency. In practice, we must always auscultate using the two options that stethoscopes offer. If a sound is better detected using the bell, it will be of low frequency. If it is better detected using the diaphragm, it will be of high frequency.
- **Configuration:** this refers to the shape of the murmur as viewed on a phonocardiogram. This characteristic is not easy to interpret using only a stethoscope and our hearing. According to this, murmurs can have a plateau, diamond, or decrescendo shape (Fig. 1).
- **Location and direction of radiation:** murmurs are described by their point of maximal intensity over the area of the heart valve at which they are loudest (Fig. 3). On the other hand, the radiation characteristics associated with the direction of blood flow responsible for the murmurs can help differentiate murmurs with a similar point of maximal intensity, such as those caused by pulmonary versus subaortic stenosis.

Box 2. SUBCHARACTERISATION OF MURMURS ACCORDING TO THE POINT OF MAXIMAL INTENSITY (PMI).

Systolic
- Early systolic or protosystolic
- Mid-systolic or mesosystolic
- Late systolic or telesystolic

Diastolic
- Early diastolic or protodiastolic
- Mid-diastolic or mesodiastolic
- Late diastolic or telediastolic

Continuous
- Holosystolic (throughout systole)
- Holodiastolic (throughout diastole)

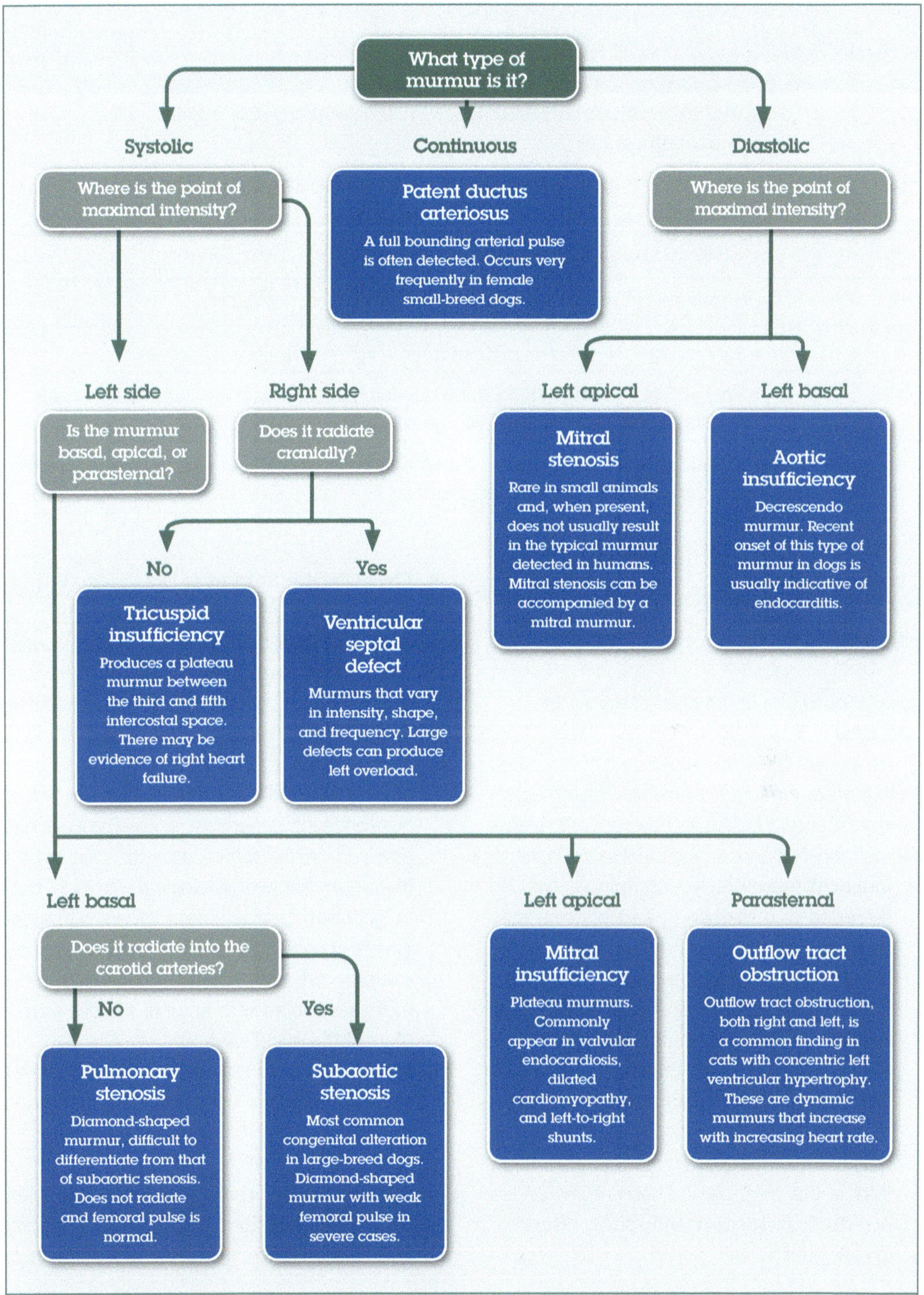

Figure 2. Characterisation of heart murmurs.

Table 1. Classification of murmurs according to intensity.

Grade	Description
I	Very soft murmur, only detectable with special effort. Only registers on a phonocardiogram.
II	Mild murmur detected within seconds of auscultation by an experienced examiner.
III	Easily audible murmur of moderate intensity.
IV	Strong murmur that does not produce vibration on palpation.
V	Very strong murmur that produces vibration on palpation.
VI	Very strong murmur that produces vibration on palpation and can be heard after separating the stethoscope from the rib cage.

As there are numerous grading scales, we will refer the murmurs as follows: murmur III/VI. This provides our colleagues with a better idea of the intensity of a given murmur.

Types of murmur

Below, we will briefly describe each of the most important murmurs.

Systolic murmurs at the base of the heart (left side)

There are five types of systolic murmurs located in this area: innocent murmurs, physiological murmurs, and those caused by subaortic stenosis, pulmonary stenosis, and atrial septal defects.

- **Innocent murmurs:** young animals with no evidence of underlying heart disease may have mild systolic murmurs (grade I to III/VI) in the left hemithorax at the base of the heart. These are typically mesosystolic and of high frequency. These murmurs are largely devoid of radiation. Although their origin is uncertain, innocent murmurs are thought to reflect increased blood flow velocity and the consequent turbulence created through the outflow tract of the ventricles.[2] These murmurs are not usually progressive and usually disappear in early adulthood.
- **Physiological murmurs:** like innocent murmurs, physiological or functional murmurs tend to be mild (grade I to III/VI), and located in the same area. They are detected in conditions of high cardiac output (e.g. hyperthyroidism, fever, pregnancy) or decreased blood viscosity (e.g. anaemia), without significant organic heart disease. They generally disappear once the underlying disease process has resolved. While some cats with mild hyperthyroidism show physiological murmurs due to increased cardiac output, others with more severe forms of this endocrinopathy may exhibit more intense and pathological murmurs associated with anterior systolic movement of the mitral valve.
- **Murmurs due to subaortic stenosis:** one of the most common congenital heart diseases in dogs is subaortic stenosis, which is the presence of a fibromuscular band just below the aortic valve. This lesion complicates left ventricular ejection, causing high-velocity and turbulent flow through the outflow tract

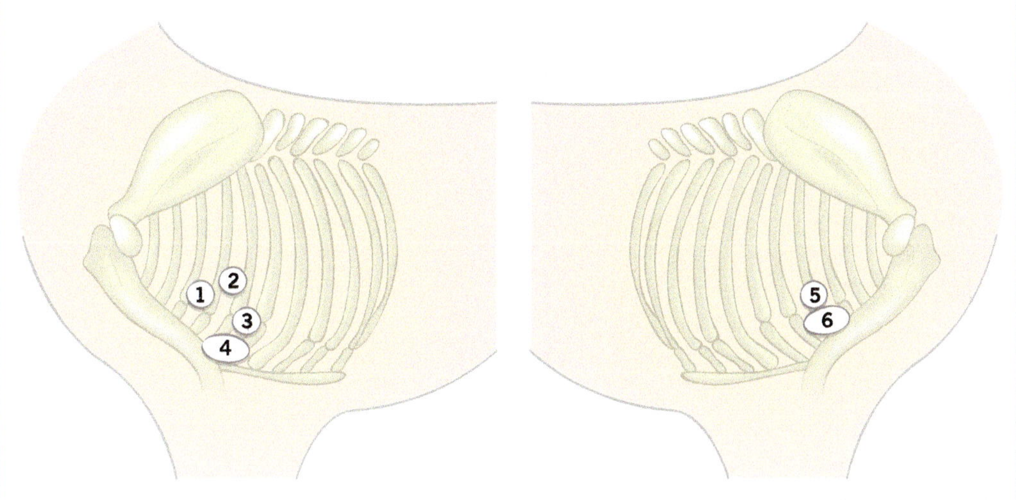

Figure 3. Points of auscultation for different murmurs. The projection areas for murmurs on the left side of the chest include the left basal region (1 and 2), the left apical region (3), and the left parasternal region (4). Murmurs originating in the pulmonary valve in dogs are generally loudest in the third intercostal space (1). Aortic valve lesions are usually most audible between the third and fourth intercostal spaces, just below the shoulder line (2), while the point of maximal intensity of mitral valve murmurs is in the fifth intercostal space, near the costochondral junction (3). Another important area for auscultation in cats is the left parasternal region (4). Heart murmurs associated with tricuspid valve disease in dogs are generally loudest in the right fourth intercostal space, near the costochondral junction (5). As with the left parasternal region, the right parasternal region (6) should be carefully auscultated in cats to detect dynamic outflow tract murmurs.

and into the aortic valve. Subaortic stenosis causes diamond-shaped murmurs of varying intensity in the left base of the heart during systole that can radiate into the right cranial chest. Mild subaortic stenosis often causes a mild systolic murmur at the left base of the heart that can be very difficult to distinguish from innocent or physiological murmurs. Moderate or severe stenosis produces a more pronounced, high-frequency systolic murmur on the left side and over the base of the heart. The most serious murmurs can radiate to the thoracic inlet along the carotid arteries and, in rare cases, may be audible at the top of the patient's head. Radiation characteristics and evaluation of the quality of the femoral pulse often help to distinguish severe subaortic stenosis (radiation to the carotid arteries with weak femoral pulses) from severe pulmonary stenosis (with only occasional radiation to the neck and normal femoral pulses).

- **Pulmonary stenosis murmurs:** the most common congenital anomaly of the pulmonary valve is valvular dysplasia, in which the leaflets of the valve fuse together. Its inability to open normally during right ventricular systole produces turbulent, high-velocity blood flow through the pulmonary valve with radiation to the pulmonary arteries. The murmurs produced during pulmonary stenosis are diamond-shaped, systolic, of variable intensity, and located in the left base of the heart.

Compared with those caused by subaortic stenosis, pulmonary stenosis murmurs do not radiate as extensively to the right cranial hemithorax or the carotid arteries. Furthermore, the quality of the femoral pulse in patients with pulmonary stenosis tends to be normal. Sometimes pulmonary stenosis can be complicated by tricuspid regurgitation and clinical signs of right heart failure. It is important to note that one of the components of tetralogy of Fallot is pulmonary stenosis, but this congenital heart defect is much more complex and is further complicated by the presence of a ventricular septal defect, juxtaposition of the aorta, and right ventricular hypertrophy.

- **Atrial septal defect murmurs:** although atrial septal defects are rare in dogs and cats, they are frequently accompanied by a diamond-shaped, mild systolic murmur at the base of the heart, on the left. This murmur is caused by the increase in volume of the right ventricle (as a consequence of left-to-right shunt; the blood then flows through a normal pulmonary valve). One possible additional auscultatory finding is fixed splitting of S_2.

Apical systolic murmurs (left side)

These are plateau-shaped systolic murmurs of variable intensity located in the apical area of the left hemithorax, and are usually due to mitral regurgitation. They vary in intensity from grade I to VI, depending on the severity of the insufficiency, the pressure gradient between the left ventricle and left atrium, the radiation of the valvular reflux, and the presence or absence of comorbid conditions (e.g. pericardial or pleural effusion, obesity, or abnormal conformation of the thorax).

TAKE NOTE!

Left apical systolic murmurs are the most common abnormalities detected on cardiac auscultation of middle-aged to senior small-breed dogs.

The mildest murmurs (grade I/VI) caused by mitral regurgitation are usually protosystolic to mesosystolic and do not mask S_1 or S_2. Detection of these murmurs requires the use of a phonocardiogram. More severe murmurs (IV to VI/VI) are usually of mixed frequency and radiate broadly in the right hemithorax (greatly complicating the diagnosis of tricuspid regurgitation). The duration usually corresponds to the entire systole (holosystolic).

Chronic degenerative valve disease is the most common cause of mitral regurgitation, although diseases that produce eccentric hypertrophy or dilation of the mitral valve annulus (e.g. dilated cardiomyopathy, left-to-right patent ductus arteriosus, ventricular septal defect) and abnormalities of the mitral valve apparatus (e.g. valve dysplasia, valvular endocarditis, or anterior systolic movement of the mitral valve) are also associated with mitral regurgitation. Therefore, a plateau-shaped left apical systolic murmur is indicative of mitral regurgitation, but is not diagnostic of the underlying disease.

Systolic murmurs originating in the right side of the heart

These are usually caused by tricuspid regurgitation or ventricular septal defects. Below, we will describe each type of murmur:

- **Tricuspid regurgitation murmurs:** the region in which tricuspid regurgitation murmurs are most easily detected on auscultation is between the third and fifth intercostal spaces, near the costochondral junction on the right hemithorax. Like mitral regurgitation, regurgitation through the tricuspid valve causes murmurs of varying intensity. The intensity and duration will depend on the systolic pressure. This murmur has a plateau shape and is commonly detected in chronic degenerative disease or valve dysplasia, dilated cardiomyopathy, and pulmonary hypertension. Unfortunately, the strong murmurs of mitral regurgitation often radiate to this area, making it very difficult to differentiate purely mitral disease from a mixed condition based on physical examination alone. Tricuspid murmurs must also be distinguished from subaortic stenosis with marked radiation to the right side and from ventricular septal defects (left-to-right).
- **Ventricular septal defect murmurs:** the murmurs that accompany these septal defects will vary depending on the location and size of the defect. Lesion severity is inversely proportional to the intensity of the murmur. Thus, large defects will produce small murmurs and vice versa. The most common murmurs, which are associated with small restrictive ventricular defects (left-to-right), are systolic with high intensity and high frequency. They are plateau shaped and their point of maximal intensity is located in the right hemithorax at the cranial level. By contrast, larger left-to-right ventricular septal defects are usually not restrictive, resulting in a mild systolic murmur. Finally, in patients with ventricular septal defects that are balanced thanks to pulmonary hypertension, flow through the defect (and hence murmur) is prevented. However, these patients usually have split S_2.[2]

Parasternal murmurs

Cats with mitral valve dysplasia or concentric left ventricular hypertrophy (e.g. patients with hypertrophic cardiomyopathy, hyperthyroidism, or systemic hypertension) may have left ventricular outflow tract obstruction. This occurs when the anterior mitral leaflet is pushed, pulled, or sucked into the outflow tract. This alteration is usually accompanied by mitral regurgitation and a left apical or sternal systolic murmur caused by high-velocity, turbulent flow through the left outflow tract. These murmurs usually intensify with tachycardia.

TAKE NOTE!

Murmurs associated with dynamic obstruction of the right ventricular outflow tract usually have characteristics very similar to those associated with dynamic obstruction of the left ventricular outflow tract, and can only be correctly differentiated using Doppler echocardiography.

Table 2. Clinical comparison between mitral valve disease and dilated cardiomyopathy in dogs.

	Mitral valve disease	Dilated cardiomyopathy
Clinical signs	Secondary to congestive heart failure: • Cough, due to pulmonary oedema. • Tachypnoea and increased respiratory effort. • Exercise intolerance and lethargy. • Syncope due to baroreceptor alterations that lead to hypotension.	Secondary to congestive heart failure: • Cough, due to pulmonary oedema. • Tachypnoea and increased respiratory effort. • Exercise intolerance and lethargy. • Syncope due to arrhythmias that can cause sudden death without previous clinical signs.
Clinical examination findings	Holosystolic or pansystolic murmur, most audible in the left apical area. Radiates dorsally and caudally and towards the right hemithorax. S_3 sometimes audible due to overload.	• Mild systolic murmur. • Normal to weak femoral pulse. • S_3 gallop rhythm.
Radiological findings	• X-rays are initially normal. Over time, left atrial dilation appears. This can lead to tracheobronchial narrowing. • Pulmonary congestion and oedema when CHF is present. Congestion often appears earlier.	Generalised cardiomegaly: • Usually begins in the left heart. • Pulmonary congestion and oedema when left CHF is present. • Pleural effusion, hepatosplenomegaly, and ascites when right CHF is present.
ECG	• Symptomatic patients: P wave >0.04 s due to atrial dilation. • High QRS due to left ventricular dilation. • Atrial arrhythmias (fibrillation). • Ventricular arrhythmias (late phases). • Tachycardia due to low cardiac output.	• Premature ventricular complexes typical in Doberman and Boxer breeds. • Atrial fibrillation in giant breeds.
Ultrasound	• Left eccentric hypertrophy. • Hyperdynamic contraction of the left heart. • Mitral regurgitation in Doppler.	Increase in diameter at the end of diastole and reduction in the shortening fraction (<25 %).

Aetiopathogenesis

Although the cause of myxomatous valvular degeneration is unknown, this disease appears to have a hereditary component in certain breeds, and its severity may be genetically determined in others. The disease is characterised by changes in cellular constituents and in the intercellular matrix of the valve apparatus (including the valve leaflets and chordae tendineae). These changes affect both the collagen content and the alignment of the collagen fibrils within the valve. The expansion of the spongy layer is characterised by changes in the proteoglycan content in this layer. Dysregulation of the extracellular matrix appears to be essential for these changes to occur. Valve interstitial cells, possibly due to post-transcriptional regulation of microsatellite RNAs, acquire properties of activated myofibroblasts, which produce proteolytic enzymes, including matrix metalloproteinases, that degrade elastin and collagen faster than inactivated valve interstitial cells can produce them.[14]

When the mitral valve leaflets become thick and twisted, they fail to close the mitral orifice during ventricular contraction, and blood leaks from the left ventricle into the left atrium. The amount that escapes depends on the pressure difference between the ventricle and atrium, the size of the gap, and the duration for which pressure is higher in the left ventricle than the left atrium. The volume of blood expelled by the left ventricle is the sum of the blood that travels to the aorta and the regurgitated blood (Fig. 4).

The **regurgitant fraction** is the relationship between ejected and regurgitated blood. This fraction may not be very large, but may be sufficient to dilate the left atrium. When this fraction reaches or exceeds 100 % (i.e. the volume of blood entering the aorta equals that which is regurgitated into the left atrium), congestion of the pulmonary vessels and pulmonary oedema will develop. At this point, cardiac output may be insufficient to maintain normal function.

Clinical signs associated with mitral insufficiency can include cough, dyspnoea, exercise intolerance, and syncope.[5–7]

Diagnostic protocol

When a patient presents with clinical signs of valvular heart disease or if a mitral murmur is detected during an annual checkup, it is advisable to recommend a cardiac examination protocol.

Below are the steps that should be followed:

1. Consultation focusing on the cardiovascular system, as described in the first part of this chapter.
2. Once this is done, perhaps the fastest, most economic, and easiest test to request is lateral and dorsoventral chest radiography (Fig. 5). In these X-rays, several parameters must be evaluated:
   - Cardiac size, relative to vertebral bodies (vertebral heart score), and estimated size of the cardiac chambers.
   - Presence of respiratory disease and/or pulmonary oedema.
   - Tracheal size.
   - Assessment of the pulmonary vessels.

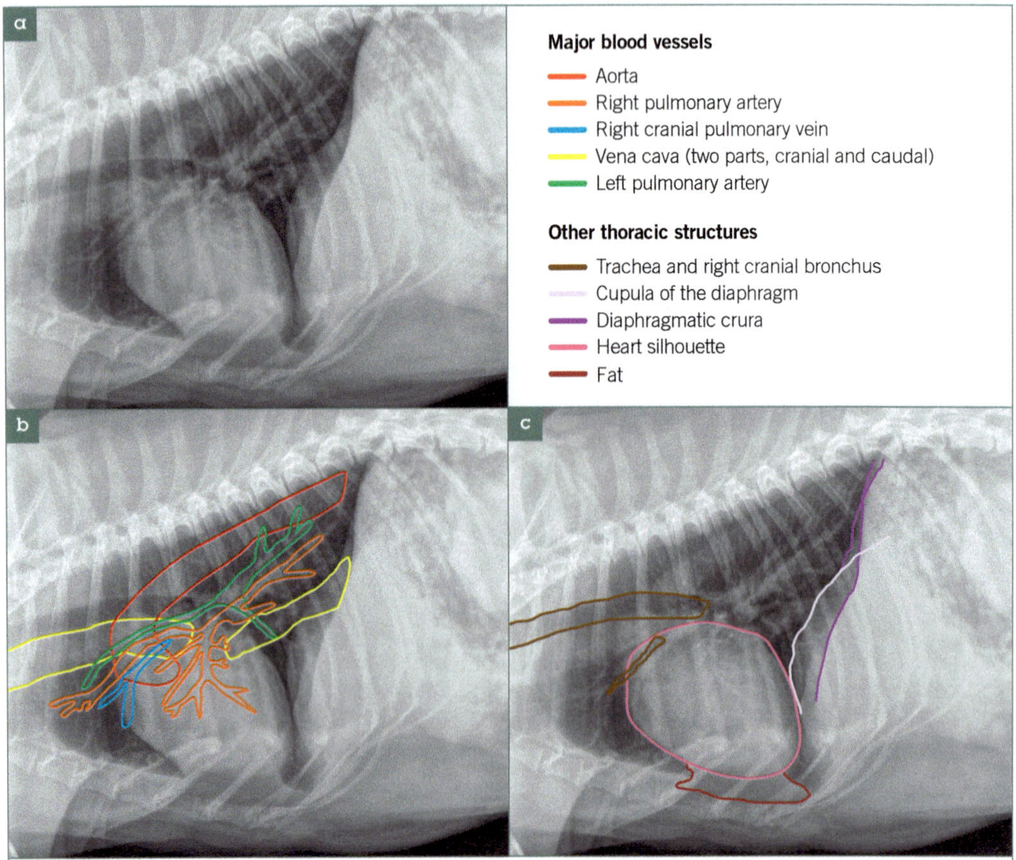

Figure 4. X-ray of a 12-year-old female German Shepherd Dog (a). Major blood vessels (b). Other thoracic structures (c).

> **TIP**
>
> If there is a risk to the life of the patient, radiography must be postponed until the patient stabilises. In these cases, it may be useful to perform rapid echocardiography or a TFAST ultrasound, even with the patient standing up. This is done not to establish a definitive diagnosis, but to determine the most appropriate treatment.

3. Whenever possible, if cardiomegaly, pulmonary oedema, or pulmonary hypertension are detected, it is advisable to perform echocardiography, ideally together with an electrocardiographic study.
4. Whenever the patient begins treatment for heart disease, it is highly recommended to measure serum levels of creatinine, albumin, and potassium, at the very least.
5. Determining blood pressure is a standard practice in both species, but is especially useful in cats given the high prevalence of arterial hypertension in this species.

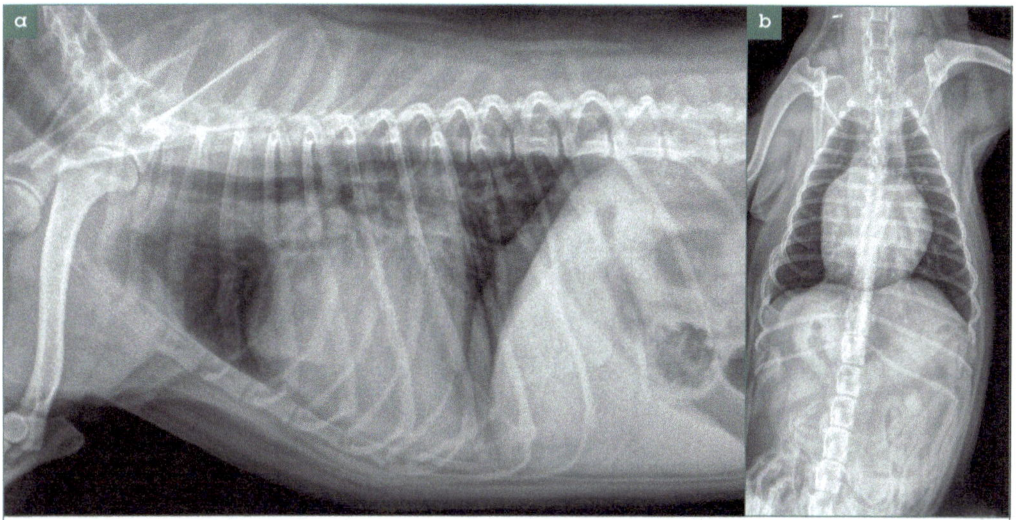

Figure 5. Lateral (a) and dorsoventral (b) chest X-rays of a dog with mitral valve disease diagnosed 3 years earlier, and treated with pimobendan, ACE inhibitors, and furosemide. An interstitial pattern is evident in the caudal area of the chest, as well as generalised cardiomegaly with elevation of the trachea and an increase in the vascular pattern (the pulmonary veins are the same size as the arteries).

Treatment of canine valvular disease

Table 3 shows the drugs most used in canine cardiology, their doses, and when and why to use them.

In 2009, the American College of Veterinary Internal Medicine (ACVIM) published their expert consensus on the treatment of canine valvular disease.[14,15] This first text,[a] as well as the 2017 revision,[b] can be consulted online. These consensus guidelines classify the patient according to their clinical status and provide corresponding treatment recommendations.

Table 4 shows the classification of patients with valvular heart disease according to the ACVIM consensus guidelines.

[a] https://doi.org/10.1111/j.1939-1676.2009.0392.x
[b] https://doi.org/10.1111/jvim.15488

Table 3. Drugs used to treat heart disease and their indications.

Drug	Dosage in dogs	Dosage in cats	Criteria for use	Effect/objective
Angiotensin converting enzyme inhibitors (ACEI)				
Benazepril	0.25–0.5 mg/kg PO every 24 h	0.25–0.5 mg/kg PO every 24 h	Dilation of the left atrium	↓ Pre- and afterload, ↓ myocardial O_2 demand, ↓ remodelling, and ↓ action of the renin–angiotensin–aldosterone system (RAAS)
Ramipril	0.125 mg/kg PO every 24 h	0.125 mg/kg PO every 24 h		
Enalapril	0.25–1 mg/kg PO every 12–24 h	0.25–0.5 mg/kg PO every 12–24 h		
Angiotensin II receptor blockers (ARBs)				
Telmisartan	-	1.5–2 mg/kg PO every 24 h	Hypertension	Systolic pressure <160 mmHg, and if possible <140 mmHg
Selective beta-blockers				
Atenolol	0.25–1 mg/kg PO every 12–24 h	6.25–12.5 mg/kg PO every 24 h	Tachycardia and dilation of the left ventricle Avoid starting during late disease stages	↓ Heart rate and ↓ myocardial oxidative stress Antiarrhythmic effect
Phosphodiesterase III inhibitors				
Pimobendan	0.5–2.5 mg/kg PO every 12 h	0.625 mg/cat PO every 12 h if <3 kg 1.25 mg/cat PO every 12 h if >3 kg	Dilation of the left ventricle	Inodilator (vasodilator and inotropic +) usually chronotropic – Improves contractility and has some antiarrhythmic effect

Table 3. Drugs used to treat heart disease and their indications (cont'd).

Drug	Dosage in dogs	Dosage in cats	Criteria for use	Effect/objective
Loop diuretics (administer the lowest possible dose for maintenance)				
Furosemide	0.25–2 mg/kg PO every 12–24 h (maintenance) 2–8 mg/kg IV every 1–6 h (acute treatment)	0.25–2 mg/kg PO every 12–24 h (maintenance) 1–4 mg/kg IV every 2–6 hours (acute treatment)	Pulmonary oedema	↑ Urine production, bronchodilation and venous dilation (if IV)
Torasemide	0.1–0.6 mg/kg PO every 24 h	0.13–0.25 mg/kg PO every 24–48 h	Pulmonary oedema	↑ Urine production
Thiazides				
Hydrochlorothiazide	1–4 mg/kg PO every 12 h	1–4 mg/kg PO every 12–24 h	Acute or refractory pulmonary oedema	↑ Urine production
Peripheral vasodilators				
Nitroglycerine	0.6–1 cm of 2 % ointment applied to the skin inside the ear every 6–12 h Also available in patches	0.6 cm of 2 % ointment applied to the skin inside the ear every 6–12 h	Acute or refractory pulmonary oedema	Peripheral vein dilation
Ca^{2+} channel blockers				
Diltiazem	0.5–1.5 mg/kg PO every 8 h 1–4 mg/kg PO every 12 h in slow-release formulations	1.75–2.5 mg/kg PO every 8 h, or 7.5–15 mg/cat PO every 8 h 10 mg/kg PO every 24 h in slow-release formulations	Atrial fibrillation and supra-ventricular tachycardia	↓ Heart rate

Table 4. Classification of heart failure according to the ACVIM consensus statement.

Grade	Mitral diseases in dogs	Myocardial diseases in cats
Stage A	Breeds at high-risk but without heart abnormalities (Cavalier King Charles Spaniel and other predisposed breeds without murmur). **Treatment not recommended.**	Breeds at high-risk but without heart abnormalities (Maine Coon, Ragdoll). **Treatment not recommended.**
Stage B	**B1:** asymptomatic dogs without cardiac remodelling or with mild remodelling. **Treatment not recommended.**	**B1:** asymptomatic cats with low risk of impending congestive heart failure (CHF) or aortic thromboembolism (ATE).* **Treatment not recommended.**
	B2: asymptomatic dogs with moderate-to-severe cardiac remodelling. **Start treatment with pimobendan and moderate sodium restriction.**	**B2:** asymptomatic cats at increased risk of impending CHF or ATE.* **Start treatment with clopidogrel ± other anticoagulant therapies. Treatment with atenolol can be started if atrial fibrillation or ectopic ventricular complexes are present.**
Stage C	Patients with current or past clinical signs of heart failure. May require hospitalisation for stabilisation.	Patients that have developed clinical signs of CHF or ATE, even if these have resolved with treatment.
Stage D	Patients with clinical signs of severe heart failure refractory to standard treatment.	Patients that have developed clinical signs of CHF or ATE refractory to standard treatment.

* In cats, atrial size is often used to differentiate risk level B1 from B2.

WHAT IS THE CURRENT STATE OF CARDIAC BIOMARKERS?

Currently two types of markers are used: markers of cellular integrity (troponins or cTnI) and markers of myocardial function (natriuretic peptides or NT-proBNP). The former allow us to determine whether loss of integrity or necrosis of the myocyte membrane has occurred. The latter allow us to determine whether there has been an alteration in myocardial function. Nowadays, these are mainly used in cases in which it is difficult to discern heart disease from respiratory disease.

Rapid NT-proBNP tests can be performed in the emergency room in cats with dyspnoea using plasma or pleural fluid diluted 1:1 with saline to increase specificity.

Hypertrophic cardiomyopathy (HCM) or hypertrophic cardiomyopathy phenotype in cats

The first expert consensus guidelines for the classification, diagnosis, and management of feline cardiomyopathy were published very recently.[16]

This is the most common form of heart disease in cats, with a prevalence of 15 %. Although it was initially thought that prevalence did not increase with age, we now know that it does, reaching up to 29 %, even after excluding patients with hyperthyroidism and arterial hypertension.[17]

Certain cat breeds (Maine Coon, Ragdoll, Persian, Bengal, Sphynx, British Shorthair, Norwegian Forest Cat, and Burmese) are thought to be predisposed to this cardiomyopathy. However, although a sarcomeric genetic mutation (MyBPC3) has been detected in the Maine Coon, the prevalence of this mutation (35–42 %) is not in line with the phenotypic prevalence of this disease in this breed. Moreover, although the role of nongenetic factors and epigenetic factors is unknown, they may help explain the discrepancies between the prevalence of genetic mutations and that of disease phenotypes.

Clinical signs

The clinical picture of HCM is not particularly notable, and most cats are brought to the veterinary clinic when the disease has already caused lung oedema, pleural effusion, or aortic thromboembolism. These cats are clearly dyspnoeic and should be handled in a manner that minimises stress as much as possible.

Table 5. Drugs useful to treat and combat thromboembolism and hypercoagulability in cats.

Anticoagulant	Dosage
Clopidogrel	18.75 mg/cat PO every 24 h
Aspirin	10–20 mg/cat PO every 72 h
Low-molecular-weight heparin (enoxaparin)	1–1.5 mg/kg SC every 12–24 h

Physical examination

Cats with HCM usually present with a holosystolic murmur on the left side or in the right sternal area (80 %). Not all patients will have a murmur, nor will all murmurs be of the same intensity. Many cats tend to have a gallop rhythm. However, detection of this rhythm is not easy due to the tachycardia that patients tend to present when they arrive at the clinic.

Additional tests

Radiography is not usually very useful for diagnosis of HCM, as cardiomegaly will not be present in all cats with this disease (Fig. 6), at least in the laterolateral projection. The ventrodorsal or dorsoventral projections may reveal a bulge in the left atrium. This atrial bulge corresponds to the radiological sign known as a "valentine heart".[18] Nonetheless, radiography is very useful for the diagnosis of pulmonary hypertension and pulmonary oedema (Fig. 7).

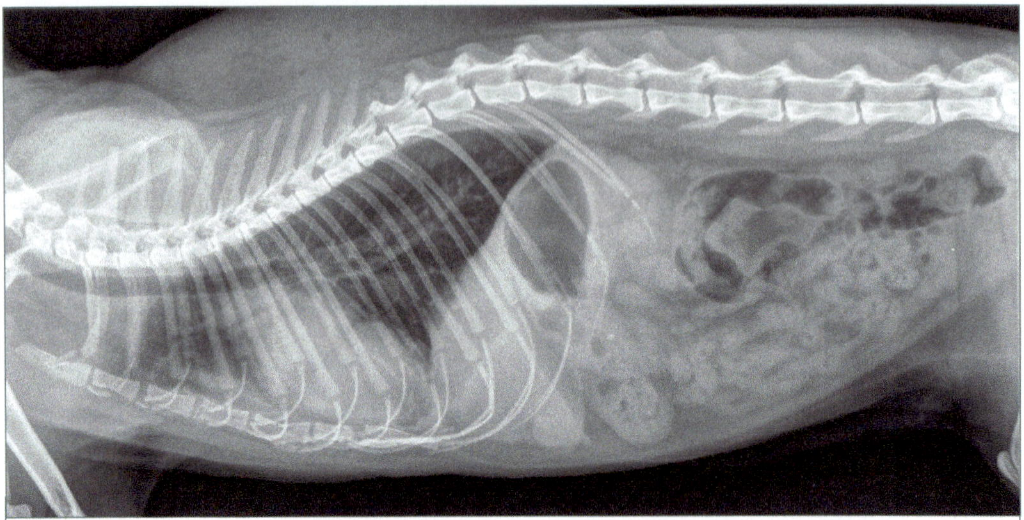

Figure 6. Cat with hypertrophic cardiomyopathy and marked cardiomegaly. X-ray taken under sedation. The appearance of the interscapular zone is due to subcutaneous fluid therapy.

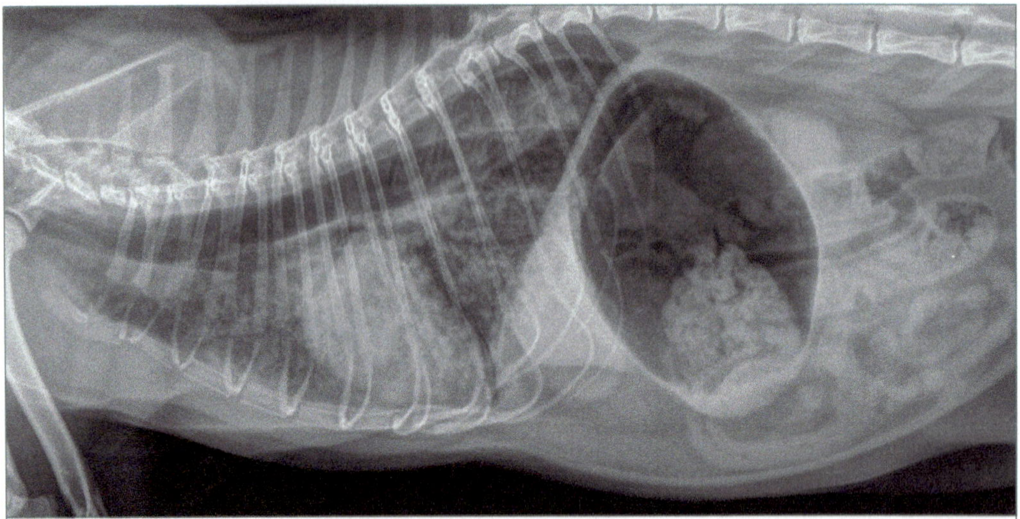

Figure 7. Cat with hypertrophic cardiomyopathy. Severe pulmonary oedema and significant dilation of the left atrium are evident. At the time the X-ray was taken, the patient had aortic thromboembolism.

How to interpret a chest X-ray

Radiography enables the detection of cardiomegaly at a lower cost than any other diagnostic tool. The problem with chest X-rays is knowing how to interpret them correctly and extracting the maximum information. For multiple reasons, this is not achieved as often as it should be. At least four important points should be borne in mind and noted in the patient's medical history.

Before beginning, we must know how to correctly perform a chest X-ray. Posture, timing of respiration, and the settings used are essential to obtain reliable readings from radiographs.

To determine whether a chest X-ray has been taken in adequate conditions, we must look at certain details:

- **Lateral projection:** the dorsal spinous process of the thoracic vertebra must be aligned with the scapula. The forelimbs should be extended forward to avoid overlap with the cranial thorax. The dorsal heads of the ribs should be superimposed on or slightly above the vertebral bodies. Finally, exposure should take place during inspiration, ensuring maximum separation between the caudal cardiac margin and the cupula of the diaphragm.
- **Dorsoventral projection:** the thoracic vertebrae should be aligned with and superimposed upon the silhouette of the heart. In turn, the spinous processes of all thoracic vertebrae should be aligned with the vertebral bodies. It is important to perform the exposure during the final phase of inspiration. If this is done correctly, the cardiac silhouette will be separated from the cupula of the diaphragm.

The following parameters should be evaluated in all cardiac X-rays:

- **Vertebral size (vertebral heart score or Buchanan index):** in a lateral X-ray, the long axis of the heart is measured following a line running from the ventral part of the left main bronchus (at the tracheal bifurcation) to the apex of the left ventricle. This line is superimposed over the vertebral column beginning at the cranial edge of the fourth thoracic vertebra. The length of the heart is calculated as the number of thoracic vertebrae that this line spans. The maximum short perpendicular axis is measured and superimposed the same way. Breed-specific studies have been performed to eliminate breed-associated variation in heart size (Box 4).
- **Presence of respiratory disease and/or pulmonary oedema:** lung oedema is relatively easy to diagnose in dogs, since it usually appears as a loss of definition in the caudal edge of the cardiac silhouette in lateral and (more notably) dorsoventral projections. Feline pulmonary oedema can be more difficult to diagnose, as it can present with a number of different patterns, from a diffuse pattern (like in dogs) to a patchy pattern.[19]
- **Tracheal size:** this parameter is used to diagnose hypoplasia or tracheal collapse. In the lateral projection we must calculate the relationship between the size of the trachea at the thoracic inlet and the thoracic inlet itself. This is determined at the point of entry into the thorax by measuring the lumen, not the external diameter. This measurement must be completely perpendicular to the longitudinal axis of the trachea. The thoracic inlet is measured from the ventral aspect of the vertebral column, at the midpoint of the first rib, to the dorsal aspect of the sternal manubrium at its thinnest point (Table 6).

Box 4. HEART SIZE WITH RESPECT TO VERTEBRAL SIZE ACCORDING TO BREED AND SPECIES.

Dogs in general: 8.5–10.5

Cats in general: 7.5 ± 0.3

Doberman: 10 ± 0.6

Boxer: 11.6 ± 0.8

Cavalier King Charles: 10.6 ± 0.5

German Shepherd Dog: 9.7 ± 0.7

Labrador Retriever: 10.8 ± 0.6

Whippet: 11 ± 0.5

Yorkshire Terrier: 9.7 ± 0.5

- **Pulmonary vessel size:** the pulmonary artery and vein should be approximately the same size. In the lateral projection, the artery and vein of the right cranial pulmonary lobe should not exceed the diameter of the narrowest proximal portion of the fourth rib. In the dorsoventral projection, the artery and vein of the caudal pulmonary lobes should be the same size as the 9th rib at the point where they intersect.

Echocardiography

Echocardiography is the gold standard for the diagnosis of this condition. The most common echocardiographic findings are:

- Thickening of the left ventricular wall in diastole (>5–6 mm, according to different sources) (Fig. 8).
- Left atrial dilation: left atrial to aortic diameter (LA:Ao) ratio >1.5:1. If this ratio reaches 2:1, the dilation is considered severe.
- Anterior systolic movement of the mitral valve.

Table 6. Description of the relationship between tracheal size and the thoracic inlet in different breeds.

		Tracheal diameter:thoracic inlet ratio
Dog breeds*	Meso- and dolichocephalic	0.21 ± 0.03
	Brachycephalic	0.16 ± 0.03
	Bulldog	0.11 ± 0.03
Cat breeds**	Domestic shorthair	0.18
	Persian	0.20

* Hayward N, Schwarz T, Weisse C. The trachea. In: Schwarz T, Johnson V, eds. *BSAVA Manual of Canine and Feline Thoracic Imaging*, 2008, pp. 213–27.
** Hammond G et al. Radiographic measurements of the trachea in domestic shorthair and Persian cats. *J Feline Med Surg*, 2011, 13(12):881–4.

Treatment

Treatment of HCM depends on the phase in which the cat is and, mainly, on its clinical signs. Thus, in a patient with CHF it may not be useful to start treatment with a beta-blocker, but instead with pimobendan (an unregistered drug that appears to help in some cases of CHF).

In general, cats with HCM can be treated according to the stage and their specific needs using beta-blockers, ACEIs, angiotensin II receptor blockers (ARBs), diuretics, and anticoagulants, among others (Table 5). Table 3 summarises the drugs most commonly used in cardiology, and their doses.

Feline hypertension

Feline arterial hypertension is becoming more prevalent. This is due to progressive aging of the feline population, increasing prevalence of different diseases that promote hypertension, and greater ease of measurement of this fundamental but often overlooked parameter (Box 5 and Table 7).

Regulation of blood pressure (the underlying physiology)

Blood pressure is regulated by a series of neuroendocrine mechanisms. These regulate pressure to maintain cardiac output and volume and blood supply to the body. The sympathetic and parasympathetic nervous systems control heart rate and myocardial contractility, as well as the resistance that the blood vessels pose to the passage of blood, via their effects on vascular smooth muscle.

Arterial baroreceptor reflex

Blood pressure is monitored by baroreceptors located in the aorta and in the carotid arteries. These receptors detect variations in pressure. This information is sent to the brainstem, which responds by transmitting different responses to the heart and vessels.

A drop in pressure increases sympathetic tone while reducing parasympathetic tone. This demonstrates how the two components of the autonomic nervous system work in perfect harmony. An increase in sympathetic tone implies

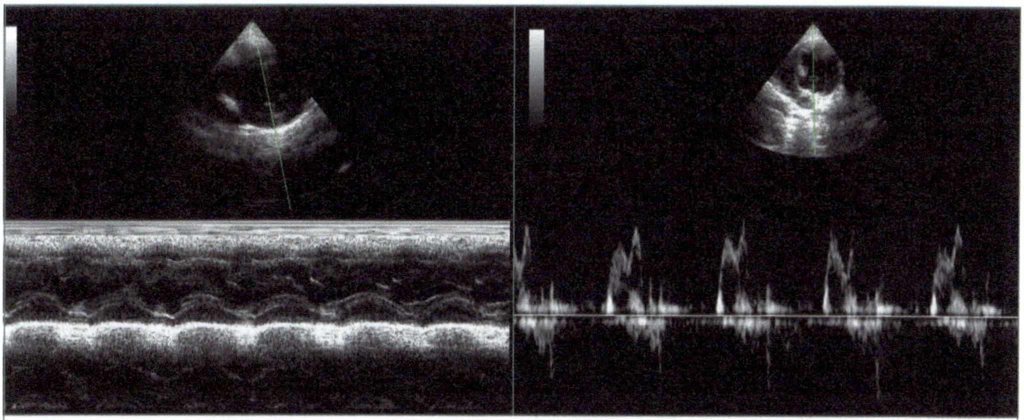

Figure 8. Echocardiograms from a cat with hypertrophic cardiomyopathy. The free wall of the left ventricle can be seen. The measurement obtained from this wall was 7.1 mm.

Box 5. CAUSES OF FELINE HYPERTENSION.

Kidney disease (20–65 % of cats with CKD)
Hyperthyroidism
Primary hyperaldosteronism
Acromegaly
Hyperadrenocorticism
Pheochromocytoma
Polycythaemia
Increased intracranial pressure
Essential, idiopathic, primary, or familial

an increase in heart rate and contraction of vascular smooth muscle (increasing resistance) in nonessential organs (e.g. skin).

The reflex occurs quickly, enabling rapid resolution of decreases in pressure. This allows for adaptation of blood pressure in response to changes in posture.

Atrial receptor reflex

These receptors detect changes in atrial volume. Like the baroreceptor reflex, perception of a decrease in atrial volume by atrial receptors is transmitted to the CNS, which in turn increases sympathetic tone. This reflex also induces an endocrine response, stimulating the secretion of antidiuretic hormone (ADH) from the pituitary gland and renin from the kidney, and increasing the thirst sensation via the hypothalamus. These three mechanisms act in concert to increase blood volume and therefore increase blood pressure.

Figure 9 depicts the function of the renin–angiotensin–aldosterone system.

Treatment

Treatment is based on diagnosis of the primary cause. However, we must establish a pharmacological regimen so that the patient does not develop sequelae due to hypertension. In feline medicine, amlodipine is the treatment of choice for arterial hypertension, and telmisartan, an ARB, has recently been authorised for this indication at doses higher than those used to treat proteinuria. Amlodipine is a calcium channel blocker that acts upon the smooth muscle of blood vessels and has practically no cardiac effect, while telmisartan blocks receptors for angiotensin II, a potent vasoconstrictor. In both cases, by relaxing the vascular muscle, the vessels dilate and blood pressure drops.

The goal of this treatment is to keep systolic blood pressure <160 mmHg initially and, if possible, to keep it <140 mmHg without inducing signs of hypotension such as weakness, syncope, tachycardia, or systolic blood pressure <120 mmHg.

The starting dose of amlodipine is 0.625 mg per cat every 24 hours. If insufficient, this dose can be doubled.

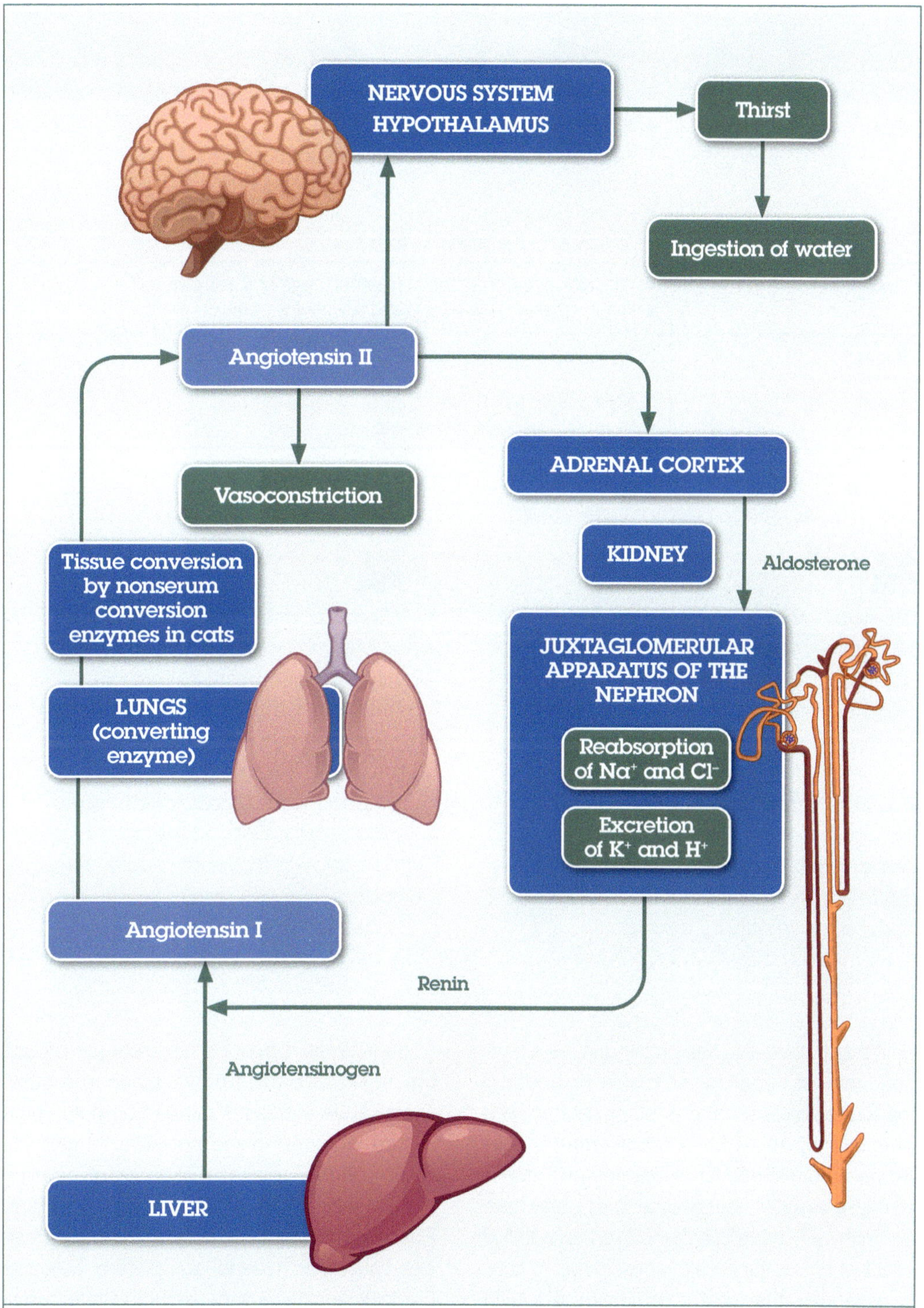

Figure 9. Functioning of the renin–angiotensin–aldosterone system.

Table 7. Consequences of high blood pressure.

Target organ	Consequences
Eye	• Hypertensive retinopathy • Vitreous (hyphaema) or retinal haemorrhage • Retinal oedema • Retinal detachment • Tortuosity of the retinal vessels
CNS	• Vascular accidents due to haemorrhage or thrombus • Hypertensive encephalopathy/cerebral oedema
Kidney	Progression of glomerulosclerosis and/or proteinuria
Heart	• Myocardial hypertrophy (rarely causes CHF) • Murmurs and gallop rhythms

TIP

The starting dose of amlodipine can be varied depending on the size of the patient, the severity of hypertension (a blood pressure value of 170 mmHg is not the same as one of 240 mmHg), and the extent of damage to target organs (Table 7). On some occasions a dose of 2.5 mg/cat every 12 or 24 hours may be required. These increases should be made progressively every 7–15 days under strict veterinary control.

TIP

When treating cats with ACEIs or ARBs it is necessary to ensure that the patient is well hydrated. Thus, in case of uraemic crisis treatment should be suspended. It should be noted that ACEIs are not effective hypotensives in cats, in contrast to dogs. If the dose needs to be increased, renal parameters, potassium levels, and hydration status should be monitored.

If that patient also has proteinuria, as a consequence of either hypertension or underlying kidney disease, and is being treated with amlodipine, an ACEI or telmisartan should be co-administered at antiproteinuric doses (1 mg/kg every 24 hours; higher doses may have an antihypertensive effect and exert an additive effect when combined with amlodipine). In cats, benazepril is the most commonly used ACEI (0.25 mg/kg every 24 hours).

Sometimes it may be necessary to reduce the heart rate to improve blood pressure. Tachycardia increases cardiac output, which in turn increases blood pressure. In cats the most common disease capable of causing hypertensive tachycardia is hyperthyroidism. Pheochromocytoma, although rare in cats, can also cause this hypertensive picture. Selective β_1 blockers can be very useful in these cases. The most commonly used in cats is atenolol, at doses of 6.25–12.5 mg/cat every 24 hours. Atenolol is normally chosen for its selectivity (avoiding the bronchoconstriction caused by other nonselective beta-blockers) and its simple, once-a-day dosing regimen. As described for the previous two drugs, treatment should begin with a low dose, which is then adjusted based on the observed effect.

IN WHICH FELINE PATIENTS SHOULD BLOOD PRESSURE BE MEASURED?

Cats >8 years of age

With chronic kidney disease

With neurological disease

With vision problems (especially those with blindness, hyphaema, or retinal detachment)

With hyperthyroidism

With heart murmur

With persistent hypokalaemia (possible cases of primary hyperaldosteronism)

ACTION TO BE TAKEN DEPENDING ON PATIENT'S BLOOD PRESSURE

If the pressure is <140 mmHg, the patient is normotensive: **do not treat**.

If the pressure is 140–160 mmHg, the patient may be normotensive or prehypertensive: **reassess in 3 months**.

If the pressure is 160–180 mmHg and there is no evidence of target organ damage: **reassess in 15–30 days**.

If the pressure is >180 mmHg: **treat with amlodipine**.

THE OWNER'S PERSPECTIVE

As with almost all **chronic diseases**, owners of affected pets tend to suffer from progressive **fatigue**. Combating these feelings can be as difficult as treating heart disease itself.

Each owner **has a different understanding of their pet's quality of life and lifestyle**. While one owner may take a nocturnal cough very seriously, another may pay no heed whatsoever to cardiac cachexia in their pet.

Clearly explaining the **diagnostic process, treatment, and evolution** of the disease can help provide the owner **with a better understanding** of their pet's care needs.

KEY POINTS VETERINARY PRACTITIONERS SHOULD BEAR IN MIND

Valvular heart diseases are **very common in dogs**, and although less so in cats, **they are more common than some may think**. **Annual checkups** in senior patients are an ideal tool for **early diagnosis** of these diseases.

In cats, systemic diseases that end up altering the heart are usually more frequent than primary heart diseases. Assessment of **blood pressure and thyroid hormone levels** should be performed in these patients at least **once a year from the age of 8, and biannually from the age of 10–12**.

These patients are usually treated with **multiple medications**. Providing ample **explanation** about drug dosage and creating a **monitoring system** managed by auxiliary veterinary staff **will improve owner compliance**.

The availability of **cardiac markers** in recent years allows us **to assess cardiac distress** in asymptomatic patients without performing a more costly echocardiographic examination. In owners with economic limitations, these tests are particularly interesting, given their considerably lower cost. Once alterations in these markers are detected, echocardiography will be mandatory.

Box 1. CANINE COGNITIVE ASSESSMENT SCALE (developed by CAWEC for Purina).

If you've noticed changes in multiple behavioural categories, be sure to talk to your vet about the health of your dog's aging brain.

Date: ______________________

Owner's name: ______________ Dog's name: ______________

Age: ________ Sex: Male ▢ Female ▢ Neutered/spayed: Yes ▢ No ▢

Breed: ______________ Weight: ______________

Body condition (1–9): ______________ Current diet: ______________

Medications, dosage, and frequency of administration: ______________

The following questionnaire is designed to evaluate the possible changes in the behaviour and mental activity of your dog due to ageing.

Please indicate the correct score for each behaviour. Describe only what you have seen in the last 6 months. If for any reason you are unable to answer a question, please leave it blank.

Please indicate how often your dog shows each of the following behaviours:

0	1	2	3
Never	**Once a month**	**Once a week**	**Almost every day**

D Disorientation

Multiply the score by 2 | Score

1. Stays looking at a fixed point (e.g. corner, wall, floor, drinking bowl).
2. Does not remember the way back home.
3. Gets stuck between objects or furniture, and is unable to get out.
4. Stays on the wrong side of the door (i.e. the hinge) while waiting to exit, or goes to the wrong door.
5. Does not respond to certain stimuli to which it used to respond (e.g. doorbell, loud noises).
6. Does not give any signal when it wants to go outside, when it used to do this.

I Altered social interactions

7. Does not recognise (or seems not to recognise) family members or acquaintances.
8. Does not recognise (or seems not to recognise) other known dogs.
9. Shows more signs of fear (e.g. ears back, low body posture, avoiding contact) or aggressiveness (e.g. growls, shows teeth, bites) than it used to.

S Changes in the sleep–wake cycle

Score

10. Walks during the night (for no apparent reason), when it did not used to do this.
11. Vocalises (barks, whines, howls) during the night (for no apparent reason), when it did not used to do this.

H Alteration of learning (house soiling)

12. Urinates and/or defecates in inappropriate places, when it did not used to do it.
13. Has trouble responding to previously learned commands.

A Alteration of activity levels

14. Is less active and/or playful than before.
15. Shows repetitive behaviours (e.g. chases own tail, hunts "invisible flies", etc.).
16. Walks without apparent purpose.

A Anxiety

17. Shows signs of anxiety when separated from its owner (e.g. trembles, salivates excessively, moans or barks, does not eat, becomes agitated, etc.) that were not previously evident, or were less intense.

Once this form is completed, **your vet will help you** to interpret the results and to establish the most appropriate management strategy for your dog, if necessary.

Total

Interpretation of the final score*

0–7	8–40	41–69
Normal aging	Mild cognitive impairment	Severe cognitive impairment

* This scale has been validated by CAWEC in a sample of 100 dogs, and significantly discriminates between normal aging and mild cognitive impairment. This sample did not include any dogs with severe cognitive impairment.

Another change that often attracts the attention of owners of pets with CDS is a loss of their pet's normal rhythm. In general, a family will have some form of routine, to which the pet adapts, waking up, lying down, eating, and playing accordingly. As CDS progresses, this routine is lost, and the animal may eat at different times, plays less often and at "odd" times, and alter its sleep–wake pattern, although in general affected animals tend to sleep more. Some owners describe their pets as being "out of sync".

Treatment

Treatment of this condition must be comprehensive. Ideally, it should consist of providing the owner with the appropriate information and medication.

Correct information for the owner

Owners of pets that wake up in the middle of the night howling or meowing often become exhausted and angry. This is further exacerbated in cases in which animals appear to unlearn basic hygiene habits. It is important to be patient and to simply and clearly explain to the owner what is likely occurring, and what steps should be taken to establish diagnosis and treatment. In terms of treatment, it is important to be aware of what can be done and what the owner's expectations should be, emphasising that they are precisely this: expectations. It may even take some effort to convince an owner that their pet's condition is not "normal", and can be improved despite the animal's advanced age.

Medication

There are many psychotropic drugs used in human medicine that can also be used in small animals. Below, we will describe those that have been studied and exert demonstrated effects.

Selegiline

This irreversible monoamine oxidase inhibitor (MAOI) increases the duration of action of dopamine at nerve endings. Two MAOs are found in dogs and cats: A (more abundant in the liver and gastrointestinal tract) and B (more common in neurons, where it mediates catecholamine metabolism). Selegiline has much higher affinity for MAO-B, and does not affect MAO-A at therapeutic doses. It can be administered to dogs (for which it is authorised in the United States and the United Kingdom) and cats.[16] The starting dose is usually 0.25–0.5 mg/kg every 24 hours, administered in the morning. If there is no noticeable improvement after a month, the dose can be increased to 0.5–1 mg/kg (lower doses are optimal in cats). Extreme caution should be exercised when administering a MAOI to a patient, as toxicity can occur if combined with a selective serotonin reuptake inhibitor (SSRI) such as fluoxetine or paroxetine or with a tricyclic antidepressant (TCA) such as clomipramine or amitriptyline. Certain authors recommend a rest or washout period to avoid the risk of combined administration. Thus, the washout period between a MAOI and a SSRI or TCA should be at least 2 weeks. When switching from a SSRI or TCA to a MAOI, this period should be extended to 5 weeks. These drugs can be erroneously prescribed in combination, as many CDS patients also experience anxiety. It is important to remember that selegiline also exerts an anxiolytic effect, which often makes the use of other anxiolytics unnecessary, and also decreases the formation of free radicals by inhibiting dopamine metabolism.

Toxicity caused by excessive serotonin levels is known as serotonin syndrome (see box on next page).

SEROTONIN SYNDROME

This syndrome can appear due to the administration of drugs that mimic the effect of serotonin or reduce its metabolism. Combined administration of these products increases the effects of serotonin in the patient's CNS. The clinical signs of this syndrome, in order of prevalence, are: vomiting, diarrhoea, seizures, hyperthermia, hyperaesthesia, depression, mydriasis, vocalisation, death, blindness, hypersalivation, dyspnoea, ataxia/paresis, disorientation, hyperreflexia, and coma.

Treatment in these cases usually consists of symptomatic (antiemetics, anticonvulsants, fluid therapy) and antiserotonergic therapies (Table 2). The most commonly used drugs are cyproheptadine (1.1 mg/kg PO in dogs and 2 mg/cat PO) or chlorpromazine (0.1–1 mg/kg IV, IM, or SC). In cases in which cyproheptadine cannot be administered orally, one tablet can be diluted in saline and administered rectally. The dosing interval will depend on the patient's condition, but is typically in the range of every 4–6 hours. Intensive treatment is usually required for 12–24 hours. If the patient has tachycardia, the drug of choice is propranolol (0.1–0.2 mg/kg every 8 hours in dogs and 2.5–10 mg/cat every 12 hours, PO), owing to its mild antiserotonergic action.

Table 2. Serotonergic potential of various drugs.[17]

High	Moderate	Low
• Amitriptyline • Clomipramine • Dexfenfluramine • Dextromethorphan • Fenfluramine • Fluoxetine • Fluvoxamine • Imipramine • Isocarboxazid • Lithium • Methylenedioxymethamphetamine • Meperidine/pethidine • Moclobemide • Paroxetine • Phenelzine • Selegiline • Sertraline • Tranylcypromine • Venlafaxine	• Buspirone • Desipramine • Doxepin • L-DOPA • Nortriptyline • Trazodone • Drugs like cocaine and LSD	• Amantadine • Bromocriptine • Bupropion • Carbamazepine • Codeine • Melatonin • Mirtazapine • Nefazodone • Pentazocine • Pergolide • Tramadol

Nicergoline

This agent is a nonselective α-adrenergic antagonist that causes cerebral vasodilation and increases neuronal metabolism. Activity in senior dogs can increase by up to 75 %. It can be administered in dogs and cats at a dose of 0.25–0.5 mg/kg every 24 hours.[18]

Propentofylline

This xanthine derivative exerts a multitude of effects that may be useful for the treatment of this disease. However, there are no studies that support its use with a high level of scientific evidence. It is a phosphodiesterase and adenosine reuptake inhibitor. It is a mild bronchodilator and a cerebral vasodilator. It helps red blood cells to deform more easily, allowing them to pass through narrow capillaries. It is also thought to exert an antiplatelet effect, preventing the development of thrombi. It is administered at doses of 12.5 mg/cat per day[18] and 2.5–5 mg/kg every 12 hours in dogs.

Adrafinil

This enhancer of noradrenergic function is a prodrug that is metabolised to modafinil. It improves mental state and helps maintain a correct sleep–wake rhythm. The noradrenergic system regulates the maintenance of alertness, improving the capacity for attention, memory, and learning. In short, patients treated with this drug are more awake. It appears to exert neuroprotective effects. Laboratory studies have shown that this drug has some potential to improve cognitive signs in treated patients.[19] Similarly, field studies have reported improved locomotion in treated dogs, in the absence of stereotypy, at a dose of 20 mg/kg.[20] A study from 2000 compared the use of nicergoline, propentofylline, and adrafinil, and concluded that adrafinil produced better outcomes in terms of increased activity.[21]

Nutraceuticals and diets

Various nutraceuticals and nutritional supplements have been approved for use in dogs and cats with CDS. This group includes many antioxidants and mitochondrial cofactors to aid the elimination of free radicals and improve the ability of neurons to obtain energy. In fact, oxidative damage and low levels of vitamin E have been observed in the brains of the dogs with CDS.[22,23]

A double-blind study found that a diet containing sufficient levels of vitamins E and C, beta-carotene, selenium, DL-α-lipoic acid, various flavonoids and carotenoids, and L-carnitine, as well as high levels of ω-3 fatty acids, improved cognitive performance in dogs.[24] Many of these nutrients have more than one function; however, combined administration appears to exert a synergistic effect against CDS in dogs. There are a multitude of simple and complex nutraceuticals available for both dogs and cats. **S-adenosylmethionine (SAMe)** is a molecule made up of methionine and ATP and found in all living cells. It is particularly abundant in the liver and brain. Its best known function is to assist the action of methyltransferase in methylation reactions, and it is required for the synthesis and inactivation of neurotransmitters such as norepinephrine, serotonin, and dopamine.[25,26] In addition, through transulphurisation demethylated SAMe is metabolised to glutathione, one of the most potent antioxidants present in mammals.[27] This product has been tested in double-blind studies in dogs and has shown promising efficacy.[28]

Another double-blind, multicentre placebo study conducted in 2006 found that dogs given a commercial supplement complex containing ω-3 fatty acids (EPA/DHA), vitamin C, N-acetylcysteine, vitamin E, L-carnitine, lipoic acid, coenzyme Q_{10}, phosphotidylserine, and selenium showed significant improvements in disorientation, social interaction, and house soiling. Improvements were also observed in the sleep–wake pattern, although this effect was not significant.[29]

The same antioxidant complex is available for cats, the difference being that it does not contain lipoic acid. This powerful antioxidant has been shown to be more toxic in cats than in other mammals, and can cause hepatocellular toxicity with a maximum tolerated dose of less than 30 mg/kg in this species.[30]

There are no cat studies comparable to those performed in dogs. However, the experience with this antioxidant complex shows that the effects are very similar to those seen in dogs.

A recent promising study has shown that the combination of fish oil, B vitamins, antioxidants (including vitamin C, vitamin E, and selenium), and arginine improves goal-oriented behaviour, decision making, problem solving, planning, organisation, and sequential tasks in senior dogs.[31] An earlier study showed that in cats a similar compound adapted to this species containing antioxidants, B vitamins, arginine, and fish oil also had positive effects and delayed the onset of clinical signs of CDS.[32]

Ketogenic diets with medium-chain triglycerides (MCTs) have also been shown to successfully combat CDS in dogs. It appears that the metabolism of glucose, the brain's main energy source, becomes less efficient with aging. The consequent decrease in energy in neurons can cause memory loss, slower learning, and reduced attention. Providing neurons with an alternative energy source, such as ketone bodies derived from the breakdown of MCTs, appears to help mitigate brain glucose hypometabolism in these patients.[33]

Finally, in 2018, a prospective, randomised, double-blind study demonstrated that the combination of a MCT-supplemented diet with fish oil, antioxidants, arginine, and B vitamins improved clinical indicators of CDS in dogs. These improvements were evident during the first month after switching to the new diet.[34]

Vestibular system involvement in senior animals

Before focusing on conditions that affect the vestibular system of senior animals, we will first review the underlying anatomy.

The vestibular system is the most important for maintaining balance. Basically it is a proprioceptive system that, together with the general proprioceptive information and the visual system, maintains the correct orientation of the organism with respect to gravitational forces.[35–38] In addition, it coordinates body posture and eye position relative to the position or movement of the head. Given these important roles, dysfunction in this system understandably leads to alterations in gait, head posture, and eyeball movement.[35,36]

Basic anatomy of the vestibular system

Traditionally, the vestibular system has been divided clinically into peripheral and central systems (Figs. 1 and 2). This division is purely diagnostic: we should not think of this system as two separate parts, but rather as a well-integrated system that is artificially divided for the purpose of locating lesions.

The peripheral portion is located in the inner ear and consists of receptors, nerve ganglia, and peripheral axons of the vestibular branch of the VIII cranial nerve (vestibulocochlear nerve). The components of the central vestibular system include the vestibular nucleus located in the medulla oblongata and the vestibular projections to the cerebellum, spinal cord, and rostral part of the brainstem.[35,36]

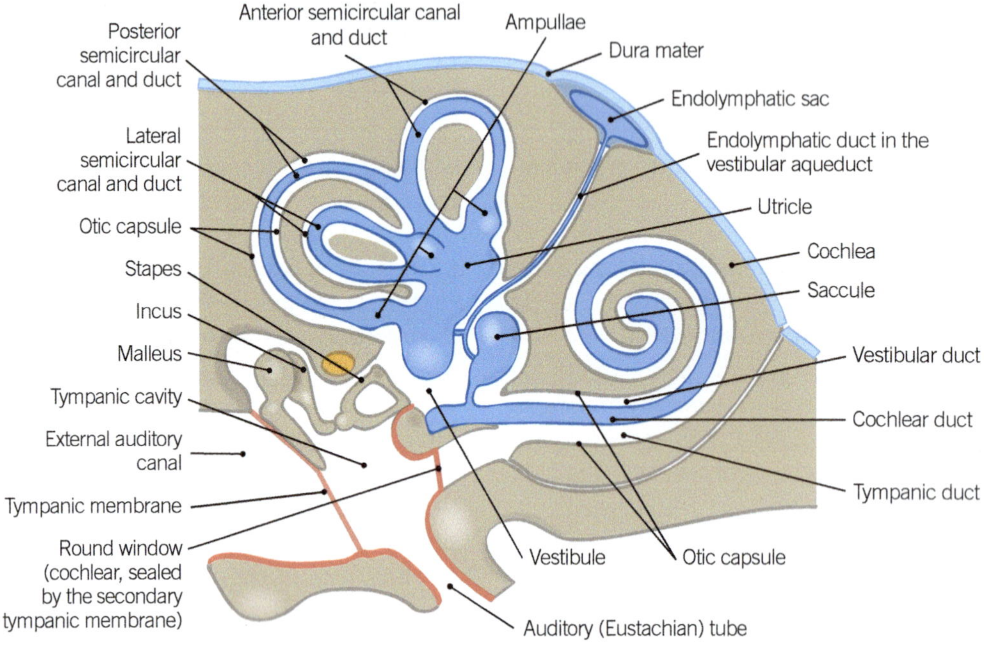

Figure 1. Schematic diagram of the bony and membranous labyrinths of the peripheral vestibular system.

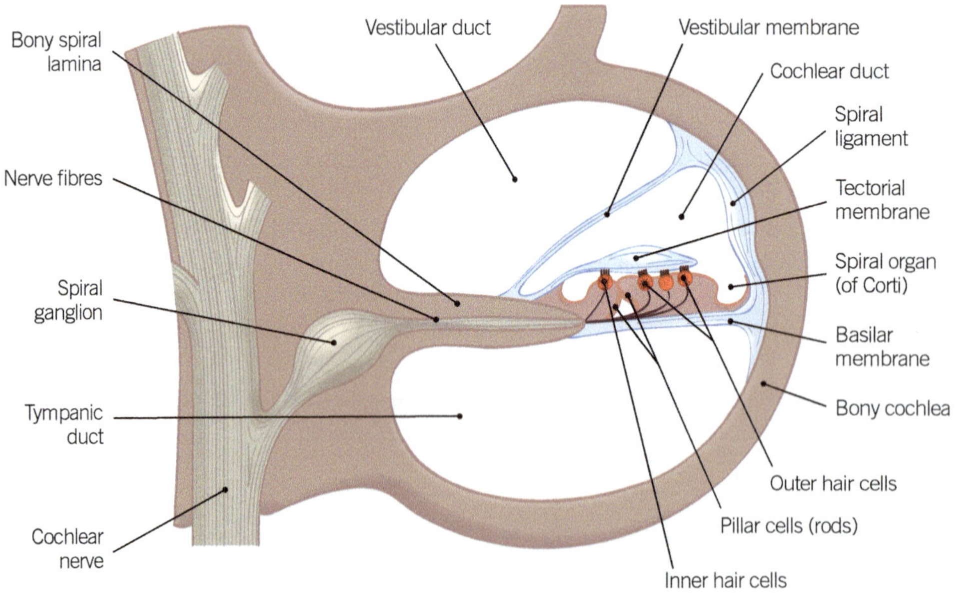

Figure 2. Schematic diagram depicting a cross section of the spiral of the cochlea.

Peripheral vestibular system

Closely related to the auditory apparatus, the peripheral part of the system is located in the petrous portion of the temporal bone (better known as the inner ear). This system consists of two parts, one of which acts as a container and another that constitutes the content. The bony labyrinth (container) is divided into three regions: the semicircular canals, the vestibule, and the cochlea. The lumen of these structures is filled with perilymph. The membranous labyrinth (content) is made up of four structures: the semicircular ducts, utricle, saccule, and cochlear duct. Thus, the semicircular canals contain the semicircular ducts, the vestibule contains the utricle and the saccule, and finally the cochlear duct is located within the cochlea. The lumen of these structures is filled with endolymph. The semicircular ducts are oriented in such a way as to form right angles with one another, thereby enabling the collection of information in three spatial planes.[36]

At the end of each membranous semicircular canal is a terminal dilation called the ampulla. The ampulla contains hair-like cells that act as mechanoreceptors. The hairs on each ampulla are perfectly aligned to form what is known as the crista ampullaris. The tonic activity of these hair cells depends on the movement of the endolymph, which alters neural signalling. The dendrites of the neurons of the vestibular branch of the VIII cranial nerve establish synapses with these hair cells. There are three types of receptors on the crista ampullaris that respond initially to acceleration, deceleration, and rotation.[35,36] The semicircular canals are organised in such a way that movement in one plane activates vestibular neurons in one crista ampullaris and simultaneously inhibits neurons in the semicircular canal on the opposite side of the head.

These are not the only receptors found in this structure.

Maculae are receptors located in the utricle and the saccule. The macula of the saccule is oriented in a vertical plane, while that of the utricle is oriented in a horizontal plane. The surface of each macula is covered by hair-like neuroepithelial cells. These cells form synapses with vestibular neurons. The function of these maculae is to maintain static equilibrium and respond to linear acceleration.[36,37] The axons of the vestibular branch of the VIII cranial nerve project through the internal acoustic meatus, while the bodies of the vestibular bipolar axons are located in the vestibular ganglion, which is located in the petrous portion of the temporal bone (Fig. 3).[39]

Central vestibular system

After passing through the internal acoustic meatus, the vestibular axons project to the lateral aspect of the medulla oblongata, where most will terminate in the vestibular nuclei. Axons that do not terminate in these nuclei are directed to the flocculonodular lobe of the cerebellar cortex and medulla through the cerebellar peduncle.[36,39] There are four vestibular nuclei on either side of the midline of the lateral wall of the fourth ventricle forming the vestibular trigone. The neurons in these nuclei are interneurons, which generally exert excitatory influences on local interneurons in other parts of the CNS. The most important features of the central vestibular system, from a clinical point of view, are the three points to which these projections from the vestibular nucleus extend:

- **Projections to the spinal cord:** the vestibulospinal tract is the main projection that descends from the vestibular nuclei in the medulla oblongata to all segments of the spinal cord in the ipsilateral ventral funiculus, where it influences motor neuron activity. This influence is mediated by segmental interneurons, which stimulate the ipsilateral extensor muscles and inhibit the flexors.

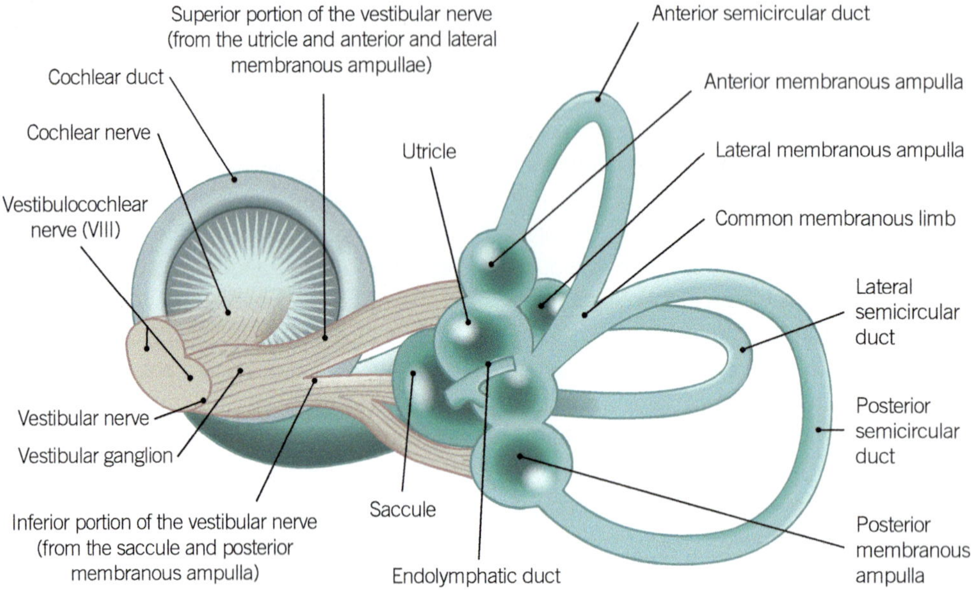

Figure 3. Schematic diagram showing peripheral vestibular innervation.

On the opposite side of the body, the contralateral extensor muscles are inhibited.

TAKE NOTE!

Activation of the vestibular system increases ipsilateral muscle tone and inhibits contralateral muscle tone, as well as extension reflexes.

These pathways contribute to the coordination of motor activity of the extremities, neck, and trunk in response to head movement. In summary, a unilateral vestibular lesion suppresses or diminishes the tonic activity of vestibular neurons on the same side, resulting in unopposed stimulation of the vestibulospinal tract on the unaffected side and a consequent tilt of the head and body towards the side of the lesion.

- **Brainstem projections:**
  - **Medial longitudinal fascicle:** this bundle ascends from the vestibular nuclei in the medulla oblongata to synapse with lower motor neurons in the motor nuclei of the cranial nerves III, IV, and VI.[37,39] This pathway mediates the coordination of eye movement as the head changes position. It is also part of the pathway responsible for physiological nystagmus, which is induced when evaluating the vestibulo-ocular reflex.
  - **Reticular formation and vomiting centre:** some axons of the vestibular nucleus project to the vomiting centre within the reticular formation. This pathway explains why vomiting is induced by motion sickness and vestibular disease.
  - **Conscious perception of balance:** in animals, the afferent pathways that mediate conscious perception of vestibular dysfunction remain poorly understood, but

are thought to ascend through junction centres in the thalamus to the temporal cerebral cortex.[38]

- **Cerebellar projections:** some of the vestibular axons that exit the vestibular ganglion and nuclei project towards the vestibulocerebellar zone (flocculonodular lobe and fastigial nucleus) through the caudal cerebellar peduncle.[40] These axons maintain coordination not only of the eyes, but also the neck, trunk, and extremities relative to head movements, and when the head is static.

Clinical signs in small animals

Diseases that affect any of the components of the vestibular system, whether central or peripheral, are usually accompanied by a set of clinical signs that are detectable with the naked eye, or can be easily provoked during the neurological examination. These clinical signs are listed below, along with the associated pathophysiology (Table 3).

- **Head tilt:** this is a postural abnormality resulting from the unilateral loss of antigravity muscle tone in the neck region. The degree of head tilt can vary, and is not necessarily linked to the prognosis. The deviation can range from a few degrees, which is intermittently evident, to as much as 45°. Normally, the ventral most ear indicates the side of the lesion. Thus, if the right ear is facing down, the lesion will be on the right side. Unfortunately, this is not always so straightforward. In cases of paradoxical central vestibular lesions, the affected side does not coincide with the ventral ear. In such cases,

Table 3. Clinical differentiation of vestibular problems according to clinical findings.

Clinical sign	Peripheral vestibular system	Central vestibular system
Head tilt	Towards the side of the lesion	Towards either side
Pathological nystagmus	• Fast phase towards the unaffected side • Horizontal or rotary • Direction not altered by change of head position	• Vertical, horizontal, or rotary • Direction of nystagmus can be altered by varying the position of the head
Postural reactions	Normal	Deficits ipsilateral to the lesion
Conscious proprioception	Normal	Deficits ipsilateral to the lesion
Cranial nerve deficits	± deficits in VII cranial nerve ipsilateral to the lesion	± deficits in V and XII cranial nerves ipsilateral to the lesion
Horner syndrome*	± postganglionic	± preganglionic (very unusual)
Level of consciousness	Normal, although confusion may be observed in acute cases	From normal to comatose

* Horner syndrome includes ptosis, myosis (produces anisocoria), and enophthalmia, with protrusion of the third eyelid.

the presence of unilateral deficiencies in other cranial nerves can also serve as an indicator of the side on which the lesion is located.

- **Nystagmus:** this is the involuntary, rhythmic movement of the eyeballs. This movement can be physiological or pathological, and is in fact a very common finding in small animal veterinary practice. Nystagmus is characterised by uneven directional movement, and is sometimes referred to as jerk nystagmus. Typically, nystagmus consists of a slow phase and a fast phase. The type of nystagmus is characterised based on the fast phase, together with the axis (horizontal, vertical, or rotary); e.g. left horizontal nystagmus.

TAKE NOTE!

The slow phase of horizontal nystagmus occurs in the opposite direction to the side on which the lesion is located, and constitutes a compensatory phase of eye movement. Conversely, the fast phase occurs in the same direction as the head movement. Vertical nystagmus always indicates central involvement.

From a general clinical point of view, it is important to be able distinguish physiological from pathological nystagmus:

- **Physiological nystagmus:** this is observed in normal animals after inducing rotation of the head. This produces a jerk nystagmus in the plane of rotation, with a rapid phase that occurs in the direction of the rotational movement. The slow phase will be in the opposite direction. This nystagmus is usually provoked during the neurological examination to demonstrate the vestibulo-ocular reflex. The function of this reflex is to maintain image stability on the retina to optimise functioning of the visual system.[37]
- **Pathological nystagmus:** this can in turn be subclassified as spontaneous or positional. Spontaneous nystagmus occurs when the head is still or in a neutral posture. By contrast, positional nystagmus occurs when the patient is placed in certain positions (e.g. supine).[35,36] In general, spontaneous nystagmus is detectable only for a brief period, as it is rapidly compensated for by voluntary visual fixation.[35,36,38]

- **Vestibular or positional strabismus:** this is a phenomenon that manifests as a ventral or ventrolateral deviation of the eyeball. This results in an increase in the dorsal exposure of the sclera when the neck and head are extended. This positional strabismus resolves when the head returns to a neutral position.
- **Vestibular ataxia:** animals with vestibular ataxia often lean, fall, roll, or circle towards the side of the lesion. This circling usually occurs within a small radius (i.e. describing a small circle). The most important feature of vestibular ataxia is its asymmetric nature. The head and trunk may sway, often forcing the animal to maintain a base-wide stance.

Idiopathic peripheral vestibular syndrome

This is also known as geriatric vestibular syndrome or vestibular neuritis. All these terms describe the same group of clinical signs.

Idiopathic peripheral vestibular syndrome is the second most common cause of peripheral vestibular dysfunction in dogs.[41] Furthermore, it is a very common cause of sudden-onset unilateral vestibular dysfunction, which usually consists of head tilt, ataxia, or nystagmus (horizontal and rotary) in both dogs and cats. Although this condition can affect dogs of any age, senior dogs seem to be more predisposed.

TAKE NOTE!

Idiopathic vestibular syndrome is very rare in dogs under 5 years of age. If a patient with vestibular signs is less than 5 years of age, it is unlikely to have this syndrome.

In both species, this clinical picture exclusively affects the vestibular system. Affected animals should never show signs of facial nerve palsy or postganglionic Horner syndrome. In cases of very sudden onset, affected animals may roll, fall, or even vomit.

TAKE NOTE!

This syndrome can be confused by owners and veterinary surgeons with an epileptoid disorder, as the patient makes a pedalling-like motion when trying to get back up. The difference is that the patient does not lose consciousness upon falling and lacks neurological sequelae, which would be expected after epileptic episodes lasting this long.

Idiopathic peripheral vestibular disease in cats differs slightly to the form observed in dogs. First, it can appear in cats of any age and it seems to have a higher incidence in animals with outdoor access. In the United States, a seasonal pattern has been established: in the eastern states more cases appear in summer and fall. These cases can be bilateral, but they are still cases of peripheral vestibular disease.[35,36,42]

Idiopathic peripheral vestibular syndrome is diagnosed by excluding other causes of peripheral vestibular dysfunction (Fig. 4 and Table 4). Imaging tools are very useful for this task (Fig. 5) and usually reveal no alterations in animals with idiopathic involvement. While the origin of this disease is unknown, it is often compared to human vestibular neuritis, and can be caused by various viral antigens.[37,38]

Treatment

Although there are many potential treatments, none have demonstrated a clear positive effect. Therefore, treatment is usually symptomatic:

- **Antiemetics:** high-dose maropitant (2–8 mg/kg PO every 24 hours) has been shown to exert a significant antiemetic effect against vomiting caused by motion sickness. Although not authorised for this indication, toxicological studies carried out before its commercialisation have shown a very high therapeutic index. Other products such as dimenhydrinate (4–8 mg/kg PO every 24 hours) can also be helpful.
- **Anxiolytics:** in animals with marked anxiety, diazepam (0.5–2.2 mg/kg PO every 8–12 hours) can be used in dogs and

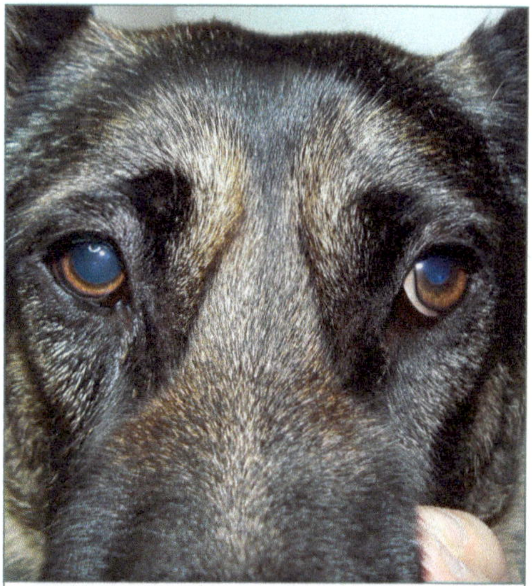

Figure 4. Dog with anisocoria caused by vestibular syndrome due to otitis.

Table 4. Common causes of peripheral vestibular disease in dogs and cats.

Category	Specific diseases	Dogs	Cats
Congenital	Congenital vestibular disease	×	×
Metabolic	Hypothyroidism	×	
Neoplastic	• Primary atrial tumour • Vestibular neurofibroma	×	×
Infectious/inflammatory	• Otitis media and interna (OMI) (Fig. 4) • Naso- or oropharyngeal polyps	× ×	× ×
Idiopathic	Idiopathic vestibular syndrome (vestibular neuritis)	×	×
Trauma	Inner ear trauma	×	×
Toxic	Ototoxic medications (topical and systemic)	×	×

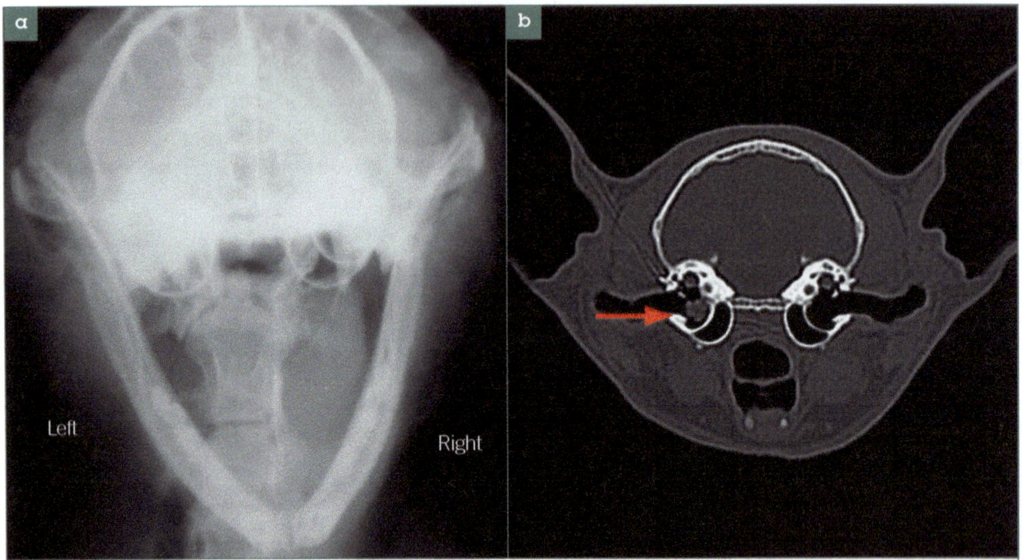

Figure 5. X-ray (a) and computed tomography (CT) scan (b) of a cat with vestibular syndrome due to a polyp. The X-ray did not demonstrate major changes in radiodensity, but the CT scan showed the presence of a polyp of inflammatory origin in the right bulla that could be removed. Images courtesy of Juanjo Vega, Hospital Felino Ventas, Madrid (Spain).

alprazolam in both cats and dogs (cats, 0.125–0.25 mg/kg PO every 12 hours; dogs, 0.05–0.1 mg/kg PO every 8–24 hours). In cats it is better not to administer diazepam orally to avoid liver necrosis.[43] This is a rare side effect that seems to be associated only with its oral administration in this species. It seems impossible to know in advance which cat will develop necrosis after diazepam administration and which will not.

If this drug is used orally, it is important to have full cooperation from the owner and excellent communication. Affected cats typically present with ataxia, anorexia, and lethargy within the first 4 days of starting treatment, and jaundice develops shortly thereafter. These initial clinical signs may be due to the action of diazepam itself; for this reason it is recommended to evaluate transaminase levels on the first and fourth days. If any increase in the concentrations of these enzymes is observed, it is advisable to stop the treatment.

- **Treatment of occult OMI:** empirical treatment with broad-spectrum systemic antibiotics may be reasonable in cases of suspected OMI. However, this treatment should not replace a thorough otoscopic examination and a skull X-ray to assess pneumatisation of the tympanic bullae. In cases in which antibiotics are used, those that better penetrate the bone and accumulate in the white blood cells are usually the most indicated (lincosamides and fluoroquinolones), as these characteristics ensure that the antibiotic reaches the affected area in adequate concentrations.
- **Anti-inflammatories:** there are no studies showing that the administration of NSAIDs or corticosteroids improves clinical signs or shortens the duration of the clinical picture. It is therefore important to be vigilant, as it is easier to aggravate occult OMI with corticosteroid treatment than to improve the clinical signs.

After the onset of clinical signs, affected animals usually improve within 3–5 days and usually recover within 3 weeks. Unfortunately, head tilt can be a permanent sequela, or can take much longer to resolve. Animals that are helped and encouraged to walk appear to compensate for vestibular dysfunction earlier than those that do not exercise.

TIP

Patients with this syndrome may experience recurrence in the future. This is something about which the owner should be notified so that they can prepare accordingly.

Degenerative myelopathy

Degenerative myelopathy (DM) is an axonal medullary disease that produces progressive paraparesis.[44] Because it is more prevalent in certain breeds it has been proposed that it may be hereditary. Very recently, a genetic mutation has been detected in at least two of these breeds (Box 2).[45] The average age of onset of this disease is 9 years, and there is no apparent sexual predisposition.

Clinical signs

This unusual spinal disease causes progressive loss of the passage of neural information. Affected dogs present with progressive and asymmetric ataxia. Signs of loss of proprioception appear first, while spinal reflexes are present or increased. Over time, significant to severe muscle atrophy develops. The patellar reflex may be diminished or absent (Fig. 7).

TAKE NOTE!

The absence of spinal hyperaesthesia is a key clinical feature in suspected cases of this disease (unlike discopathies or spinal tumours).

Box 2. BREEDS PREDISPOSED TO DEGENERATIVE MYELOPATHY.

- German Shepherd Dog
- Boxer
- Pembroke Welsh Corgi
- Standard Poodle
- Collie
- Irish Setter (Fig. 6)
- Rhodesian Ridgeback
- Chesapeake Bay Retriever

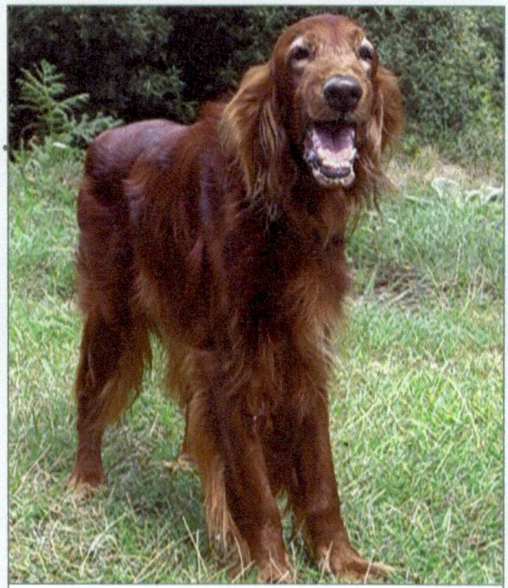

Figure 6. Irish Setter with degenerative myelopathy. This dog had clinical signs for 3 years, and was ultimately unable to stand.

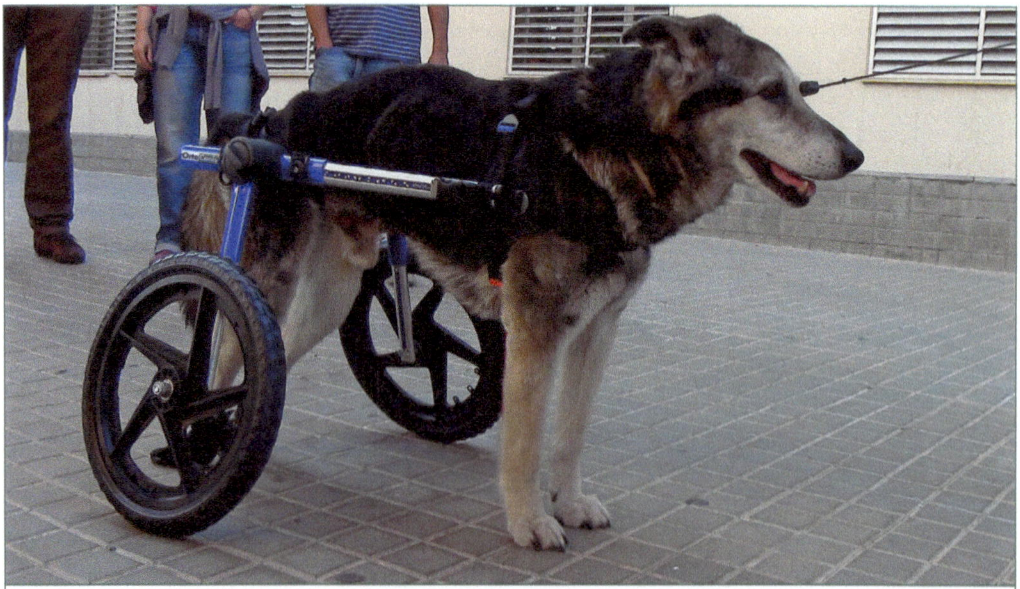

Figure 7. Dog in a wheelchair. Dogs with spinal degeneration typically require orthopaedic systems like that shown in the photograph. Image courtesy of Ortocanis.com.

Diagnosis

DM is diagnosed by exclusion, as there is no test to directly identify the disease.

Plain or contrast X-rays show no compressive abnormalities or bone lesions compatible with other diseases (discospondylitis, bone or spinal tumours). Neither MRI nor CT reveal lesions compatible with other diseases. Cerebrospinal fluid analysis is normal or reveals an increase in protein concentration. Definitive diagnosis is established by necropsy of the CNS.

TIP

It is important to rule out the presence of metabolic diseases that cause neuropathies (e.g. hypothyroidism), as this can lead to confusion.

Treatment

There is no treatment to cure or even delay the progression of DM. Because spinal lesions in DM occur more frequently in the thoracic area, possibly due to the reduced blood irrigation of this part of the spinal cord, treatment with drugs that improve nerve irrigation (e.g. propentofylline) is an option, but does not hold much promise. Combinations of antioxidants, such as those used for CDS, can also be administered to attempt to slow disease progression (although their efficacy for this indication has not been demonstrated).

While awaiting the development of more effective treatments, current care consists of physiotherapy and nursing to avoid loss of muscle mass, pressure ulcers, and urine scald.

The prognosis is poor and paraplegia appears between 6 and 9 months after diagnosis.

For further information on this disease, the reader can consult the bibliography.[44–46]

THE OWNER'S PERSPECTIVE

Chronic neurological diseases are highly exasperating for owners. They may not understand how their pet, without leaving the house, can develop a serious neurological disease for which there may be no clear treatment. **Trust** and **transparent communication** are vital. If necessary, we can seek advice from a specialist in neurology and request imaging tests such as computed tomography or magnetic resonance imaging.

These chronic neurological diseases **can improve** very slowly in some cases, often slower than the owner expects. **Calls from the auxiliary veterinary team** to check on the patient's progression and the owner's mood can help **preserve our good image** and maintain the **trust** that the owner has placed in our centre.

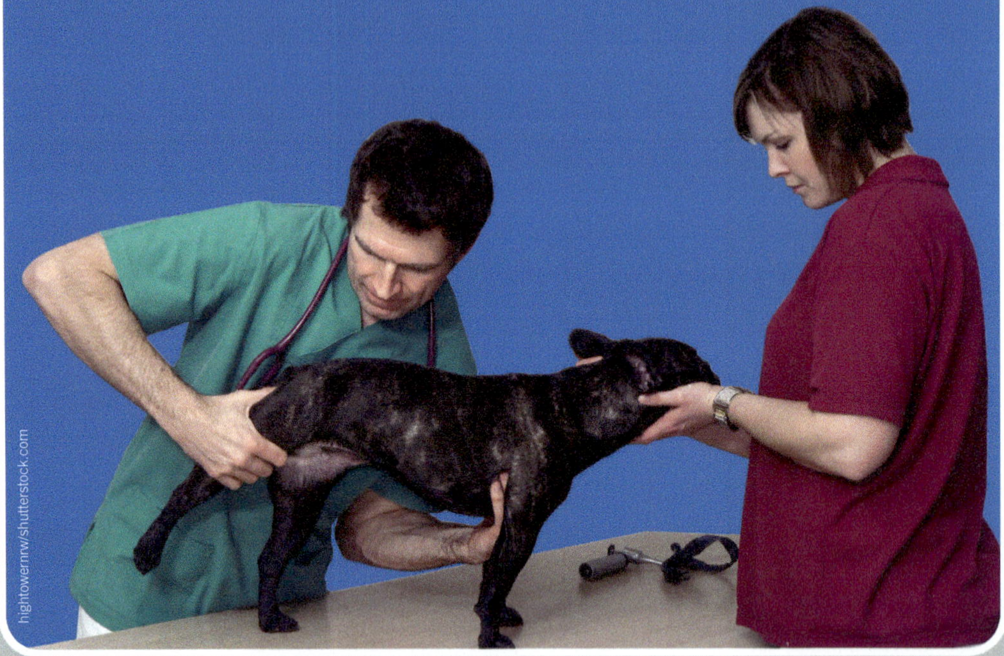

KEY POINTS VETERINARY PRACTITIONERS SHOULD BEAR IN MIND

Many veterinary surgeons are **very pessimistic** in these cases owing to the advanced **age** of the patients and the **poor prognosis** of many of these diseases. However, thanks to **physiotherapy and rehabilitation techniques**, as well as unconventional therapies such as **acupuncture**, many of these animals maintain an acceptable quality of life. **Ultimately, it is up to the owner to decide** what they do or don't want for their animal.

These owners can take up a lot of the veterinary surgeon's time, especially at the beginning, as they need **advice** on whether to continue, whether to euthanise, and how to navigate the line between selfishness and ethics. **Clear information from the** veterinary surgeon **explaining what to expect and not to expect** in these cases can help the owner, without making the decision for them. The owners may not want us to decide for them.

By anticipating what may happen, the veterinary surgeon can **reassure the owner** that they have chosen the right veterinary clinic, **and prove their worth as advisors** on the health of their pet. Once this is achieved, we must leverage this trust to proceed with the **diagnostic protocol**. Without this, no clear diagnosis can be established, and we cannot reach any definitive conclusion.

14 Health plans in senior animals

We have already extensively discussed the prevalence rates of a multitude of diseases that affect senior cats and dogs. At this point, it goes without saying that prevention is the best weapon to fight disease, and all the more so in the case of diseases of senior patients, for which treatment is often limited to palliative therapy or delaying disease progression. If we are all in agreement on this fact, how can it be that most veterinary centres do not have established senior health plans?

Note that we refer here to centres with established health plans, not those that have designed plans but then fail to advertise them correctly. Regardless, the result is the same: a plan that either has not been developed or is not properly advertised is useless. So what are we waiting for? For the client and pet owner to ask us? If this has ever happened to you, as a veterinary surgeon and entrepreneur, you may have felt embarrassed to be asked for a service that you should already provide. Let's not dwell further on excuses: we hope that this chapter will help you to set up the first health plan for senior patients in your centre. If you already have such a plan but for whatever reason do not advertise it, this chapter will outline the tools that we have used to overcome the reluctance of veterinary surgeons, assistants, and receptionists and ensure that all involved are convinced that what we are selling is better health, and not some strategy to further milk our clients, as some continue to believe.

The aim of this chapter is to provide some useful tips on how to design and establish a health plan in our centre. This will depend to some degree on the culture in a given country around how people pay for healthcare and medicine, whether human or veterinary. For example, in Spain there is still not really a culture of purchasing medical insurance for pets, probably because the national health system is paid for by the taxpayer, whether or not all are aware of this fact. In other countries, the situation is almost the opposite. So, take the advice provided in this chapter as a humble proposal from a country with little tradition of preventive medicine.

Approach to the senior health programme

In the following pages we will describe the creation of a senior pet health plan step by step.

Step 1: who is it for? (internal level)

To establish a plan, which is a product after all, the first thing we must decide is the profile of the patient at which it is aimed. We must therefore begin by defining to ourselves and all who work in our centre exactly what constitutes a senior dog or cat. As seen throughout the chapters of this book, there is little agreement on this topic, and it is therefore best that the entire team is in agreement to avoid confusion.

Step 2: how to inform the owner (in reception)

Once we have established which pets are considered senior, we must communicate this to their owners. To this end, it can be helpful to provide a **poster** or **age chart** so that pet owners can determine whether their dogs or cats are already within this age range. Personally, we feel that these more passive measures allow interested owners to take the first step, and not feel coerced into doing so. When the owners actively inquire at the reception of the clinic, it is also useful to have some **brochures** available to inform them about the different prevalences of diseases of senior patients, as well as the importance of early diagnosis and adequate control. We believe that these brochures should not contain very detailed or complicated information: the most effective, in our experience, are those that present the owner with a series of generic questions. The owner, who will understand that these issues pertain to their pet, should be invited to ask for more information during the consultation with the veterinary surgeon.

The role of the assistants and receptionists is essential at this point, as they tend to interact more with the client.

> **TAKE NOTE!**
>
> The health plan must be explained by assistants and receptionists in a generic way, while pointing out that there are variations within the same programme and that the plan will be tailored specifically and appropriately to each pet.

Step 3: how to present the health plan (during the consultation)

Here, we will not discuss clients who are already receptive to or completely against the idea of a health plan. Ideally, unless someone on the veterinary care team makes a serious mistake, there should be no problem in successfully selling a health plan to an already convinced owner. On the other hand, no matter what we do, a client who is completely against the idea is unlikely to change their mind. Below we will describe how we handle cases of clients who are only moderately receptive. Note that this is the protocol used in our clinics, but any method that yields positive results is valid. These results should be two-fold: get the patient to enter the health plan and also retain the owner (Figs. 1 and 2).

The first thing to remember is that, despite the cultural differences between countries, very few clients will directly consult for a checkup of their senior pet. For this reason, the first thing the veterinary surgeon should do is examine the patient and address and resolve the main reason for the owner's visit to the clinic. Only then will we be ready to explain to them what a health plan designed specifically for their pet would consist of (Table 1).

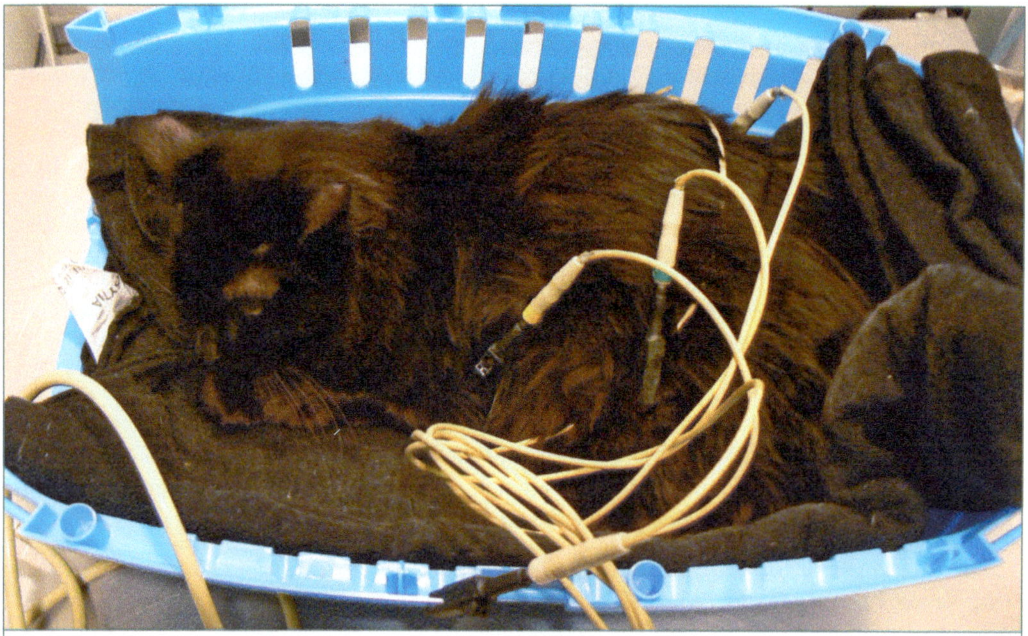

Figure 1. Performing an electrocardiogram on a cat as part of a senior health plan.

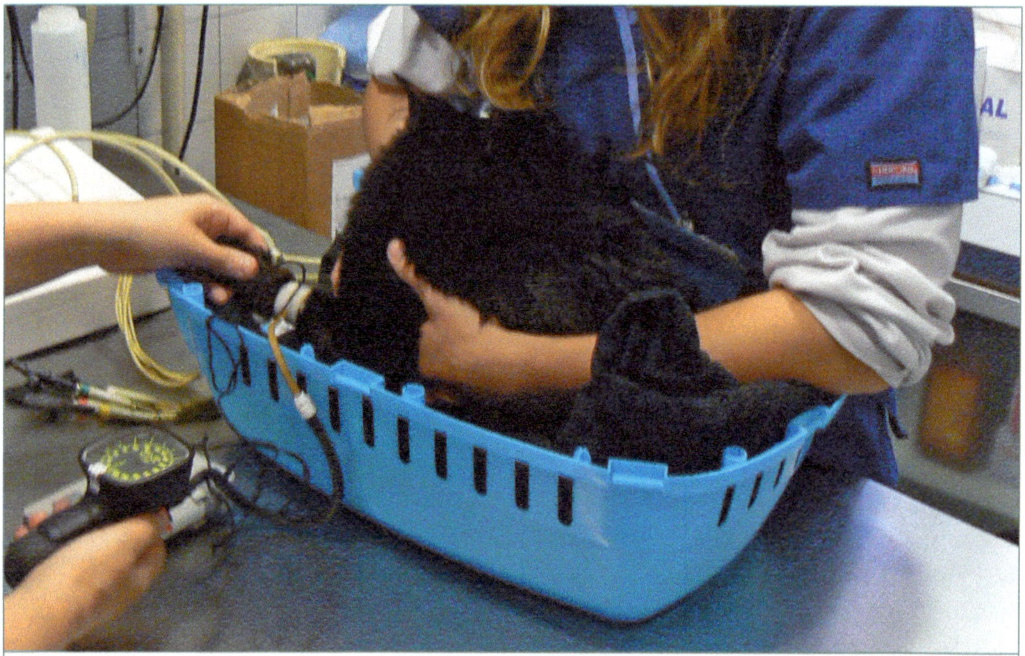

Figure 2. Blood pressure measurement in the cat from the previous figure.

Table 1. Benefits of a senior health plan: some effects of the passage of time and their consequences in small animals.

Type of alteration	Effects	Consequences
Renal	Decreased kidney weight and glomerular filtration rate, tubular atrophy.	Accumulation of nitrogenous products, anaemia, dehydration, etc.
Hepatic	Decreased number of hepatocytes, increased liver fibrosis, reduced detoxification capacity.	Decreased production of clotting factors, increased portal pressure, accumulation of toxins in the circulation.
Metabolic	Decreased basal metabolism, which in many cases causes weight gain and decline of other systems: cardiovascular, osteoarticular, and/or endocrine. Reduced activity.	Decreased lean mass:muscle mass ratio. Appearance of insulin resistance. Joint pain/osteoarthritis.
Immunological	Decreased phagocytic and chemotactic capacity of neutrophils. Reduction of lymphocyte function (not lymphocyte number).	Increase in the prevalence of infections: respiratory, urinary (pyelonephritis), cholangiohepatitis.
Gastrointestinal	Reduced capacity to digest/absorb certain nutrients.	Nutritional imbalances, diarrhoea or pasty stools.
Cardiovascular	Increased valvular fibrosis, reduced cardiac function.	Appearance of murmurs, exercise intolerance. Arrhythmias.

These health plans can be as extensive or complex as we wish: since all systems in the patient's body are affected by the passage of time, none should be excluded. At this stage, budget sheets (Table 2) can help us to demonstrate how each patient's prevention plan will be truly personalised, and how the price compares with the cost of each of the individual services included.

TIP

It can be helpful to design the health plan in front of the owner, in order to emphasise the level of personalisation. This conveys the message that each patient is considered unique, both by the owner and the clinician.

Table 2. Example of a budget sheet for a health plan for a senior dog or cat.

Type of clinical evaluation		Standard price	Selected tests	Final price
Examination	Ophthalmic Neurological Osteoarticular	€100	×	€85
Blood tests	Basic	€100	×	€85
	Bile acids	€30		
	Ionogram	€26	×	€22.1
	Blood gases	€26	×	€22.1
	Coagulogram	€50		
	Hormones • Total T_4 • Cortisol	 €30 €30	×	€25.5
Urinalysis		€30	×	€25.5
Culture		€50		
Chest X-ray (two projections)		€82	×	€69.7
Abdominal ultrasound		€85		
Total price of the selected tests			€394	€334.9 (savings of €55.1 = 15 % discount)

Step 4: take advantage of the moment

During our daily practice, we may have the opportunity to offer these services using a more medical than commercial approach. If we avail of these opportunities, we can convince an owner to invest more and better in their pet. This fourth step can be applied in different clinical settings, where an increase in the added value of the health plan can be essential.

- **Dental prophylaxis:** many owners are reluctant to incur the expense associated with a health plan. For this reason, it may be helpful to use the health plan to perform a more complete preanaesthetic checkup before a dental prophylaxis. As already mentioned in the chapter on orodental diseases, many owners feel apprehension or even panic about the anaesthesia necessary to perform this procedure. This provides a good excuse to evaluate the pet's general health, while decreasing the anaesthetic risk. This lends the health plan an added value that the client may not have previously perceived (Fig. 3).

- **To obtain baseline readings in asymptomatic patients:** measuring baseline haematological and biochemical parameters is useful for future comparisons, before the animal undergoes any changes in its health status. In the case of purebred animals, it is useful to be aware of the prevalence rates of the diseases to which they are most susceptible. For all other animals, we should bear in mind the diseases that most commonly affect senior animals in general.
- **Patients that need a checkup, but whose owners are reluctant:** implementing a health plan for patients that have been showing signs compatible with hyperadrenocorticism or hyperthyroidism for months or years could allow us to finally establish a diagnosis. When designing tailor-made health plans, we can use this moment to demonstrate our knowledge of the patient's medical history, explaining what tests we would perform to finally clear up doubts. In general, health plans should only be offered to healthy animals. However, it can also be helpful to offer them to owners of pets showing signs of chronic disease. If a diagnosis is established, it may be easier to convince the owner that their animal's disease can be treated and that the improvement in their quality of life will be worth the cost of the regular checkups offered as part of the health plan (Fig. 4).

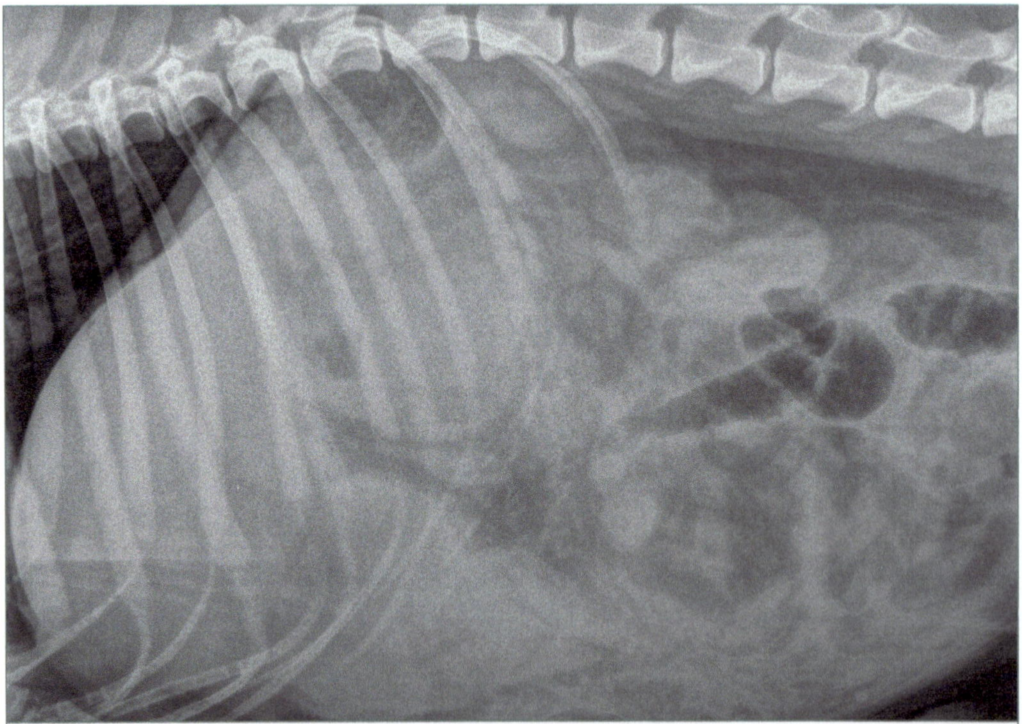

Figure 3. Lateral X-ray of the abdomen of a Golden Retriever taken as part of a senior health plan. The patient had a splenic hemangiosarcoma that was detected by chance. It died 3 months after excision of this tumour due to metastasis to the liver and pancreas.

Step 5: calculate the price of the health plan

Although we may think that the price is the most important aspect for the owner, it is not the main determinant of the decision to authorise testing. Let's not fool ourselves; price is undoubtedly an important element in this type of decision, but it is definitely not the most important. To better illustrate this point, we will provide an example using the so-called mental anchor technique (see next page).

Step 6: closing the deal

If all has gone according to plan, it is now time to specify and agree on when and how to proceed. Here, it is best to involve the clinic's auxiliary personnel once again, as the owner may feel unduly pressured if we do this ourselves. To avoid this situation, and to put the client more at ease, we can let them choose, together with the auxiliary personnel, the optimal moment to begin the health plan.

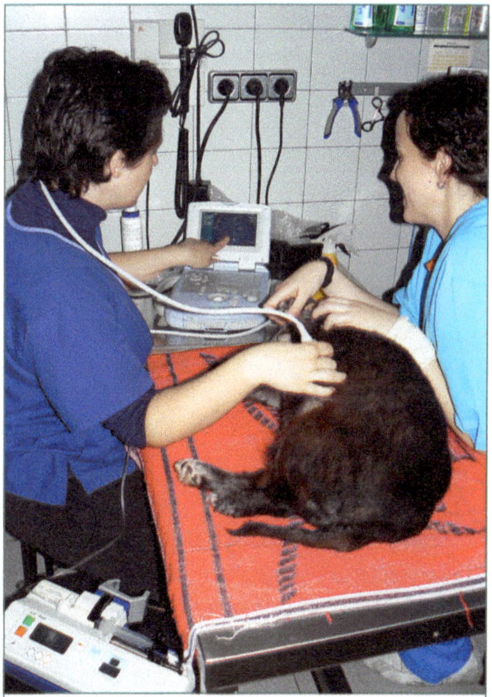

Figure 4. Performing an abdominal ultrasound in a 15-year-old dog with chronic pancreatitis. Adrenal tumours were detected during the course of the examination.

TIP

Auxiliary personnel should be trained to insist only up to a certain point: in the event that an owner changes their mind, the staff should be flexible enough to propose an alternative plan. This plan B could consist of a series of scheduled reminder calls, e.g. will we call you at the end of the month? (before payday); will we call you in June or December? (before the extra pay); how about we call you next month and that way we can devise a plan to spread out expenses?

Helpful advice in difficult situations

When developing and presenting a health plan certain obstacles will always arise. Below we will describe some of the obstacles that we have encountered in our centres over the last 10 years.

Team consensus

The first step is to ensure that all veterinary surgeons/technicians working in a given centre are on the same page. It is very common for all personnel to have different ideas about what is or is not necessary in a certain case. One issue on which staff members tend to disagree is the price that should be charged for services that are more or less essential.

PRACTICAL EXAMPLE OF THE MENTAL ANCHOR TECHNIQUE

This technique can be used in all cases in which there is a dilemma regarding the price of the services to be provided. Economists and marketing experts have long known that a buyer tends to choose the intermediate price when given three options.

How can we use this to our advantage? Put simply, we must be clear about what tests we want to perform on a patient. Let's take a typical example, which is summarised for greater ease of interpretation: a 10-year-old dog whose owner is only moderately convinced. We will design a tailored health plan for this patient. First, we need to think about what a patient of that age requires:

- Complete blood count, 6 basic biochemical tests, urinalysis, and a chest X-ray.
  We estimate that comes to a total cost of €150.

Once this is established, we repeat the process twice: once using broader strokes and a second time applying a greater level of complexity:

- Basic: 5 biochemical tests and a chest X-ray.
  Price: €100.
- Advanced: complete blood count, 8 basic biochemical tests, ionogram, urinalysis with urine protein:creatinine ratio, and a chest X-ray.
  Price: €200.

The objective here is not to perform tests that the patient does not need, but to choose or prioritise those that are required to obtain more information, are of greater prognostic value, or facilitate the selection of subsequent therapies.

Most of our clients will choose the €150 option, as they feel that it provides the best return on their money without spending excessively. Few opt for the most economic option, for various reasons (including, "what will the vet think if I get the cheapest option for my pet").

As the head of a clinic, the first step before offering health plans is to present it to all staff and provide them with the necessary tools to support this strategy. Obviously, the final decision lies with the director; however, personnel who are convinced of the value of a product, and not forced or obliged to push it, will be better motivated to sell it. This is, after all, the goal of our policy.

Clarity and transparency

Some veterinary surgeons and assistants worry that selling this type of product will result in the loss of the owner's trust. This feeling is very common, especially when a clinic starts to lay the foundations of a preventive medicine approach, beyond vaccination programmes. For those accustomed to selling curative or palliative medicine, such "ethical" problems tend not to arise.

In our centres this issue became a major obstacle, and so we decided to do the following: we conducted a survey to determine the value that clients attached to different aspects of the health plan. We found that the veterinary surgeon's ability to explain themselves, their level of sincerity, and the price (or the feeling of being offered an overall discount), in that order, were the aspects valued the most. Based on this information, we proposed the following approach:

- **The veterinary surgeon's ability to explain themselves:** to work on this aspect, we created fictitious situations in which we played the role of the veterinary surgeons or the owner. This helped team members with poorer communication skills to better cope with the questions or complaints often received from unconvinced owners.
- **The veterinary surgeon's level of sincerity, or lack thereof:** to address this issue, we exhaustively examined the main diseases of senior pets, as well as the benefits of diagnosing them early and the consequences of not doing so. We focused primarily on survival in two distinct scenarios: when the appropriate protocol is followed and when it is not. We created brochures and electronic presentations to explain this in the clinic.
- **The feeling of being offered an overall discount:** we used a spreadsheet to calculate the overall cost of the services included in the plan. Then, following preestablished criteria, we established a graded system, for example: a 7 % discount on the official price is applied to health plans costing €100–€150; a 10 % discount to those costing €150–€200; and a 15 % discount to those over €200. These percentages can obviously vary: each centre will need to do their own calculations to ensure that the plans are profitable (see Table 2).

The target customer

Deciding the type of client to whom the plan will be presented is fundamental. In our opinion, plans should only be actively proposed to clients known to be somewhat receptive. Thus, plans should be proposed to the 20 % of clients that spend the most. For all others, it may be sufficient to passively promote health plans in the waiting room or by sending emails that direct the client to our website. If these clients are interested, they will actively seek out further information. This way, we avoid several common inconveniences at the same time:

- We avoid the "encyclopaedia seller effect"; i.e. creating the impression that we are attempting to sell the client a product that does not interest them.
- We avoid making our staff feel like salespeople.
- We will avoid a mutual feeling (on the part of both the owner and the veterinary surgeon) of wasting time. This can be a problem in itself: a veterinary surgeon may feel obliged to inform the owner about a health plan even though the waiting room is full of other clients. If the owner inquires about a health plan, a brief visit can be arranged in which we explain everything in a more detailed and relaxed way, at a time that suits both the veterinary surgeon and the client. Conversely, if we take advantage of an annual vaccination appointment to discuss the pros and cons of aging with the client, we cannot ask them to return another day to discuss the issue more calmly.

Bibliography

Chapter 1. Ageing in small animals

1. Blanco Moreno Á et al. Real per capita health spending by age and sex in Spain (1998–2008): changes and effects on public healthcare expenditure projections. *Gac Sanit*, 2013, 27(3):220–5.
2. Rodes Texidor J, Guardia Massó J. *Biología del envejecimiento*. Editorial Masson, 1997, pp. 3472–5.
3. Salgado A, Guillén F. *Manual de geriatría*. Barcelona, Editorial Salvat, 1990, pp. 1–17.
4. Migliaccio E et al. The p66shc adaptor protein controls oxidative stress response and life span in mammals. *Nature*, 1999, 402:309–13.
5. Olovnikov AM. A theory of marginotomy. The incomplete copying of template margin in enzymic synthesis of polynucleotides and biological significance of the phenomenon. *J Theor Biol*, 1973, 41(1):181–90.
6. Greider CW, Blackburn EH. Identification of a specific telomere terminal transferase activity in Tetrahymena extracts. *Cell*, 1985, 43(2 Pt 1):405–13.
7. Hoskins JD. Preventive health program for dogs. *Comp Cont Educ Pract Vet*, 1988, 9:187–92.

Chapter 2. Nutrition in elderly patients

1. Harper EJ. Changing perspectives on aging and energy requirements: aging and digestive function in humans, dogs and cats. *J Nutr*, 1998, 128(12 Suppl):2632S–5S.
2. Laflamme DP et al. Effect of age on maintenance energy requirements and apparent digestibility of canine diets. *Compendium*, 2000, 22(9 Suppl):113.
3. Elia M. The inter-organ flux of substrates in fed and fasted man, as indicated by arterio-venous balance studies. *Nutr Res Rev*, 1991, 4:3–31.
4. Kealy RD. Factors influencing lean body mass in aging dogs. *Comp Contin Educ Pract Vet*, 1999, 21(suppl):34–7.
5. Pérez Camargo G. Cat nutrition: what is new in the old? *Compen Contin Educ Pract Vet*, 2004, 26(Suppl 2A):5–10.
6. Armstrong PJ, Lund EM. Changes in body composition and energy balance with aging. *Vet Clin Nutr*, 1996, 3:83–96.
7. Finco DR et al. Effects of aging and dietary protein intake on uninephrectomized geriatric dogs. *Am J Vet Res*, 1994, 55:1282–90.
8. Finco DR. Effects of dietary protein intake on renal functions. *Vet Forum*, 1999, 16:34–44.
9. Finco DR. Effects of dietary protein and phosphorus on the kidney of dogs. *Proceedings of the Waltham/OSU Symposium*, Vernon, CA, Kal Kan Foods Inc., 1992, pp. 39–41.
10. Wannemacher RW, McCoy JR. Determination of optimal dietary protein requirements of young and old dogs. *J Nutr*, 1966, 88:66–74.
11. McMurray DN. Effect of moderate protein deficiency on immune function. *Compend Contin Educ Pract Vet*, 1999, 21:21–4.
12. Yoshino K et al. IgE responses in mice fed moderate protein deficient and high protein diets. *J Nutr Sci Vitaminol (Tokyo)*, 2003, 49(3):172–8.

58. Graham PA et al. Influence of a high fiber diet on glycemic control and quality of life in dogs with diabetes mellitus. *J Small Anim Nutr*, 2002, 43:67–73.
59. Hagander B et al. Dietary fiber decreases fasting blood glucose levels and plasma LDL concentration in noninsulin-dependent diabetes mellitus patients. *Am J Clin Nutr*, 1988, 47:852–8.
60. Kimmel SE et al. Effects of insoluble and soluble dietary fiber on glycemic control in dogs with naturally occurring insulin-dependent diabetes mellitus. *J Am Vet Med Assoc*, 2000, 216:1076–81.
61. Fleeman LM, Rand JS, Markwell PJ. Lack of advantage of high-fibre, moderate-carbohydrate diets in dogs with stabilised diabetes. *J Small Anim Pract*, 2009, 50:604–14.
62. Nelson RW et al. Effect of dietary insoluble fiber on control of glycemia in cats with naturally acquired diabetes mellitus. *J Am Vet Med Assoc*, 2000, 216:1082–8.
63. Frank G et al. Use of a high protein diet in the management of feline diabetes mellitus. *Vet Ther*, 2001, 2:238–46.
64. Bennett N et al. Comparison of a low carbohydrate-low fiber diet and a moderate carbohydrate-high fiber diet in the management of feline diabetes mellitus. *J Feline Med Surg*, 2006, 8(2):73–84.
65. Linn T et al. Effect of dietary protein intake on insulin secretion and glucose metabolism in insulin-dependent diabetes mellitus. *J Clin Endrocrinol Metab*, 1996, 81:3938–43.
66. Peters AL, Davidson MB. Protein and fat effects on glucose responses and insulin requirements in subjects with insulin-dependent diabetes mellitus. *Am J Clin Nutr*, 1993, 58:555–60.
67. Freyse EJ et al. Increased urea synthesis in insulin-dependent diabetic dogs maintained normoglycemic: effect of portal insulin administration and food protein content. *Diabetes*, 1996, 45:667–74.

Chapter 3. Pharmacological treatment of geriatric patients

1. Ambrose PJ. Altered drug action with aging. *Health Notes*, 2003, 1(7):12–9.
2. Riviere J. Dosage adjustments in renal disease. In: *Comparative Pharmacokinetics: Principles, Techniques and Applications*. Ames, Iowa State University Press, 1999, pp. 283–95.
3. St Peter WL, Redic-Kill KA, Halstenson CE. Clinical pharmacokinetics of antibiotics in patients with impaired renal function. *Clin Pharmacokinet*, 1992, 22(3):169–210.
4. Turnheim K. Drug dosage in the elderly. Is it rational? *Drugs Aging*, 1998, 13(5):357–79.
5. Tumer N, Scarpace PJ, Lowenthal DT. Geriatric pharmacology: basic and clinical considerations. *Annu Rev Pharmacol Toxicol*, 1992, 32:271–302.
6. Muhlberg W, Platt D. Age-dependent changes of the kidneys: pharmacological implications. *Gerontology*, 1999, 45(5):243–53.
7. Dieppe P et al. Balancing benefits and harms: the example of nonsteroidal anti-inflammatory drugs. *BMJ*, 2004, 329(7456):31–4.
8. Burkholder WJ. Dietary considerations for dogs and cats with renal disease. *J Am Vet Med Assoc*, 2000, 216(11):1730–4.
9. Rowland M, Benet LZ, Graham GG. Clearance concepts in pharmacokinetics. *J Pharmacokinet Biopharm*, 1973, 1(2):123–36.
10. Haney SL. Drug use in renal failure. *Crit Care Nurs Clin N Am*, 2002, 14(1):77–80.
11. Rubin SI. Chronic renal failure and its management and nephrolithiasis. *Vet Clin N Am Small Anim Pract*, 1997, 27(6):1331–54.

12. Nagode LA, Chew DJ, Podell M. Benefits of calcitriol therapy and serum phosphorus control in dogs and cats with chronic renal failure. Both are essential to prevent of suppress toxic hyperparathyroidism. *Vet Clin N Am Small Anim Pract*, 1996, 26(6):1293–330.
13. Reidenberg MM, Drayer DE. Alteration of drug-protein binding in renal disease. *Clin Pharmacokinet*, 1984, 9(Suppl 1):18–26.
14. Reidenberg MM, Drayer DE. Effects of renal disease upon drug disposition. *Drug Metab Rev*, 1978, 8(2):293–302.
15. Reidenberg MM, Drayer DE. Drug therapy in renal failure. *Annu Rev Pharmacol Toxicol*, 1980, 20:45–54.
16. Lefebvre HP, Laroute V, Alvinerie M. The effect of experimental renal failure on tolfenamic acid disposition in the dog. *Biopharm Drug Dispos*, 1997, 18(1):79–91.
17. Sica DA. Pharmacotherapy in congestive heart failure: drug absorption in the management of congestive heart failure: loop diuretics. *Congest Heart Fail*, 2003, 9(5):287–92.
18. Burkholder WJ. Age-related changes to nutritional requirements and digestive function in adult dogs and cats. *J Am Vet Med Assoc*, 1999, 215(5):625–9.

Chapter 4. Anaesthesia in elderly patients

1. Harvey RC, Paddleford RR. Management of geriatric patients. A common occurrence. *Vet Clin North Am Small Anim Pract*, 1999, 29(3):683–99.
2. Dodman NH, Seeler DC, Court NH. Aging changes in the geriatric dog and their impact on anesthesia. *Compend Cont Educ Pract Vet*, 1984, 6:1106–12.
3. Fisch C. Electrocardiogram in the aged: an independent marker of heart disease? *Am J Med*, 1981, 70(1):4–6.
4. Owens W. The geriatric patient-physiology of aging. *Proceedings of the American Society of Anesthesiologists*, Saint Louis, 1985, pp. 1–4.
5. Knudson RJ et al. Effect of aging alone on mechanical properties of the normal adult human lung. *J Appl Physiol*, 1977, 43(6):1054–62.
6. Robinson NE, Gillespie JR. Lung volumes in aging beagle dogs. *J Appl Physiol*, 1973, 35(3):317–21.
7. Pontoppidan H, Beecher HK. Progressive loss of protective reflexes in the airway with the advance of age. *JAMA*, 1960, 174:2209–13.
8. Greenblatt DJ, Sellers EM, Shader RI. Drug therapy: drug disposition in old age. *N Engl J Med*, 1982, 306(18):1081–8.
9. Marshall M. Capnography in dogs. *Compend Cont Educ Pract Vet*, 2004, 26(10):761–77.
10. Brodbelt DC, Hammond R, Tuminaro D. Risk factors for anaesthetic-related death in referred dogs. *Vet Rec*, 2006, 158(16):563–4.
11. Tobias KM, Marioni-Henry K, Wagner R. A retrospective study on the use of acepromazine maleate in dogs with seizures. *J Am Anim Hosp Assoc*, 2006, 42(4):283–9.
12. McConnell J, Kirby R, Rudloff E. A retrospective study on the use of acepromazine maleate in dogs with seizures. *J Vet Emerg Crit Care*, 2007, 17(3): 262–7.
13. Crowell-Davis SL. Benzodiazepines: pros and cons for fear and anxiety. *Compend Cont Educ Pract Vet*, 2008, 30(10):526–9.
14. Jones DJ, Stehling LC. Cardiovascular responses to diazepam and midazolam maleate in the dog. *Anesthesiology*, 1979, 51(5):430–4.
15. Murray T. Amino acid neurotransmitters: glutamate, GABA, and the pharmacology of benzodiazpines. In: Crowell-Davis SL, Murray T, eds. *Veterinary Psychopharmacology*. Ames, Blackwell Publishing, 2006, pp. 25–33.

15. McCune S. Caged cats: avoiding problems and providing solutions. *Newsletter of the Companion Animal Behaviour Therapy Study Group*, 1994, 7:33–40.
16. Fox MW. *Laboratory Animal Husbandry*. London, State University of New York Press, 1986.
17. Wolfle TL. Policy, program and people: the three P's to well-being. In: Mench JA, Krulisch L, eds. *Canine Research Environment*. Bethesda, Scientists Center for Animal Welfare, 1990, pp. 41–7.
18. DeLuca AM, Kranda KC. Environmental enrichment. *Lab Anim*, 1992, 21:38–44.
19. Holmes RJ. Environmental enrichment for confined dogs and cats. The TG Hungerford refresher course for veterinarians. In: *Proceedings from the Postgraduate Committee in Veterinary Science*, University of Sydney, Australia, 1993, 214:191–7.
20. Loveridge GG. Provision of environmentally enriched housing for cats. *Anim Technol*, 1994, 45:69–87.
21. Loveridge GG, Horrocks LJ, Hawthorne AJ. Environmentally enriched housing for cats when housed singly. *Anim Welf*, 1995, 4:135–41.
22. Tuber DS et al. Dogs in animal shelters: problems suggestions and needed expertise. *Psychtr Sci*, 1999, 10:379–86.
23. Gourkow N, Fraser D. The effect of housing and handling practices on the welfare behaviour and selection of domestic cats (*Felis sylvestris catus*) by adopters in an animal shelter. *Anim Welf*, 2006, 15:371–7.
24. Kessler MR, Turner DC. Stress and adaptation of cats (*Felis silvestris catus*) housed singly, in pairs and in groups in boarding catteries. *Anim Welf*, 1997, 6:243–54.
25. Lore RK, Eisenberg FB. Avoidance reactions of domestic dogs to unfamiliar male and female humans in a kennel setting. *Appl Anim Behav Sci*, 1986, 15:262–6.
26. Wells DL, Hepper PG. The influence of environmental change on the behaviour of sheltered dogs. *Appl Anim Behav Sci*, 2000, 68:151–62.
27. Wells DL, Hepper PG. Prevalence of behaviour problems in dogs purchased from an animal rescue shelter. *Appl Anim Behav Sci*, 2000, 69:55–65.
28. Soennichsen S, Chamove AS. Responses of cats to petting by humans. *Anthrozoos*, 2002, 15:258–65.
29. Feuerstein N, Terkel J. Interrelationships of dogs (*Canis familiaris*) and cats (*Felis catus L.*) living under the same roof. *Appl Anim Behav Sci*, 2008, 113:150–65.
30. Ellis SL. Environmental enrichment: practical strategies for improving feline welfare. *J Fel Med Surg*, 2009, 11(11):901–12.
31. DeLuca AM, Kranda KC. Environmental enrichment in a large animal facility. *Lab Anim*, 1992, 21:38–44.
32. Shepherdson DJ, Mellen JD, Hutchins M. *Second Nature: Environmental Enrichment for Captive Animals*. London, Smithsonian Institution Press, 1998.
33. Wells DL. The influence of toys on the behaviour and welfare of kennelled dogs. *Anim Welfare*, 2004, 13(3):367–73.
34. Hubrecht RC. A comparison of social and laboratory environmental enrichment methods for laboratory housed dogs. *Appl Anim Behav Sci*, 1993, 37:345–61.
35. De Monte M, Le Pape G. Behavioural effects of cage enrichment in single-caged adult cats. *Anim Welf*, 1997, 6:53–66.
36. Hall SL, Bradshaw JWS, Robinson IH. Object play in adult domestic cats: the roles of habituation and disinhibition. *Appl Anim Behav Sci*, 2002, 79:263–71.

37. Denenberg S. Cat toy play trial: a comparison of different toys. *Proceedings of the Annual Scientific Symposium of Animal Behaviour, American Veterinary Society of Animal Behaviour*, Denver, CO, 2003.
38. Case LP. *The Cat: Its Behavior Nutrition and Health*. Ames, Iowa State Press, 2003.
39. Hall SL, Bradshaw JWS. The influence of hunger on object play by adult domestic cats. *Appl Anim Behav Sci*, 1998, 58:143–50.
40. Gourkow N. *The Emotional Life of Cats: A Manual for Improving the Psychological Well-being of Shelter Cats*. Canada, British Columbia Society for the Prevention of Cruelty to Animals, 2003.
41. Hawkins KR. *Stress, Enrichment and Welfare of Domestic Cats in Rescue Shelters*. PhD diss. University of Bristol, UK, 2005.
42. Overall KL, Dyer D. Enrichment strategies for laboratory animals from the viewpoint of clinical veterinary behavioural medicine: emphasis on cats and dogs. *ILAR J*, 2005, 46:202–16.
43. McCune S. Enriching the environment of the laboratory cat-a review. *Proceedings of the 2nd International Conference on Environmental Enrichment*. Copenhagen, 1995, pp. 103–17.
44. Wells DL, Graham L, Hepper PG. The influence of auditory stimulation on the behaviour of dogs housed in a rescue shelter. *Anim Welf*, 2002, 11:385–93.
45. Graham L, Wells DL, Hepper PG. The influence of olfactory stimulation on the behavior of dogs housed in a rescue shelter, *Appl Anim Behav Sci*, 2005, 91(1–2):143–53.
46. Hart BL. Feline behaviour: olfaction and feline behaviour. *Feline Pract*, 1977, 7:8–10.
47. Bowen J, Heath S. *Behaviour Problems in Small Animals: Practical Advice for the Veterinary Team*. Elsevier Health Sciences, 2005, p. 58.
48. Mills D. Pheromonatherapy: theory and applications. *In Pract*, 2005, 27:368–73.
49. Landsberg G. Therapeutic options for cognitive decline in senior pets. *J Am Anim Hosp Assoc*, 2006, 42(6):407–13.
50. Conclusiones de la mesa redonda entre los grupos de especialidad GRETCA-GEMFE [Conclusions of the roundtable between the ethology and animal behaviour (GRETCA) and feline medicine (GEMFE) specialty groups], GTA-AVEPA Congress, Cordoba (Spain), March 2012.
51. Wells DL. A review of environmental enrichment for kennelled dogs, *Canis familiaris*. *App Anim Behav Sci*, 2004, 85:307–17.
52. Shyan-Norwalt MR. Caregiver perceptions of what indoor cats do "for fun". *J Appl Anim Welf Sci*, 2005, 8:199–209.
53. Ellis SLH, Wells DL. The influence of visual stimulation on the behaviour of cats housed in a rescue shelter. *Appl Anim Behav Sci*, 2008, 113:166–74.

Chapter 6. Chronic pain. Arthrosis

1. Merskey H, Bogduk N. *Classification of Chronic Pain: Descriptions of Chronic Pain Syndromes and Definitions of Pain Terms*. Seattle, IASP Press, 1994.
2. Kroenke K, Krebs EE, Bair MJ. Pharmacotherapy of chronic pain: a synthesis of recommedations from systematic reviews. *Gen Hosp Psychiatry*, 2009, 31:206–19.
3. Pain Facts and Figures: Web site of the American Pain Foundation. www.painfoundation.org. Accessed March 2011.
4. Von Korff M, Dunn KM. Chronic pain reconsidered. *Pain*, 2008, 138:267–76.

5. Willard F. Basic mechanisms of pain. In: Audette JF, Bailey A, eds. *Integrative Pain Medicine: The Science and Practice of Complementary and Alternative Medicine in Pain Management.* Totowa, NJ, Humana Press, 2008, pp. 19–62.
6. Chuck A et al. The willingness to pay for reducing pain and pain-related disability. *Value Health*, 2009, 12(4):498–506.
7. Apkarian AV, Baliki MN, Geha PY. Towards a theory of chronic pain. *Prog Neurobiol*, 2009, 87:81–97.
8. Green SA. Chronic pain: pathophysiology and treatment implications. *Topics Comp Anim Med*, 2010, 25:5–9.
9. Pozzi A, Muir WW, Traverso F. Prevention of central sensitization and pain by N-metyl-D-aspartate receptor antagonists. *J Am Vet Med Assoc*, 2006, 228:53–60.
10. Stanfa L et al. Cholecystokinin and morphine analgesia: variations on a theme. *Trends Pharmacol Sci*, 1994, 15: 65–6.
11. Sparkes HA et al. ISFM/AAFP consensus guidelines: long-term use of NSAIDs in cats. *J Feline Med Surg*, 2010, 12(7):521–38.
12. Papich MG. An update on nonsteroidal anti-inflammatory drugs (NSAIDs) in small animals. *Vet Clin Small Anim*, 2008, 38:1243–66.
13. Papich MG. Pharmacologic considerations for opiate and nonsteroidal anti-inflammatory drugs. *Vet Clin North Am Small Anim Pract*, 2000, 30:815–37.
14. Lees P et al. Pharmacodynamics and pharmacokinetics of nonsteroidal anti-inflammatory drugs in species of veterinary interest. *J Vet Pharmacol Ther*, 2004, 27(6):479–90.
15. Lees P et al. PK-PD integration and PK-PD modeling of nonsteroidal anti-inflammatory drugs: principles and applications in veterinary pharmacology. *J Vet Pharmacol Ther*, 2004, 27(6):491–502.
16. Savides MC, Oehme FW, Nash SL. The toxicity and biotransformation of single doses of acetaminophen in dogs and cats. *Toxicol Appl Pharmacol*, 1984, 74(1):26–34.
17. KuKanich B, Lascelles BDX, Papich MG. Pharmacokinetics of morphine and plasma concentrations of morphine-6-glucuronide following morphine administration to dogs. *J Vet Pharmacol Ther*, 2005, 28(4):371–6.
18. Dohoo SE, Tasker RA. Pharmacokinetics of oral morphine sulfate in dogs: a comparison of sustained release and conventional formulation. *Can J Vet Res*, 1997, 61(4):251–5.
19. Aragon CL et al. Pharmacokinetics of an immediate and extended release oral morphine formulation utilizing the spheroidal oral drug absorption system in dogs. *J Vet Pharmacol Ther*, 2009, 32(2):129–36.
20. Findlay JW, Jones EC, Welch RM. Radioimmunoassay determination of the absolute oral bioavailabilities and O-demethylation of codeine and hydrocodone in the dog. *Drug Metab Dispos*, 1979, 7(5):310–4.
21. Yeh SY, Woods LA. Excretion of codeine and its metabolites by dogs, rabbits and cats. *Arch Int Pharmacodyn Ther*, 1971, 191(2):231–42.
22. Kukanich B et al. The effects of inhibiting cytochrome P450 3A, p-glycoprotein, and gastric acid secretion on the oral bioavailability of methadone in dogs. *J Vet Pharmacol Ther*, 2005, 28(5):461–6.
23. Maiante AA et al. Comparison of the cardio-respiratory effects of methadone and morphine in conscious dogs. *J Vet Pharmacol Ther*, 2009, 32(4):317–28.
24. KuKanich B, Papich MG. Pharmacokinetics of tramadol and the metabolite O-desmethyltramadol in dogs. *J Vet Pharmacol Ther*, 2004, 27(4):239–46.

25. Giorgi M et al. Pharmacokinetic and urine profile of tramadol and its major metabolites following oral immediate release capsules administration in dogs. *Vet Res Commun*, 2009, 33(8):875–85.
26. Giorgi M et al. Pharmacokinetic evaluation of tramadol and its major metabolites after single oral sustained tablet administration in the dog: a pilot study. *Vet J*, 2009, 180(2):253–5.
27. Mathews KA. Neuropathic pain in dogs and cats: if only they could tell us if they hurt. *Vet Clin North Am Small Anim Pract*, 2008, 38(6):1365–414.
28. Siao KT et al. Pharmacokinetics of amantadine in cats. *J Vet Pharmacol Ther*, 2011, 34(6):599–604.
29. Norkus C et al. Pharmacokinetics of oral amantadine in greyhound dogs. *J Vet Pharmacol Ther*, 2015, 38(3):305–8.
30. Lamont LA. Adjuntive analgesic therapy in veterinary medicine. *Vet Clin North Am Small Anim Pract*, 2008, 38(6):1187–203.
31. Bokerawa M et al. Reistin, an adipoline with potent proinflammatory properties. *J Immunol*, 2005, 174:5789–95.
32. Vuolteenaho K et al. Leptin enhances synthesis of proinflammatory mediators in humans osteoarthritis cartilage mediator role of NO in leptin-induced PGE2, IL-6 and IL-8 production. *Mediators Inflamm*, 2009, 2009:345838.
33. Jonhston SA, McLaughlin RM, Budsbers SC. Nonsurgical management of osteoarthritis in dogs. *Vet Clin North Am Small Anim Pract*, 2008, 38(6):1449–70.
34. Aragon CL, Hofmeister EH, Budsberg SC. Systematic review of clinical trials of treatments for osteoarthritis in dogs. *J Am Vet Med Assoc*, 2007, 230(4):514–21.
35. Canapp SO Jr et al. Scintigraphic evaluation of dogs with acute synovitis after treatment with glucosamine hydrochloride and chondroitin sulfate. *Am J Vet Res*, 1999, 60(12):1552–7.
36. Adebowale A et al. The bioavailibility and pharmacokinetics of glucosamine hydrochloride and low molecular chondroitin sulfate after single and multiple doses to Beagle dogs. *Biopharm Drug Dispos*, 2002, 23:217–25.
37. Lerman RH et al. Nutritional approach for relief of joint discomfort: a 12-week, open-case series and illustrative case report. *Integr Med (Encinitas)*, 2015, 14(5):52–61.
38. Tong T et al. Chicken type II collagen induced immune balance of main subtype of helper T cells in mesenteric lymph node lymphocytes in rats with collagen-induced arthritis. *Inflamm Res*, 2010, 59(5):369–77.
39. Gencoglu H et al. Undenatured type II collagen (UC-II) in joint health and disease: a review on the current knowledge of companion animals. *Animals (Basel)*, 2020, 10(4):697.
40. Bauer JE. Responses of dogs to dietary omega-3 fatty acids. *J Am Vet Med Assoc*, 2007, 231(11):1657–61.
41. Roudebush P, Davenport DJ, Novotny BJ. The use of nutraceuticals in cancer therapy. *Vet Clin North Am Small Anim Pract*, 2004, 34(1):249–69.
42. Ogilvie GK. Interventional nutrition for the cancer patient. *Clin Tech Small Anim Pract*, 1998, 13(4):224–31.
43. Biondo PD, Brindley DN, Sawyer MB. The potential for treatment with dietary long-chain polyunsaturated n-3 fatty acids during chemotherapy. *J Nutr Biochem*, 2008, 19(12):787–96.
44. Altinel L et al. Treatment with unsaponifiable extracts of avocado and soybean increases TGF-beta1 and TGF-beta2 levels in canine joint fluid. *Tohoku J Exp Med*, 2007, 211(2):181–6.

45. Boileau C et al. Protective effects of total fraction of avocado/soybean unsaponifiables on the structural changes in experimental dog osteoarthritis: inhibition of nitric oxide synthase and matrix metalloproteinase-13. *Arthritis Res Ther*, 2009, 11(2):R41.
46. Kapatkin AS et al. Effects of electrostimulated acupuncture on ground reaction forces and pain scores in dogs with chronic elbow joint arthritis. *Am Vet Med Assoc*, 2006, 228(9):1350–4.
47. Sluka KA. Osteoarthritis and rheumatoid arthritis. In: Sluka KA, ed. *Mechanisms and Management of Pain for the Physical Therapist*. Seattle, IASP Press, 2009.
48. Sartini I, Giorgi M. Grapiprant: a snapshot of the current knowledge. *J Vet Pharmacol Ther*, 2021, 44(5):679–88.
49. Enomoto M et al. Anti-nerve growth factor monoclonal antibodies for the control of pain in dogs and cats. *Vet Rec*, 2019, 184(1):23.

Chapter 7. Orodental problems in elderly animals

1. Holmstrom SE et al. AAHA dental care guidelines for dogs and cats. *J Am Anim Hosp Assoc*, 2005, 41(5):277–83.
2. Floyd MR. The modified Triadan system: nomenclature for veterinary dentistry. *J Vet Dent*, 1991, 8(4):18–9.
3. Verstraete FJM, Kass PH, Terpak CH. Diagnostic value of full-mouth radiography in dogs. *Am J Vet Res*, 1998, 59:686–91.
4. Verstraete JM, Kass PH, Terpak CH. Diagnostic value of full mouth radiology in cats. *Am J Vet Res*, 1998, 59:692–5.
5. Brodbelt D. Perioperative mortality in small animal anaesthesia. *Vet J*, 2009, 182(2):152–61.
6. Peddle GD et al. Association of periodontal disease, oral procedures, and other clinical findings with bacterial endocarditis in dogs. *J Am Vet Med Assoc*, 2009, 234:100–7.
7. Davé S, Van Dyke T. The link between periodontal disease and cardiovascular disease is probably inflammation. *Oral Dis*, 2008, 14:95–101.
8. Niemiec BA. Periodontal disease. *Top Companion Anim Med*, 2008, 23:72–80.
9. Pavlica Z et al. Periodontal disease burden and pathological changes in organs of dogs. *J Vet Dent*, 2008, 25:97–105.
10. Wilson W et al. Prevention of infective endocarditis. Guidelines from the American Heart Association: a guideline from the American Heart Association-Rheumatic Fever, Endocarditis and Kawasaki Disease Committee, Council on Cardiovascular Disease in the Young, and the Council on Clinical Cardiology, Council on Cardiovascular Surgery and Anesthesia, and the Quality of Care and Outcomes Research Interdisciplinary Working Group. *J Am Dent Assoc*, 2008, 139 Suppl:3S–24S.
11. Tou SP, Adin DB, Castleman WL. Mitral valve endocarditis after dental prophylaxis in a dog. *J Vet Intern Med*, 2005, 19:268–70.
12. Strom BL et al. Dental and cardiac risk factors for infective endocarditis. A population-based, case-control study. *Ann Intern Med*, 1998, 129:761–9.

Chapter 8. Chronic kidney disease

1. Brown SA. Renal dysfunction in small animals. *Merck Veterinary Manual*, 2013, accessed November 1, 2021. https://www.merckvetmanual.com/urinary-system/noninfectious-diseases-of-the-urinary-system-in-small-animals/renal-dysfunction-in-small-animals

2. Guyton MD, Hall J. *Fisiología humana y mecanismos de las enfermedades*, [Human Physiology and Mechanisms of Disease] 6th ed. Havana, 1996.
3. Pérez Camargo G. Cat nutrition: what is new in the old? *Compen Contin Educ Pract Vet*, 2004, 26(Suppl 2A):5–10.
4. Adams LG et al. Correlation of urine protein/creatinine ratio and twenty-four-hour urinary protein excretion in normal cats and cats with surgically induced chronic renal failure. *J Vet Intern Med*, 1992, 6(1):36–40.
5. Syme HM. Proteinuria in cats. Prognostic marker or mediator? *J Feline Med Surg*, 2009, 11(3):211–8.
6. Lulich JP, Osborn CA. Feline renal failure: questions, answers, questions. *Compend Cont Educ Pract Vet*, 1992, 2:127–52.
7. Adin CA et al. Antegrade pyelography for suspected ureteral obstruction in cats: 11 cases (1995–2001). *J Am Vet Med Assoc*, 2003, 222(11):1576–81.
8. Kyles AE, Hardie EM, Wooden BG. Clinical, clinicopathologic, radiographic and ultrasonographic abnormalities in cats with ureteral calculi: 163 cases (1984–2002). *J Am Vet Med Assoc*, 2005, 226(6):932–6.
9. Barr FJ, Holt PE, Gibbs C. Ultrasonographic measurement of normal renal parameters. *J Small Anim Pract*, 1990, 31(4):180–4.
10. Langston C et al. Diagnosis of urolithiasis. *Compend Cont Educ Pract Vet*, 2008, 30(8):447–55.
11. Shiroma JT et al. Effect of reproductive status on feline renal size. *Vet Radiol Ultrasound*, 1999, 40(3):242–5.
12. d'Anjou M. Kidneys and ureters. In: Penninck D, d'Anjou M, eds. *Atlas of Small Animal Ultrasonography*. Ames, Blackwell Publishing, 2008, pp. 339–64.
13. Reusch CE et al. Ultrasonography of the parathyroid glands as an aid in differentiation of acute and chronic kidney failure in dogs. *J Am Vet Med Assoc*, 2000, 217(12):1849–52.
14. Lees GE, Cianciolo RE, Clubb FJ Jr. Renal biopsy and pathologic evaluation of glomerular disease. *Top Companion Anim Med*, 2011, 26(3):143–53.
15. Vaden SL. Renal biopsy of dogs and cats. *Clin Tech Small Anim Pract*, 2005, 20:11–22.
16. Vaden SL. Renal biopsy. How and why. In: *2000 Scientific Proceedings, 18th Annual Veterinary Medical Forum*, American College of Veterinary Internal Medicine, Seattle, WA, 2000, pp. 675–6.
17. Polzin DJ, Osborne CA, Ross S. Tratamiento basado en la evidencia de la nefropatía crónica [Evidence-based management of chronic kidney disease]. In: Bonagura JD, Twedt DC, eds. *Kirk Terapéutica veterinaria actual*. Elsevier Saunders, 2009, chap. 190, pp. 872–82.
18. Plantinga EA et al. Retrospective study of the survival of cats with acquired chronic renal insufficiency offered different commercial diets. *Vet Rec*, 2005, 157(7):185–7.
19. Brown SA. Oxidative stress and chronic kidney disease. *Vet Clin North Am Small Anim Pract*, 2008, 38(1):157–66.
20. Brown SA et al. Beneficial effects of chronic administration of dietary omega-3 polyunsaturated fatty acids in dogs with renal insufficiency. *J Clin Lab Med*, 1998, 131:447–55.
21. Lees GL et al. Assessment and management of proteinuria in dogs and cats: 2004 ACVIM Forum consensus statement (small animal). *J Vet Intern Med*, 2005, 19:377–85.
22. Maschio G et al. Effect of angiotensin-converting enzyme inhibitor benazepril on the progression of chronic renal insufficiency. *N Engl J Med*, 1996, 334:939–45.

23. Brown SA et al. Effects of the angiotensin converting enzyme inhibitor benazepril in cats with induced renal failure. *Am J Vet Res*, 2001, 62:375–83.
24. King JN et al. Tolerability and efficacy of benazepril in cats with chronic kidney disease. *J Vet Intern Med*, 2006, 20:1054–64.
25. Mizutani H et al. Evaluation of the clinical efficacy of benazepril in the treatment of chronic renal insufficiency in cats. *J Vet Intern Med*, 2006, 20:1074–9.
26. Grauer GF. Canine glomerulonephritis: new thoughts on proteinuria and treatment. *J Small Anim Pract*, 2005, 46(10):469–78.

Chapter 9. Liver problems in geriatric patients

1. Johnson SE. Portal hypertension. Part I. Pathophysiology and clinical consequences. *Compend Contin Educ Pract Vet*, 1987, 9:741–8.
2. Johnson SE. Portal hypertension. Part II. Clinical assessment and treatment. *Compend Contin Educ Pract Vet*, 1987, 9:917–25.
3. Crawford MA et al. Chronic active hepatitis in 26 Doberman pinschers. *J Am Vet Med Assoc*, 1985, 187(12):1343–50.
4. Thornburg LP, Rottinghaus G. What is the significance of hepatic copper values in dogs with cirrhosis? *Vet Med*, 1985, 80:50–4.
5. Thornburg LP, Rottinghaus G, Gage H. Chronic liver disease associated with high hepatic copper concentration in a dog. *J Am Vet Med Assoc*, 1986, 188(10):1190–1.
6. Brewer GJ et al. Use of zinc acetate to treat copper toxicosis in dogs. *J Am Vet Med Assoc*, 1992, 201(4):564–8.
7. Center SA. The jaundiced cat. *Proceedings of the Feline Medicine Symposium*, 1997, p. 41.
8. van den Ingh TSGAM et al. Morphological classification of biliary disorders of the canine and feline liver. In: WSAVA Liver Standardization Group. *WSAVA Standards for Clinical and Histological Diagnosis of Canine and Feline Liver Diseases*. WB Saunders, 2006, pp. 61–76.
9. Hoskins JD. Liver disease in the geriatric patient. *Vet Clin North Am Small Anim Pract*, 2005, 35(3):617–34.
10. Armstrong PJ, Weiss DJ, Gagne JM. Inflammatory liver disease. In: August JR, ed. *Consultations in Feline Internal Medicine*. Philadelphia, WB Saunders, 1997, pp. 68–78.
11. Bunch SE. Hepatobiliary diseases in the cat, In: Couto CG, Nelson RW, eds. *Small Animal Internal Medicine*. Saint Louis, Mosby, 1998, pp. 510–28.
12. Mehler SJ et al. Variables associated with outcome in dogs undergoing extrahepatic biliary surgery: 60 cases (1988–2002). *Vet Surg*, 2004, 33(6):644–9.
13. Mayhew PD et al. Choledochal tube stenting for decompression of the extrahepatic portion of the biliary tract in dogs: 13 cases (2002–2005). *J Am Vet Med Assoc*, 2006, 228(8):1209–14.
14. Savary-Bataille KCM et al. Percutaneous ultrasound-guided cholecystocentesis in healthy cats. *J Vet Intern Med*, 2003, 17(3):298–303.
15. Day DG. Feline cholangiohepatitis complex. *Vet Clin North Am Small Anim Pract*, 1995, 25(2):375–85.
16. Flatland B et al. Liver aspirate from a Shar Pei dog. *Vet Clin Pathol*, 2007, 36(1):105–8.
17. Niewold TA et al. Familial amyloidosis in cats: Siamese and Abyssinian AA proteins differ in primary sequence and pattern of deposition. *Amyloid*, 1999, 6(3):205–9.
18. Beatty JA et al. Spontaneous hepatic rupture in six cats with systemic amyloidosis. *J Small Anim Pract*, 2002, 43(8):355–63.

19. Sprague WS et al. Hemochromatosis secondary to repeated blood transfusions in a dog. *Vet Pathol*, 2003, 40(3):334–7.
20. Harvey JW. Pathogenesis, laboratory diagnosis, and clinical implications of erythrocyte enzyme deficiencies in dogs, cats, and horses. *Vet Clin Pathol*, 2006, 35(2):144–56.
21. Lowe AD et al. Clinical, clinicopathological and histological changes observed in 14 cats treated with glucocorticoids. *Vet Rec*, 2008, 162(24):777–83.
22. Schaer M, Ginn PE. Iatrogenic Cushing's syndrome and steroid hepatopathy in a cat. *J Am Anim Hosp Assoc*, 1999, 35(1):48–51.
23. Badylak SF, Van Vleet JF. Sequential morphologic and clinicopathologic alterations in dogs with experimentally induced glucocorticoid hepatopathy. *Am J Vet Res*, 1981, 42(8):1310–8.
24. Thornburg LP, Simpson S, Digilio K. Fatty liver syndrome in cats. *J Am Anim Hosp Assoc*, 1982, 18:397–400.
25. Biller DS, Kantrowitz B, Miyabayashi T. Ultrasonography of diffuse liver disease. A review. *J Vet Intern Med*, 1992, 6(2):71–6.
26. Meyer D, French T. The liver. In: Cowell R, Tyler R, eds. *Diagnostic Cytology of the Dog and Cat*. Goleta, CA, American Veterinary Publications, 1989, p. 189.
27. Strombeck D, Guilford W. *Small Animal Gastroenterology*. Davis, CA, Stonegate Publishing, 1990.
28. Boer HH, Nelson RW, Long GG. Colchicine therapy for hepatic fibrosis in a dog. *J Am Vet Med Assoc*, 1984, 185(3):303–5.
29. Byrne KP. Metabolic epidermal necrosis—hepatocutaneous syndrome. *Vet Clin North Am Small Anim Pract*, 1999, 29(6):1337–55.
30. McNeil PE. The underlying pathology of the hepatocutaneous syndrome: a report of 18 cases. In: Ihrke PJ, Mason IS, White SD, eds. *Advances in Veterinary Dermatology*, vol. 2. New York, Pergamon Press, 1993, p. 113.
31. Gross TL et al. Glucagon-producing pancreatic endocrine tumors in two dogs with superficial necrolytic dermatitis. *J Am Vet Med Assoc*, 1990, 197(12):1619–22.
32. Torres SM et al. Resolution of superficial necrolytic dermatitis following excision of a glucagon-secreting pancreatic neoplasm in a dog. *J Am Anim Hosp Assoc*, 1997, 33(4):313–9.
33. Yoshida M et al. A case report of superficial necrolytic dermatitis in a beagle dog with diabetes mellitus. *Toxicol Pathol*, 1996, 24(4):498–501.
34. Strombeck DR. Clinicopathologic features of primary and metastatic neoplastic disease of the liver in dogs. *J Am Vet Med Assoc*, 1978, 173(3):267–9.
35. Cullen JM, Popp JA. Tumors of the liver and gall bladder. In: Meuten DJ, ed. *Tumors in Domestic Animals*. Ames, Iowa State Press, 2002, pp. 483–508.
36. Hammer AS, Sikkema DA. Hepatic neoplasia in the dog and cat. *Vet Clin North Am Small Anim Pract*, 1995, 25(2):419–35.
37. Thamm DH. Hepatobiliary tumors. In: Withrow SJ, MacEwen EG, eds. *Small Animal Clinical Oncology*. Philadelphia, WB Saunders, 2001, pp. 327–34.
38. Patnaik AK, Hurvitz AI, Lieberman PH. Canine hepatic neoplasms: a clinicopathological study. *Vet Pathol*, 1980, 17(5):553–64.
39. Morrell CN, Volk MV, Mankowski JL. A carcinoid tumor in the gallbladder of a dog. *Vet Pathol*, 2002, 39(6):756–8.
40. Patnaik AK. A morphologic and immunocytochemical study of hepatic neoplasms in cats. *Vet Pathol*, 1992, 29(5):405–15.

41. Post G, Patnaik AK. Nonhematopoietic hepatic neoplasms in cats: 21 cases (1983–1988). *J Am Vet Med Assoc*, 1992, 201(7):1080–2.
42. Lawrence HJ, Erb HN, Harvey HJ. Nonlymphomatous hepatobiliary masses in cats: 41 cases (1972 to 1991). *Vet Surg*, 1994, 23(5):365–8.
43. Patnaik AK et al. Canine hepatocellular carcinoma. *Vet Pathol*, 1981, 18(4):427–38.
44. Košovský JE et al. Results of partial hepatectomy in 18 dogs with hepatocellular carcinoma. *J Am Anim Hosp Assoc*, 1989, 25:203–6.
45. Liptak JM et al. Massive hepatocellular carcinoma: surgical outcome in 40 dogs. *Proc Vet Cancer Soc Conf*, 2002, 22:32.
46. Patnaik AK et al. Canine bile duct carcinoma. *Vet Pathol*, 1981, 18(4):439–44.
47. Hayes HM Jr, Morin MM, Rubenstein DA. Canine biliary carcinoma: epidemiological comparisons with man. *J Comp Pathol*, 1983, 93(1):99–107.
48. Patnaik AK et al. Canine hepatic carcinoids. *Vet Pathol*, 1981, 18(4):445–53.
49. Shiga A et al. Hepatoblastoma in a dog. *J Vet Med Sci*, 1997, 59(12):1167–70.
50. Trout NJ et al. Surgical treatment of hepatobiliary cystadenomas in cats: five cases (1988–1993). *J Am Vet Med Assoc*, 1995, 206(4):505–7.
51. Nyland TG, Koblik PD, Tellyer SE. Ultrasonographic evaluation of biliary cystadenomas in cats. *Vet Radiol Ultrasound*, 1999, 40(3):300–6.
52. Willard MD, Dunstan RW, Faulkner J. Neuroendocrine carcinoma of the gallbladder in a dog. *J Am Vet Med Assoc*, 1988, 192(7):926–8.
53. Kapatkin AS et al. Leiomyosarcoma in dogs: 44 cases (1983–1988). *J Am Vet Med Assoc*, 1992, 201(7):1077–9.
54. Leifer CE et al. Hypoglycemia associated with nonislet cell tumor in 13 dogs. *J Am Vet Med Assoc*, 1985, 186(1):53–5.
55. Rogers KS. Anemia. In: Ettinger SJ, Feldman EC, eds. *Textbook of Veterinary Internal Medicine*. Philadelphia, WB Saunders, 2000, pp. 198–203.
56. Helfand SC. Platelets and neoplasia. *Vet Clin North Am Small Anim Pract*, 1988, 18(1):131–56.
57. Baatout S. Interleukin-6 and megakaryocytopoiesis: an update. *Ann Hematol*, 1996, 73(4):157–62.
58. Jelkmann W. The role of the liver in the production of thrombopoietin compared with erythropoietin. *Eur J Gastroenterol Hepatol*, 2001, 13(7):791–801.
59. McConnell MF, Lumsden JH. Biochemical evaluation of metastatic liver disease in the dog. *J Am Anim Hosp Assoc*, 1983, 19:173–8.
60. Feeney DA, Johnston GR, Hardy RM. Two-dimensional, gray-scale ultrasonography for assessment of hepatic and splenic neoplasia in the dog and cat. *J Am Vet Med Assoc*, 1984, 184(1):68–81.
61. Vörös K et al. Correlation of ultrasonographic and patho-morphological findings in canine hepatic diseases. *J Small Anim Pract*, 1991, 32(12):627–34.
62. Newell SM et al. Correlations between ultrasonographic findings and specific hepatic disease in cats: 72 cases (1985–1997). *J Am Vet Med Assoc*, 1998, 213(1):94–8.
63. Léveillé R et al. Complications after ultrasound-guided biopsy of abdominal structures in dogs and cats: 246 cases (1984–1991). *J Am Vet Med Assoc*, 1993, 203(3):413–5.
64. Barr F. Percutaneous biopsy of abdominal organs under ultrasound guidance. *J Small Anim Pract*, 1995, 36(3):105–13.
65. Fong Y, Kemeny N, Lawrence TS. Cancer of the liver and biliary tree. In: DeVita VT, Hellman S, Rosenberg SA, eds. *Cancer: Principles and Practice of Oncology*. Philadelphia, Lippincott Williams & Wilkins, 2001, pp. 1162–203.

66. Martin RA, Lanz OI, Tobias KM. Liver and biliary system. In: Slatter DH, ed. *Textbook of Small Animal Surgery*. Philadelphia, WB Saunders, 2003, pp. 708–26.
67. Tyler J. Hepatoencephalopathy. Part I. Clinical signs and diagnosis. *Compend Contin Educ Pract Vet*, 1990, 12:1060.
68. Tyler J. Hepatoencephalopathy. Part II. Pathophysiology and treatment. *Compend Contin Educ Pract Vet*, 1990, 12:1269.

Chapter 10. Endocrine problems in senior patients

1. Nelson RW. Canine diabetes mellitus. In: Ettinger SJ, Feldman EC, eds. *Textbook of Veterinary Internal Medicine*, 7th ed. Saint Louis, Saunders, 2010, pp. 1782–96.
2. Reusch C. Feline diabetes mellitus. In: Ettinger SJ, Feldman EC, eds. *Textbook of Veterinary Internal Medicine*, 7th ed. Saint Louis, Saunders, 2010, pp. 1796–816.
3. Monroe WE. Canine diabetes mellitus. In: Bonagura JD, Twedt DC, eds. *Kirk's Current Veterinary Therapy XIV*. Saint Louis, Saunders Elsevier, 2009, p. 196.
4. Manhiani MM, Cormican MT, Brands MW. Chronic sodium-retaining action of insulin in diabetic dogs. *Am J Physiol Renal Physiol*, 2011, 300(4):F957–65.
5. Behrend E et al. 2018 AAHA diabetes management guidelines for dogs and cats. *J Am Anim Hosp Assoc*, 2018, 54(1):1–21.
6. Rand JS et al. Over representation of Burmese cats with diabetes mellitus. *Aust Vet J*, 1997, 75(6):402–5.
7. Hess RS, Kass PH, Ward CR. Breed distribution of dogs with diabetes mellitus admitted to a tertiary care facility. *J Am Vet Med Assoc*, 2000, 216(9):1414–7.
8. Goossens MM et al. Response to insulin treatment and survival in 104 cats with diabetes mellitus (1985–1995). *J Vet Intern Med*, 1998, 12(1):1–6.
9. Link KR, Rand JS. Changes in blood glucose concentration are associated with relatively rapid changes in circulating fructosamine concentrations in cats. *J Feline Med Surg*, 2008, 10(6):583–92.
10. Reusch CE, Tomsa K. Serum fructosamine concentration in cats with overt hyperthyroidism. *J Am Vet Med Assoc*, 1999, 215(9):1297–300.
11. Graham PA, Mooney CT, Murray M. Serum fructosamine concentrations in hyperthyroid cats. *Res Vet Sci*, 1999, 67(2):171–5.
12. Bloom CA, Rand J. Feline diabetes mellitus: clinical use of long-acting glargine and detemir. *J Feline Med Surg*, 2014, 16(3):205–15.
13. Hess RS, Drobatz KJ. Glargine insulin for treatment of naturally occurring diabetes mellitus in dogs. *J Am Vet Med Assoc*, 2013, 243(8):1154–61.
14. Marshall RD, Rand JS, Morton JM. Glargine and protamine zinc insulin have a longer duration of action and result in lower mean daily glucose concentrations than lente insulin in healthy cats. *J Vet Pharmacol Ther*, 2008, 31(3):205–12.
15. Martin GJ, Rand JS. Pharmacology of a 40 IU/ml porcine lente insulin preparation in diabetic cats: findings during the first week and after 5 or 9 weeks of therapy. *J Feline Med Surg*, 2001, 3(1):23–30.
16. Briggs CE et al. Reliability of history and physical examination findings for assessing control of glycemia in dogs with diabetes mellitus: 53 cases (1995–1998). *J Am Vet Med Assoc*, 2000, 217(1):48–53.

17. Martin GJ, Rand JS. Comparisons of different measurements for monitoring diabetic cats treated with porcine insulin zinc suspension. *Vet Rec*, 2007, 161(2):52–8.
18. Behrend E. Canine hyperadrenocorticism. In: Feldman EC et al., eds. *Canine and Feline Endocrinology*, 4th ed. Saint Louis, Elsevier, 2015, pp. 403–5.
19. Valentin SY et al. Clinical findings, diagnostic test results, and treatment outcome in cats with spontaneous hyperadrenocorticism: 30 cases. *J Vet Intern Med*, 2014, 28(2):481–7.
20. Niessen SJ et al. Feline acromegaly: an underdiagnosed endocrinopathy? *J Vet Intern Med*, 2007, 21(5):899–905.
21. Berg RI et al. Serum insulin-like growth factor-I concentration in cats with diabetes mellitus and acromegaly. *J Vet Intern Med*, 2007, 21(5):892–8.
22. Mooney CT. Canine hyperthyroidism. In: Ettinger SJ, Feldman EC, Côté E, eds. *Textbook of Veterinary Internal Medicine*, 8th ed. Saint Louis, Elsevier, 2017, pp. 1731–42.
23. Peterson ME et al. Evaluation of serum thyroid-stimulating hormone concentration as a diagnostic test for hyperthyroidism in cats. *J Vet Intern Med*, 2015, 29(5):1327–34.
24. Greco DS. Cushing disease (pituitary-dependent hyperadrenocorticism) in animals. *Merck Veterinary Manual*, 2019, accessed April 4, 2021. https://www.merckvetmanual.com/endocrine-system/the-pituitary-gland/cushing-disease-pituitary-dependent-hyperadrenocorticism-in-animals
25. de Bruin C et al. Cushing's disease in dogs and humans. *Horm Res*, 2009, 71 Suppl 1:140–3.
26. Willeberg P, Priester WA. Epidemiological aspects of clinical hyperadrenocorticism in dogs (canine Cushing's syndrome). *J Am Anim Hosp Assoc*, 1982, 18(5):717–24.
27. Mamelak AN, Owen TJ, Bruyette D. Transsphenoidal surgery using a high definition video telescope for pituitary adenomas in dogs with pituitary dependent hypercortisolism: methods and results. *Vet Surg*, 2014, 43(4):369–79.
28. Melián C, Pérez-Alenza MD, Peterson ME. Hyperadrenocorticism in dogs. In: Ettinger SJ, Feldman EC, eds. *Textbook of Veterinary Internal Medicine*, 7th ed. Saint Louis, Saunders Elsevier, 2010, pp. 1816–40.
29. Galac S et al. Hyperadrenocorticism in a dog due to ectopic secretion of adrenocorticotropic hormone. *Domest Anim Endocrinol*, 2005, 28(3):338–48.
30. Galac S et al. ACTH-independent hyperadrenocorticism due to food-dependent hypercortisolemia in a dog: a case report. *Vet J*, 2008, 177(1):141–3.
31. Boland LA, Barrs VR. Peculiarities of feline hyperadrenocorticism: update on diagnosis and treatment. *J Feline Med Surg*, 2017, 19(9):933–47.
32. Behrend EN, Melián C. Hyperadrenocorticism in dogs. In: Rand J, ed. *Clinical Endocrinology of Companion Animals*. Ames, Wiley-Blackwell, 2013, pp. 43–64.
33. Behrend EN et al. Diagnosis of spontaneous canine hyperadrenocorticism: 2012 ACVIM consensus statement (small animal). *J Vet Intern Med*, 2013, 27(6):1292–304.
34. Forrester SD et al. Retrospective evaluation of urinary tract infection in 42 dogs with hyperadrenocorticism or diabetes mellitus or both. *J Vet Intern Med*, 1999, 13(6):557–60.
35. Feldman EC, Mack RE. Urine cortisol:creatinine ratio as a screening test for hyperadrenocorticism in dogs. *J Am Vet Med Assoc*, 1992, 200(11):1637–41.
36. Stolp R et al. Urinary corticoids in the diagnosis of canine hyperadrenocorticism. *Res Vet Sci*, 1983, 34(2):141–4.

37. Jensen AL et al. Evaluation of the urinary cortisol: creatinine ratio in the diagnosis of hyperadrenocorticism in dogs. *J Small Anim Pract*, 1997, 38(3):99–102.
38. Rijnberk A, van Wees A, Mol JA. Assessment of two tests for the diagnosis of canine hyperadrenocorticism. *Vet Rec*, 1988, 122(8):178–80.
39. Rodríguez Piñeiro MI et al. Accuracy of an adrenocorticotropic hormone (ACTH) immunoluminometric assay for differentiating ACTH-dependent from ACTH-independent hyperadrenocorticism in dogs. *J Vet Intern Med*, 2009, 23(4):850–5.
40. Bosje JT et al. Plasma concentrations of ACTH precursors correlate with pituitary size and resistance to dexamethasone in dogs with pituitary-dependent hyperadrenocorticism. *Domest Anim Endocrinol*, 2002, 22(4):201–10.
41. Feldman EC, Nelson RW, Feldman MS. Use of low- and high-dose dexamethasone tests for distinguishing pituitary-dependent from adrenal tumor hyperadrenocorticism in dogs. *J Am Vet Med Assoc*, 1996, 209(4):772–5.
42. Barrera JS et al. Evaluation of risk factors for outcome associated with adrenal gland tumors with or without invasion of the caudal vena cava and treated via adrenalectomy in dogs: 86 cases (1993–2009). *J Am Vet Med Assoc*, 2013, 242(12):1715–21.
43. Hanson JM et al. Efficacy of transsphenoidal hypophysectomy in treatment of dogs with pituitary-dependent hyperadrenocorticism. *J Vet Intern Med*, 2005, 19(5):687–94.
44. Kent MS et al. Survival, neurologic response, and prognostic factors in dogs with pituitary masses treated with radiation therapy and untreated dogs. *J Vet Intern Med*, 2007, 21(5):1027–33.
45. Clemente M et al. Comparison of non-selective adrenocorticolysis with mitotane or trilostane for the treatment of dogs with pituitary-dependent hyperadrenocorticism. *Vet Rec*, 2007, 161(24):805–9.
46. Arenas C, Melián C, Pérez-Alenza MD. Long-term survival of dogs with adrenal-dependent hyperadrenocorticism: a comparison between mitotane and twice daily trilostane treatment. *J Vet Intern Med*, 2014, 28(2):473–80.
47. Peterson ME, Johnson JG, Andrews LK. Spontaneous hyperthyroidism in the cat. *Proceedings of the American College of Veterinary Internal Medicine Forum*, 1979.
48. Peterson ME et al. Feline hyperthyroidism: pretreatment clinical and laboratory evaluation of 131 cases. *J Am Vet Med Assoc*, 1983, 183(1):103–10.
49. Prandi D et al. Hipertiroidismo felino: caso clínico [Feline hyperthyroidism: case study]. *Clínica veterinaria de pequeños animales (AVEPA)*, 1999, 19(1):23–9.
50. de la Fuente Hernández C et al. Hipertiroidismo felino apático: caso clínico [Apathetic feline hyperthyroidism: case study]. *Pequeños animales*, 2001, 30:67–77.
51. Wakeling J et al. Diagnosis of hyperthyroidism in cats with mild chronic kidney disease. *J Small Anim Pract*, 2008, 49(6):287–94.
52. Poutasse CM et al. Silicone pet tags associate tris(1,3-dichloro-2-isopropyl) phosphate exposures with feline hyperthyroidism. *Environ Sci Technol*, 2019, 53(15):9203–13.
53. Peterson M. Hyperthyroidism in cats: what's causing this epidemic of thyroid disease and can we prevent it? *J Feline Med Surg*, 2012, 14(11):804–18.
54. Wakeling J et al. Risk factors for feline hyperthyroidism in the UK. *J Small Anim Pract*, 2009, 50(8):406–14.

47. Nelson RW, Feldman EC. Pyometra. *Vet Clin North Am Small Anim Pract*, 1986, 16(3):561–76.
48. Borresen B. Pyometra in the dog—a pathophysiological investigation. I. The pyometra syndrome, a review. *Nord Vet Med*, 1975, 27(10):508–17.
49. Felmand EC. The cystic endometrial hyperplasia/pyometra complex and infertility in female dogs. In: Ettinger SJ, Feldman EC, eds. *Textbook of Veterinary Internal Medicine: Diseases of the Dog and Cat*, 5th ed. Philadelphia, WB Saunders, 2000, pp. 1549–55.
50. Feldman EC, Nelson RW. *Endocrinología y reproducción en perros y gatos* [Canine and Feline Endocrinology and Reproduction], 2th ed. Mexico, McGraw-Hill Interamericana, 2000, pp. 657–71 and 826–9.
51. Hardie EM. Life-threatening bacterial infection. *Compend Contin Educ Pract Vet*, 1995, 17(6):763–77.
52. Brady CA et al. Severe sepsis in cats: 29 cases (1986–1998). *J Am Vet Med Assoc*, 2000, 217(4):531–5.
53. Hauptman JG, Walshaw R, Olivier NB. Evaluation of the sensitivity and specificity of diagnostic criteria for sepsis in dogs. *Vet Surg*, 1997, 26(5):393–7.
54. Fontbonne A. Anti-progestins compounds in reproduction. *World Small Animal Veterinary Association World Congress Proceedings*, 2007.
55. Nak D, Nak Y, Tuna B. Follow-up examinations after medical treatment of pyometra in cats with the progesterone-antagonist aglepristone. *J Feline Med Surg*, 2009, 11(6):499–502.
56. Fieni F. Clinical evaluation of the use of aglepristone, with or without cloprostenol, to treat cystic endometrial hyperplasia–pyometra complex in bitches. *Theriogenology*, 2006, 66(6–7):1550–6.
57. Agudelo CF. Cystic endometrial hyperplasia–pyometra complex in cats. A review. *Vet Q*, 2005, 27(4):173–82.
58. Ogilvie GK, Moore AS. *Managing the Veterinary Cancer Patient: A Practice Manual*. Trenton, NJ, Veterinary Learning Systems, 1995.
59. Patnaik AK et al. Nonhematopoietic neoplasms in cats. *J Natl Cancer Inst*, 1975, 54(4):855–60.
60. Schneider R, Dorn CR, Taylor DO. Factors influencing canine mammary cancer development and postsurgical survival. *J Natl Cancer Inst*, 1969, 43(6):1249–61.
61. Overley B et al. Association between ovarihysterectomy and feline mammary carcinoma. *J Vet Intern Med*, 2005, 19(4):560–3.
62. Allen SW, Prasse KW, Mahaffey EA. Cytologic differentiation of benign from malignant canine mammary tumors. *Vet Pathol*, 1986, 23(6):649–55.
63. Jonhnston SD. Reproductive systems. In: Slatter DH, ed. *Textbook of Small Animal Surgery*, 2th ed. Philadelphia, WB Saunders, 1993, pp. 2177–200.
64. Jeglum KA, deGuzman E, Young KM. Chemotherapy of advanced mammary adenocarcinoma in 14 cats. *J Am Vet Med Assoc*, 1985, 187(2):157–60.
65. Mauldin GN et al. Efficacy and toxicity of doxorubicin and cyclophosphamide used in the treatment of selected malignant tumors in 23 cats. *J Vet Intern Med*, 1988, 2(2):60–5.
66. Doré M, Lanthier I, Sirois J. Cyclooxygenase-2 expression in canine mammary tumors. *Vet Pathol*, 2003, 40(2):207–12.
67. Greenhough A et al. The COX-2/PGE_2 pathway: key roles in the hallmarks of cancer and adaptation to the tumour microenvironment. *Carcinogenesis*, 2009, 30(3):377–86.
68. Gupta GP et al. Mediators of vascular remodelling co-opted for sequential steps in lung metastasis. *Nature*, 2007, 446(7137):765–70.

69. Harris SG et al. Prostaglandins as modulators of immunity. *Trends Immunol*, 2002, 23(3):144–50.
70. Xu XC. COX-2 inhibitors in cancer treatment and prevention, a recent development. *Anticancer Drugs*, 2002, 13(2):127–37.
71. Cuzick J et al. Aspirin and non-steroidal anti-inflammatory drugs for cancer prevention: an international consensus statement. *Lancet Oncol*, 2009, 10(5):501–7.
72. Queiroga FL et al. Cox-2 levels in canine mammary tumors, including inflammatory mammary carcinoma: clinicopathological features and prognostic significance. *Anticancer Res*, 2005, 25(6B):4269–75.
73. de M Souza CH et al. Inflammatory mammary carcinoma in 12 dogs: clinical features, cyclooxygenase-2 expression, and response to piroxicam treatment. *Can Vet J*, 2009, 50(5):506–10.
74. Heller DA et al. Cyclooxygenase-2 expression is associated with histologic tumor type in canine mammary carcinoma. *Vet Pathol*, 2005, 42(6):776–80.
75. Queiroga FL et al. Expression of Cox-1 and Cox-2 in canine mammary tumours. *J Comp Pathol*, 2007, 136(2–3):177–85.
76. Sorenmo KU et al. Evaluation of cyclooxygenase-1 and cyclooxygenase-2 expression and the effect of cyclooxygenase inhibitors in canine prostatic carcinoma. *Vet Comp Oncol*, 2004, 2(1):13–23.
77. Tremblay C et al. Induction of prostaglandin G/H synthase-2 in a canine model of spontaneous prostatic adenocarcinoma. *J Natl Cancer Inst*, 1999, 91(16):1398–403.
78. Khan KN et al. Expression of cyclooxygenase-2 in transitional cell carcinoma of the urinary bladder in dogs. *Am J Vet Res*, 2000, 61(5):478–81.
79. Pestili de Almeida EM et al. Expression of cyclo-oxygenase-2 in naturally occurring squamous cell carcinomas in dogs. *J Histochem Cytochem*, 2001, 49(7):867–75.
80. Borzacchiello G, Paciello O, Papparella S. Expression of cyclooxygenase-1 and -2 in canine nasal carcinomas. *J Comp Pathol*, 2004, 131(1):70–6.
81. Impellizeri JA, Esplin DG. Expression of cyclooxygenase-2 in canine nasal carcinomas. *Vet J*, 2008, 176(3):408–10.
82. Kleiter M et al. Expression of cyclooxygenase-2 in canine epithelial nasal tumors. *Vet Radiol Ultrasound*, 2004, 45(3):255–60.
83. Khan KN et al. Expression of cyclooxygenase-2 in canine renal cell carcinoma. *Vet Pathol*, 2001, 38(1):116–9.
84. Borzacchiello G, Russo V, Russo M. Immunohistochemical expression of cyclooxygenase-2 in canine ovarian carcinomas. *J Vet Med A Physiol Pathol Clin Med*, 2007, 54(5):247–9.
85. Boria PA et al. Evaluation of cisplatin combined with piroxicam for the treatment of oral malignant melanoma and oral squamous cell carcinoma in dogs. *J Am Vet Med Assoc*, 2004, 224(3):388–94.
86. Mullins MN et al. Cyclooxygenase-2 expression in canine appendicular osteosarcomas. *J Vet Intern Med*, 2004, 18(6):859–65.
87. Rossmeisl JH Jr et al. Cyclooxygenase-2 (COX-2) expression in canine intracranial meningiomas. *Vet Comp Oncol*, 2009, 7(3):173–80.
88. Millanta F et al. COX-2 expression in canine and feline invasive mammary carcinomas: correlation with clinicopathological features and prognostic molecular markers. *Breast Cancer Res Treat*, 2006, 98(1):115–20.

89. Sayasith K, Sirois J, Doré M. Molecular characterization of feline COX-2 and expression in feline mammary carcinomas. *Vet Pathol*, 2009, 46(3):423–9.
90. Beam SL et al. An immunohistochemical study of cyclooxygenase-2 expression in various feline neoplasms. *Vet Pathol*, 2003, 40(5):496–500.
91. Hayes A et al. COX-1 and COX-2 expression in feline oral squamous cell carcinoma. *J Comp Path*, 2006, 135(2–3):93–9.
92. Hayes AM et al. Survival of 54 cats with oral squamous cell carcinoma in United Kingdom general practice. *J Small Anim Pract*, 2007, 48(7):394–9.
93. Newman SJ, Mrkonjich L. Cyclooxygenase-2 expression in feline pancreatic adenocarcinomas. *J Vet Diagn Invest*, 2006, 18(6):590–3.
94. Mohammed SI et al. Expression of cyclooxygenase-1 and 2 in naturally-occurring canine cancer. *Prostaglandins Leukot Essent Fatty Acids*, 2004, 70(5):479–83.
95. Morris JS, Dobson JM, Bostock DE. Use of tamoxifen in the control of canine mammary neoplasia. *Vet Rec*, 1993, 133(22):539–42.
96. Chang CC et al. Evaluation of hormone receptor expression for use in predicting survival of female dogs with malignant mammary gland tumors. *J Am Vet Med Assoc*, 2009, 235(4):391–6.
97. Akkoc A, Inan S, Sonmez G. Matrix metalloproteinase (MMP-2 and MMP-9) and steroid receptor expressions in feline mammary tumors. *Biotech Histochem*, 2012, 87(4):312–9.
98. Millanta F et al. Steroid hormone receptors in normal, dysplastic and neoplastic feline mammary tissues and their prognostic significance. *Vet Rec*, 2006, 158(24):821–4.
99. Chon E et al. Safety evaluation of combination toceranib phosphate (Palladia®) and piroxicam in tumour-bearing dogs (excluding mast cell tumours): a phase I dose-finding study. *Vet Comp Oncol*, 2012, 10(3):184–93.
100. Mitchell L, Thamm DH, Biller BJ. Clinical and immunomodulatory effects of toceranib combined with low-dose cyclophosphamide in dogs with cancer. *J Vet Intern Med*, 2012, 26(2):355–62.

Chapter 12. Senior cardiovascular disease

1. Sisson DD, Ettinger SJ. The physical examination. In: Fox PR, Sisson DD, Moise NS, eds. *Textbook of Canine and Feline Cardiology: Principles and Clinical Practice*, 2th ed. Philadelphia, PA, WB Saunders, 1999, pp. 46–64.
2. Braunwald E. Physical examination of the heart and circulation. In: Zipes DP et al., eds. *Braunwald's Heart Disease: A Textbook of Cardiovascular Medicine*, 7th ed. Philadelphia, PA, Elsevier Saunders, 2005, pp. 77–106.
3. Detweiler DK, Patterson DF. Abnormal heart sounds and murmurs of the dog. *J Small Anim Pract*, 1967, 8:193–205.
4. Lehmkuhl LB, Ware WA, Bonagura JD. Mitral stenosis in 15 dogs. *J Vet Intern Med*, 1994, 8:2–17.
5. Buchanan JW. Valvular disease (endocardiosis in dogs). *Adv Vet Sci Comp Med*, 1979, 21:75–99.
6. Detweiler DK, Patterson DF. The prevalence and types of cardiovascular diseases in dogs. *Ann NY Acad Sci*, 1965, 127:481–93.
7. Detweiler DK et al. The natural history of acquired cardiac disability in the dog. *Ann NY Acad Sci*, 1968, 147:318–29.

8. Tidholm A et al. Canine idiopathic dilated cardiomyopathy. Part I: aetiology, clinical characteristics, epidemiology and pathology. *Vet J*, 2001, 162:92–107.
9. Haggstrom J, Duelund Pedersen H, Kvart C. New insights into degenerative mitral valve disease in dogs. *Vet Clin N Am Small Anim Pract*, 1998, 28:1057–62.
10. Haggstrom J et al. Chronic valvular disease in the Cavalier King Charles Spaniel in Sweden. *Vet Rec*, 1992, 131:549–53.
11. Haggstrom J, Kvart C, Hansson K. Heart sounds and murmurs: changes related to severity of chronic valvular disease in the Cavalier King Charles Spaniel. *J Vet Intern Med*, 1995, 9:75–85.
12. Kvart C, Haggstrom J, Pedersen HD. ACE inhibitors in dogs with subclinical chronic mitral insufficiency [in Dutch]. *Tijdschr Diergeneeskd*, 2003, 128:76–7.
13. Kvart C et al. Efficacy of enalapril for prevention of congestive heart failure in dogs with myxomatous valve disease and asymptomatic mitral regurgitation. *J Vet Intern Med*, 2002, 16:80–8.
14. Keene BW et al. ACVIM consensus guidelines for the diagnosis and treatment of myxomatous mitral valve disease in dogs. *J Vet Intern Med*, 2019, 33(3):1127–40.
15. Atkins C et al. Guidelines for the diagnosis and treatment of canine chronic valvular heart. *J Vet Intern Med*, 2009, 23(6):1142–50.
16. Luis Fuentes V et al. ACVIM consensus statement guidelines for the classification, diagnosis, and management of cardiomyopathies in cats. *J Vet Intern Med*, 2020, 34(3):1062–77.
17. Payne JR, Brodbelt DC, Luis Fuentes V. Cardiomyopathy prevalence in 780 apparently healthy cats in rehoming centres (the CatScan study). *J Vet Cardiol*, 2015, 17 Suppl 1:S244–57.
18. Oura TJ et al. A valentine-shaped cardiac silhouette in feline thoracic radiographs is primarily due to left atrial enlargement. *Vet Radiol Ultrasound*, 2015, 56(3):245–50.
19. Benigni L, Morgan N, Lamb CR. Radiographic appearance of cardiogenic pulmonary oedema in 23 cats. *J Small Anim Pract*, 2009, 50(1):9–14.

Chapter 13. Most frequent neurological problems in senior patients

1. Crowell-Davis SL. Cognitive dysfunction in senior pets. *Compend Contin Educ Vet*, 2008, 30(2):106–8.
2. Neilson JC et al. Prevalence of behavioral changes associated with age-related cognitive impairment in dogs. *J Am Vet Med Assoc*, 2001, 218(11):1787–91.
3. Porter VR et al. Frequency and characteristics of anxiety among patients with Alzheimer's disease and related dementias. *J Neuropsychiatry Clin Neurosci*, 2003, 15(2):180–6.
4. Dimakopoulos AC, Mayer RJ. Aspects of neurodegeneration in the canine brain. *J Nutr*, 2002, 132(6 Suppl 2):1579S–82S.
5. Landsberg G, Araujo JA. Behavior problems in geriatric pets. *Vet Clin North Am Small Anim Pract*, 2005, 35(3):675–98.
6. Shigenaga MK, Hagen TM, Ames BN. Oxidative damage and mitochondrial decay in aging. *Proc Natl Acad Sci U S A*, 1994, 91(23):10771–8.
7. Roudebush P et al. Nutritional management of brain aging in dogs. *J Am Vet Med Assoc*, 2005, 227(5):722–8.
8. Hardy JA, Higgins GA. Alzheimer's disease: the amyloid cascade hypothesis. *Science*, 1992, 256(5054):184–5.

9. Dickson DW et al. Correlations of synaptic and pathological markers with cognition of the elderly. *Neurobiol Aging*, 1995, 16(3):285–98; discussion 298–304.
10. Hardy J. A hundred years of Alzheimer's disease research. *Neuron*, 2006, 52(1):3–13.
11. Head E, Milgram N, Cotman CW. Neurobiological methods of aging in the dog and other vertebrate species. In: Hof PR, Mobbs CV, eds. *Functional Neurobiology of Aging*. San Diego, CA, Academic Press, 2000, pp. 457–68.
12. Selkoe DJ et al. Conservation of brain amyloid proteins in aged mammals and humans with Alzheimer's disease. *Science*, 1987, 235(4791):873–7.
13. Blümcke I et al. Cellular pathology of hilar neurons in Ammon's horn sclerosis. *J Comp Neurol*, 1999, 414(4):437–53.
14. Burkhart KK et al. Alterations in tau phosphorylation in rat and human neocortical brain slices following hypoxia and glucose deprivation. *Exp Neurol*, 1998, 154(2):464–72.
15. Zhang C et al. Age-related changes of structures in cerebellar cortex of cat. *J Biosci*, 2006, 31(1):55–60.
16. Landsberg G. Feline house soiling: marking and inappropriate elimination. *Proc Atlantic Coast Vet Conf*, 1999, pp. 315–20.
17. Wismer T. Serotonin syndrome. *Proceedings of the International Veterinary Emergency and Critical Care Symposium*, 2005.
18. Overall KL. Assessing brain aging in cats. *DVM360*, 2010, accessed February 15, 2012. https://www.dvm360.com/view/assessing-brain-aging-cats
19. Milgram NW et al. Oral administration of adrafinil improves discrimination learning in aged beagle dogs. *Pharmacol Biochem Behav*, 2000, 66(2):301–5.
20. Siwak CT et al. Behavioral activating effects of adrafinil in aged canines. *Pharmacol Biochem Behav*, 2000, 66(2):293–300.
21. Siwak CT et al. Comparison of the effects of adrafinil, propentofylline and nicergoline on behavior in aged dogs. *Am J Vet Res*, 2000, 61(11):1410–4.
22. Skoumalova A et al. The role of free radicals in canine counterpart of senile dementia of the Alzheimer type. *Exp Gerontol*, 2003, 38(6):711–9.
23. Head E et al. Oxidative damage increases with age in a canine model of human brain aging. *J Neurochem*, 2002, 82(2):375–81.
24. Dodd CE et al. Can a fortified food affect the behavioral manifestations of age-related cognitive decline in dogs? *Vet Med*, 2003, 98:396–408.
25. Mischoulon D, Fava M. Role of S-adenosyl-L-methionine in the treatment of depression: a review of the evidence. *Am J Clin Nutr*, 2002, 76(5):1158S–61S.
26. Nguyen M, Gregan A. S-adenosylmethionine and depression. *Aust Fam Physician*, 2002, 31(4):339–43.
27. Bottiglieri T, Hyland K, Reynolds EH. The clinical potential of ademetionine (S-adenosylmethionine) in neurological disorders. *Drugs*, 1994, 48(2):137–52.
28. Rème CA et al. Effect of S-adenosylmethionine tablets on the reduction of age-related mental decline in dogs: a double-blinded, placebo-controlled trial. *Vet Ther*, 2008, 9(2):69–82.
29. Heath SE, Barabas S, Craze PG. Nutritional supplementation in cases of canine cognitive dysfunction—a clinical trial. *Appl Anim Behav Sci*, 2007, 105(4):284–96.
30. Hill AS et al. Lipoic acid is 10 times more toxic in cats than reported in humans, dogs or rats. *J Anim Physiol Anim Nutr (Berl)*, 2004, 88(3–4):150–6.

31. Pan Y et al. Cognitive enhancement in old dogs from dietary supplementation with a nutrient blend containing arginine, antioxidants, B vitamins and fish oil. *Br J Nutr*, 2018, 119(3):349–58.
32. Pan Y et al. Cognitive enhancement in middle-aged and old cats with dietary supplementation with a nutrient blend containing fish oil, B vitamins, antioxidants and arginine. *Br J Nutr*, 2013, 110(1):40–9.
33. Pan Y et al. Dietary supplementation with medium-chain TAG has long-lasting cognition-enhancing effects in aged dogs. *Br J Nutr*, 2010, 103(12):1746–54.
34. Pan Y et al. Efficacy of a therapeutic diet on dogs with signs of cognitive dysfunction syndrome (CDS): a prospective double blinded placebo controlled clinical study. *Front Nutr*, 2018, 5:127.
35. Thomas WB. Vestibular dysfunction. *Vet Clin North Am Small Anim Pract*, 2000, 30(1):227–49.
36. de Lahunta A, Glass E. Vestibular system: special proprioception. In: *Veterinary Neuroanatomy and Clinical Neurology*, 3rd ed. Saint Louis, Saunders/Elsevier, 2009, pp. 319–47.
37. Angelaki DE, Cullen KE. Vestibular system: the many facets of a multimodal sense. *Annu Rev Neurosci*, 2008, 31:125–50.
38. Brandt T, Strupp M. General vestibular testing. *Clin Neurophysiol*, 2005, 116(2):406–26.
39. Evans HE, Kitchell RL. Cranial nerves and cutaneous innervation of the head. In: Evans HE, Miller ME, eds. *Miller's Anatomy of the Dog*, 3rd ed. Philadelphia, WB Saunders, 1993, pp. 953–87.
40. King AS. *Physiological and Clinical Anatomy of the Domestic Mammals. Vol. 1, Central Nervous System*. New York, Oxford University Press, 1994, pp. 171–82.
41. Schunk KL, Averill DR Jr. Peripheral vestibular syndrome in the dog: a review of 83 cases. *J Am Vet Med Assoc*, 1983, 182(12):1354–7.
42. Burke EE et al. Review of idiopathic feline vestibular syndrome in 75 cats. *J Am Vet Med Assoc*, 1985, 187(9):941–3.
43. Center SA et al. Fulminant hepatic failure associated with oral administration of diazepam in 11 cats. *J Am Vet Med Assoc*, 1996, 209(3):618–25.
44. Averill DR Jr. Degenerative myelopathy in the aging German Shepherd dog: clinical and pathologic findings. *J Am Vet Med Assoc*, 1973, 162(12):1045–51.
45. Shelton GD et al. Degenerative myelopathy associated with a missense mutation in the superoxide dismutase 1 (*SOD1*) gene progresses to peripheral neuropathy in Pembroke Welsh Corgis and Boxers. *J Neurol Sci*, 2012, 318(1–2):55–64.
46. Coates JR et al. Clinical characterization of a familial degenerative myelopathy in Pembroke Welsh Corgi dogs. *J Vet Intern Med*, 2007, 21(6):1323–31.